T0226748

Pediatric Head and Neck Masses

Editors

JOHN MADDALOZZO
JEFFREY C. RASTATTER

OTOLARYNGOLOGIC CLINICS OF NORTH AMERICA

www.oto.theclinics.com

February 2015 • Volume 48 • Number 1

ELSEVIER

1600 John F. Kennedy Boulevard • Suite 1800 • Philadelphia, Pennsylvania, 19103-2899

http://www.oto.theclinics.com

OTOLARYNGOLOGIC CLINICS OF NORTH AMERICA Volume 48, Number 1
February 2015 ISSN 0030-6665, ISBN-13: 978-0-323-32668-1

Editor: Joanne Husovski
Developmental Editor: Susan Showalter

Otolaryngologic Clinics of North America (ISSN 0030-6665) is published bimonthly by Elsevier, Inc., 360 Park Avenue South, New York, NY 10010-1710. Months of issue are February, April, June, August, October, and December. Business and Editorial Offices: 1600 John F. Kennedy Blvd., Suite 1800, Philadelphia, PA 19103-2899. Customer Service Office: 6277 Sea Harbor Drive, Orlando, FL 32887-4800. Periodicals postage paid at New York, NY and additional mailing offices. Subscription prices is $365.00 per year (US individuals), $692.00 per year (US institutions), $175.00 per year (US student/resident), $485.00 per year (Canadian individuals), $876.00 per year (Canadian institutions), $540.00 per year (international individuals), $876.00 per year (international institutions), $270.00 per year (international & Canadian student/resident). Foreign air speed delivery is included in all *Clinics'* subscription prices. All prices are subject to change without notice. **POSTMASTER:** Send address changes to *Otolaryngologic Clinics of North America*, Elsevier Health Sciences Division, Subscription Customer Service, 3251 Riverport Lane, Maryland Heights, MO 63043. **Telephone: 1-800-654-2452 (U.S. and Canada); 314-447-8871 (outside U.S. and Canada). Fax: 314-447-8029. E-mail: journalscustomerservice-usa@elsevier.com (for print support); journalsonlinesupport-usa@elsevier.com (for online support).**

Reprints. For copies of 100 or more of articles in this publication, please contact the Commercial Reprints Department, Elsevier Inc., 360 Park Avenue South, New York, NY 10010-1710. Tel.: 212-633-3874; Fax: 212-633-3820; E-mail: reprints@elsevier.com.

Otolaryngologic Clinics of North America is also published in Spanish by McGraw-Hill Interamericana Editores S.A., P.O. Box 5-237, 06500 Mexico D.F., Mexico.

Otolaryngologic Clinics of North America is covered in *MEDLINE/PubMed (Index Medicus), Current Contents/Clinical Medicine, Excerpta Medica, BIOSIS, Science Citation Index,* and *ISI/BIOMED.*

PROGRAM OBJECTIVE

The goal of the *Otolaryngologic Clinics of North America* is to provide information on the latest trends in patient management, the newest advances; and provide a sound basis for choosing treatment options in the field of otolaryngology.

TARGET AUDIENCE

All practicing physicians and healthcare professionals who provide patient care to otolaryngologic patients.

LEARNING OBJECTIVES

Upon completion of this activity, participants will be able to:
1. Discuss medical imaging of pediatric head and neck lesions.
2. Recognize lesions of the pediatric skull base and nasal, intraoral and lingual lesions, lesions of the maxilla and mandible, as well as congenital lesions of epithelial lesions.
3. Review the management of tumors and masses of the head and neck in children.

ACCREDITATION

The Elsevier Office of Continuing Medical Education (EOCME) is accredited by the Accreditation Council for Continuing Medical Education (ACCME) to provide continuing medical education for physicians.

The EOCME designates this enduring material for a maximum of 15 *AMA PRA Category 1 Credit*(s)™. Physicians should claim only the credit commensurate with the extent of their participation in the activity.

All other health care professionals requesting continuing education credit for this enduring material will be issued a certificate of participation.

DISCLOSURE OF CONFLICTS OF INTEREST

The EOCME assesses conflict of interest with its instructors, faculty, planners, and other individuals who are in a position to control the content of CME activities. All relevant conflicts of interest that are identified are thoroughly vetted by EOCME for fair balance, scientific objectivity, and patient care recommendations. EOCME is committed to providing its learners with CME activities that promote improvements or quality in healthcare and not a specific proprietary business or a commercial interest.

The planning committee, staff, authors and editors listed below have identified no financial relationships or relationships to products or devices they or their spouse/life partner have with commercial interest related to the content of this CME activity:

Matthew T. Brigger, MD, MPH; Daniel T. Ginat, MD, MS; Steven L. Goudy, MD; Kristen Helm; Susannah E. Hills, MD; Stephen R. Hoff, MD, FACS, FAAP; Brynne Hunter; Joanne Husovski; Kris R. Jatana, MD; Paul R. Krakovitz, MD; Brian D. Kulbersh, MD; Sandy Lavery; Paul Lennon, MB BCh; John Maddalozzo, MD; Vikash K. Modi, MD; Charles M. Myer III, MD; Jennifer L. Nicholas, MD; Karin P.Q. Oomen, MD, PhD; Josée Paradis, MD, MSc, FRCSC; Edward B. Penn Jr, MD; Antonio Perez-Atayde, MD; Santha Priya; J. Drew Prosser, MD; Reza Rahbar, DMD, MD; Jeffrey C. Rastatter, MD, FACS, FAAP; Gresham T. Richter, MD, FACS, FAAP; Maura E. Ryan, MD; James W. Schroeder Jr, MD, FACS, FAAP; V. Michelle Silvera, MD; Susan Showalter; Samuel J. Trosman, MD; Elizabeth Tyler-Kabara, MD, PhD; Patrick C. Walz, MD; Brian J. Wiatrak, MD; Donald Zimmerman, MD.

The planning committee, staff, authors and editors listed below have identified financial relationships or relationships to products or devices they or their spouse/life partner have with commercial interest related to the content of this CME activity:

Tord D. Alden, MD is on speakers bureau for BioMarin Pharmaceutical Inc.
Michael J. Cunningham, MD, FACS, has royalties/patents with Plural Publishing, Inc.
Paul A. Gardner, MD, is a consultant/advisor for Integra LifeSciences Corporation.
Peter J. Koltai, MD, FACS, is a consultant/advisor for Acclarent, Inc. and Medtronic, Inc.
Carl H. Snyderman, MD, MBA, is a consultant/advisor for and has stock ownership in SPIWay, LLC.
Jessica S. Stern, MD, spouse/partner has stock ownership in AbbVie Inc.

UNAPPROVED/OFF-LABEL USE DISCLOSURE

The EOCME requires CME faculty to disclose to the participants:
1. When products or procedures being discussed are off-label, unlabelled, experimental, and/or investigational (not US Food and Drug Administration [FDA] approved); and
2. Any limitations on the information presented, such as data that are preliminary or that represent ongoing research, interim analyses, and/or unsupported opinions. Faculty may discuss information about

pharmaceutical agents that is outside of FDA-approved labelling. This information is intended solely for CME and is not intended to promote off-label use of these medications. If you have any questions, contact the medical affairs department of the manufacturer for the most recent prescribing information.

TO ENROLL
To enroll in the *Otolaryngologic Clinics of North America* Continuing Medical Education program, call customer service at 1-800-654-2452 or sign up online at http://www.theclinics.com/home/cme. The CME program is available to subscribers for an additional annual fee of USD 260.

METHOD OF PARTICIPATION
In order to claim credit, participants must complete the following:
1. Complete enrolment as indicated above.
2. Read the activity.
3. Complete the CME Test and Evaluation. Participants must achieve a score of 70% on the test. All CME Tests and Evaluations must be completed online.

CME INQUIRIES/SPECIAL NEEDS
For all CME inquiries or special needs, please contact elsevierCME@elsevier.com.

Contributors

EDITORS

JOHN MADDALOZZO, MD
Pediatric Otolaryngology–Head and Neck Surgery, Professor, Division of Otolaryngology–Head and Neck Surgery, Ann & Robert H. Lurie Children's Hospital of Chicago, Northwestern University Feinberg School of Medicine, Chicago, Illinois

JEFFREY C. RASTATTER, MD, FACS, FAAP
Assistant Professor, Department of Otolaryngology–Head and Neck Surgery, Northwestern University Feinberg School of Medicine; Division of Pediatric Otolaryngology–Head and Neck Surgery, Ann & Robert H. Lurie Children's Hospital of Chicago, Chicago, Illinois

AUTHORS

TORD D. ALDEN, MD
Assistant Professor, Department of Neurological Surgery, Feinberg School of Medicine, Northwestern University; Division of Pediatric Neurosurgery, Ann & Robert H. Lurie Children's Hospital of Chicago, Chicago, Illinois

MATTHEW T. BRIGGER, MD, MPH, CDR, MC, USN
Department of Otolaryngology–Head and Neck Surgery, Naval Medical Center San Diego, San Diego, California; Assistant Professor of Surgery, Uniformed Services University of the Health Sciences, Bethesda, Maryland

MICHAEL J. CUNNINGHAM, MD, FACS
Otolaryngologist-in-Chief, Department of Otolaryngology and Communication Enhancement, Boston Children's Hospital; Professor, Department of Otology and Laryngology, Harvard Medical School, Boston, Massachusetts

PAUL A. GARDNER, MD
Associate Professor, Department of Neurological Surgery, University of Pittsburgh School of Medicine, Pittsburgh, Pennsylvania

DANIEL T. GINAT, MD, MS
Assistant Professor, Department of Radiology, Pritzker School of Medicine, University of Chicago, Chicago, Illinois

STEVEN L. GOUDY, MD
Department of Otolaryngology, Monroe Carell Jr Children's Hospital, Vanderbilt University, Nashville, Tennessee

SUSANNAH E. HILLS, MD
Division of Otolaryngology, Ann & Robert H. Lurie Children's Hospital of Chicago, Chicago, Illinois

STEPHEN R. HOFF, MD, FACS, FAAP
Department of Otolaryngology–Head and Neck Surgery, Northwestern University
Feinberg School of Medicine; Division of Pediatric Otolaryngology–Head and Neck
Surgery, Ann & Robert H. Lurie Children's Hospital of Chicago, Chicago, Illinois

KRIS R. JATANA, MD
Assistant Professor, Department of Otolaryngology–Head and Neck Surgery, Nationwide
Children's Hospital, The Ohio State University, Columbus, Ohio

PETER J. KOLTAI, MD, FACS
Professor of Otolaryngology and Pediatrics, Division of Pediatric Otolaryngology,
Lucile Packard Children's Hospital, Stanford University School of Medicine, Stanford,
California

PAUL R. KRAKOVITZ, MD
Section Head of Pediatric Otolaryngology; Professor, Head and Neck Institute, Cleveland
Clinic Foundation, Cleveland, Ohio

BRIAN D. KULBERSH, MD
Pediatric ENT Associates, Children's of Alabama, Birmingham, Alabama

PAUL LENNON, MB BCh, FRCS (ORL HNS)
Specialist Registrar, Department of Otolaryngology, Head and Neck Surgery, St. James
Hospital, Dublin, Ireland

JOHN MADDALOZZO, MD
Pediatric Otolaryngology–Head and Neck Surgery, Professor, Division of
Otolaryngology–Head and Neck Surgery, Ann & Robert H. Lurie Children's Hospital of
Chicago, Northwestern University Feinberg School of Medicine, Chicago, Illinois

VIKASH K. MODI, MD
Assistant Professor, Pediatric Otolaryngology–Head & Neck Surgery, Department of
Otolaryngology–Head & Neck Surgery, Weill Cornell Medical College, New York, New York

CHARLES M. MYER III, MD
Professor, Department of Pediatric Otolaryngology, Cincinnati Children's Hospital
Medical Center, Cincinnati, Ohio

JENNIFER L. NICHOLAS, MD, M.H.A
Assistant Professor of Radiology, Feinberg School of Medicine, Northwestern University;
Department of Medical Imaging, Ann & Robert H. Lurie Children's Hospital of Chicago,
Chicago, Illinois

KARIN P.Q. OOMEN, MD, PhD
Assistant Professor, Department of Otolaryngology–Head and Neck Surgery; Pediatric
Otolaryngology–Head and Neck Surgery, Wilhelmina Children's Hospital, University
Medical Center Utrecht, Utrecht, The Netherlands

JOSÉE PARADIS, MD, MSc, FRCSC
Former fellow of Pediatric Otolarynology, Stanford, California; Associate Professor of
Otolaryngology, Head and Neck Surgery, Division of Pediatric Otolarynoglogy, University
of Western Ontario, London, Ontario, Canada

EDWARD B. PENN Jr, MD
Department of Otolaryngology, Monroe Carell Jr Children's Hospital, Vanderbilt
University, Nashville, Tennessee

ANTONIO PEREZ-ATAYDE, MD
Director of Special Techniques, Staff Pathologist, Boston Children's Hospital, Boston; Associate Professor of Pathology, Harvard Medical School, Boston, Massachusetts

J. DREW PROSSER, MD
Fellow, Department of Pediatric Otolaryngology, Cincinnati Children's Hospital Medical Center, Cincinnati, Ohio

REZA RAHBAR, DMD, MD
Associate Otolaryngologist-in-Chief, McGill Chair in Pediatric Otolaryngology, Department of Otolaryngology and Communication Enhancement, Boston Children's Hospital, Boston; Director of Center for Airway Disorders, Co-Director, Center for Head, Neck and Skull base Tumors, Boston Children's Hospital, Boston; Associate Professor of Otology and Laryngology, Harvard Medical School, Boston, Massachusetts

JEFFREY C. RASTATTER, MD, FACS, FAAP
Assistant Professor, Department of Otolaryngology–Head and Neck Surgery, Northwestern University Feinberg School of Medicine; Division of Pediatric Otolaryngology–Head and Neck Surgery, Ann & Robert H. Lurie Children's Hospital of Chicago, Chicago, Illinois

GRESHAM T. RICHTER, MD, FACS, FAAP
Department of Otolaryngology–Head and Neck Surgery, University of Arkansas for Medical Sciences, Little Rock, Arkansas

MAURA E. RYAN, MD
Assistant Professor of Radiology, Feinberg School of Medicine, Northwestern University; Department of Medical Imaging, Ann & Robert H. Lurie Children's Hospital of Chicago, Chicago, Illinois

JAMES W. SCHROEDER Jr, MD, FACS, FAAP
Associate Professor, Departments of Otolaryngology–Head and Neck Surgery and Medical Education, Northwestern University Feinberg School of Medicine, Chicago, Illinois

V. MICHELLE SILVERA, MD
Pediatric Neuroradiologist, Childrens Hospital; Instructor in Radiology, Harvard Medical School, Boston, Massachusetts

CARL H. SNYDERMAN, MD, MBA
Professor, Department of Otolaryngology, Eye & Ear Institute, University of Pittsburgh School of Medicine; Department of Neurological Surgery, University of Pittsburgh School of Medicine, Pittsburgh, Pennsylvania

JESSICA S. STERN, MD
Assistant Professor of Radiology, Feinberg School of Medicine, Northwestern University; Department of Medical Imaging, Ann & Robert H. Lurie Children's Hospital of Chicago, Chicago, Illinois

SAMUEL J. TROSMAN, MD
Resident, Head and Neck Institute, Cleveland Clinic Foundation, Cleveland, Ohio

ELIZABETH TYLER-KABARA, MD, PhD
Assistant Professor, Department of Neurological Surgery, University of Pittsburgh School of Medicine; Division of Pediatric Neurosurgery, Children's Hospital of Pittsburgh of the University of Pittsburgh Medical Center, Pittsburgh, Pennsylvania

PATRICK C. WALZ, MD
Fellow, Class of 2013-2014, Division of Pediatric Otolaryngology, Ann and Robert H. Lurie Children's Hospital of Chicago, Northwestern University Feinberg School of Medicine, Chicago, Illinois; Assistant Professor, Department of Otolaryngology–Head and Neck Surgery, The Ohio State University, Columbus, Ohio

BRIAN J. WIATRAK, MD
Pediatric ENT Associates, Children's of Alabama, Birmingham, Alabama

DONALD ZIMMERMAN, MD
Head of Pediatric Endocrinology; Professor, Department of Pediatrics, Lurie Children's Hospital, Northwestern University Feinberg School of Medicine, Chicago, Illinois

Contents

> Branchial cleft anomalies are a common cause of congenital neck masses
> and can present as a cyst, sinus, or fistula. A comprehensive understand-
> ing of the embryologic basis of these anomalies aids in diagnosis and
> surgical excision. Fistulas tend to present at an earlier age than sinuses
> or cysts, with most lesions presenting as either a neck mass, draining si-
> nus, or recurrent infections. The eventual management of each is complete
> surgical excision, which is curative. A history of recurrent preoperative
> infections leads to a higher rate of recurrence.

> The embryology, presentation, imaging, and treatment of the thyroglossal
> duct cyst will be reviewed. Anatomic features and surgical technique to
> prevent complications and recurrence will be discussed. Included in the
> discussion will be the management of thyroglossal duct cyst malignancy
> and ectopic thyroid.

> Vascular lesions of the head and neck are complex and diverse. These include
> infantile hemangioma, venous malformations, lymphatic malformations, and
> arteriovenous malformations, among others. Vascular malformations and
> tumors display different growth patterns and require different approaches
> to treatment. Therefore, accurate diagnosis is of utmost importance. This
> article is a guide for the diagnosis and management of vascular lesions of
> the head and neck.

> Proper management of pediatric thyroid nodules is crucial to achieving
> good outcomes. It is important to obtain a thorough history, including prior
> radiation exposure and family history of thyroid cancer and any symptoms
> of hypothyroidism or hyperthyroidism. A complete physical examination
> with special attention to the thyroid gland and any cervical lymphadenop-
> athy is important. Nodules between 5 and 10 mm with risk factors (clinical
> or sonographic) and all nodules greater than 10 mm should undergo a fine-
> needle aspiration biopsy. A comprehensive center of pediatric specialists
> is the best environment for treatment of these patients.

The timely diagnosis of malignant cervical masses in children necessitates a high level of suspicion. The care of children with malignant cervical masses requires a multidisciplinary approach. Staging systems provide a basis for counseling, risk stratification, and treatment planning for children with cervical malignancies. Recent advances in molecular genetics, tumor biology, and treatment strategies are changing the management of head and neck malignancies in children.

 A video of an endoscopy demonstrating a congenital skull base lesion accompanies this article

Endoscopic endonasal skull base surgical techniques, initially developed in adult patients, are being utilized with increasing frequency in pediatric patients to treat sinonasal and skull base lesions. This article reviews the current state of endoscopic endonasal approaches to the skull base to both treat disease and reconstruct the skull base in pediatric patients. Sinonasal and skull base embryology and anatomy are reviewed as a foundation for understanding the disease processes and surgical techniques. Selected skull base pathologies and conditions that involve the pediatric skull base are also reviewed.

Pediatric maxillary and mandibular tumors offer considerable challenges to otolaryngologists, oral surgeons, pathologists, and radiologists alike. Because of the close proximity to vital structures, appropriate steps toward a definitive diagnosis and treatment plan are of paramount importance. This article reviews the most common causes of pediatric jaw masses and discusses diagnostic and therapeutic considerations and recommendations.

Teratomas and dermoid cysts are germ cell neoplasms. This article focuses on cervical and craniofacial teratomas. Presentation of these neoplasms varies in degree of severity, from cosmetic deformities to airway distress requiring emergent intervention. Nasal lesions (particularly if suspicious for a nasal dermoid) require imaging before biopsy to assess for intracranial extension. Treatment consists of airway management if respiratory distress is present, and early surgical intervention. Postoperative follow-up is required to monitor for recurrence.

The differential diagnosis in pediatric lymphadenopathy includes bacterial, viral, fungal, and idiopathic causes. A systematic approach to patient evaluation is necessary because the differential diagnosis, presentation, and work up must consider infectious, immunologic, neoplastic, and idiopathic disorders. A thorough history and examination are vital to determining the diagnosis and ruling out a malignant process.

Salivary gland neoplasms are rare in children. In infants most tumors are benign hemangiomas, with some notable exceptions, such as sialoblastomas. An asymptomatic swelling in the periauricular region is the most common presenting complaint in older children. Approximately 50% of these lesions are malignant, which dictates a thorough diagnostic evaluation by a head and neck surgeon. Surgical excision is the primary treatment modality. Prognosis is primarily determined by histopathologic findings. This review discusses neoplastic lesions of the salivary glands in children, and malignant epithelial tumors in particular.

This article explores pediatric lingual and other intraoral lesions. First the embryology and anatomy of the oral anatomy is outlined. Then the article discusses infections and inflammatory diseases, congenital malformations, benign neoplasms, and malignant tumors.

Advances in prenatal imaging in the last 20 years have enabled prenatal diagnosis of obstructive head and neck masses. These advances, coupled with improvements in maternal-fetal anesthesia, have made possible the development of the ex utero intrapartum treatment (EXIT) procedure for management of obstructive head and neck masses, during which the airway is managed in a controlled fashion while maintaining fetal circulation for oxygenation. This review addresses the preoperative and perioperative assessment and management of patients with prenatally diagnosed airway obstruction, indications and contraindications for the EXIT procedure, technical details of the procedure, and outcomes.

Defects of embryologic development give rise to a variety of congenital lesions arising from the epithelium and are among the most common congenital lesions of the head and neck in the pediatric population. This article presents several congenital lesions of epithelial origin, including congenital midline cervical cleft, pilomatrixoma, dermoid, foregut duplication cysts, and preauricular sinuses and pits. In addition, the management of these lesions is reviewed.

Medical imaging is an important tool in the evaluation and classification of pediatric head and neck masses. Such lesions may include congenital, inflammatory, infectious, vascular, or neoplastic processes. Ultrasound is often the first line modality in the workup of a neck mass in a child, followed by MRI or CT depending on the scenario. This information must be interpreted in the context of the patient's clinical history, physical examination, and demographics. The medical imaging workup of a neck mass in a child must be focused to yield the maximum information possible while minimizing the risks of radiation and sedation.

OTOLARYNGOLOGIC CLINICS
OF NORTH AMERICA

RELATED INTEREST

Magnetic Resonance Imaging of the Pediatric Neck: An Overview
Shekdar KV, Mirsky DM, Kazahaya K, and Bilaniuk LT, *Authors*
in
Magnetic Resonance Imaging Clinics of North America
August 2012 (Vol. 20, Issue 3, Pages 573–603)
Practical MR Imaging in the Head and Neck
Laurie Loevner, *Editor*
http://www.mri.theclinics.com/

NOW AVAILABLE FOR YOUR iPhone and iPad

OTOLARYNGOLOGIC CLINICS
OF NORTH AMERICA

FORTHCOMING ISSUES

April 2015
Sleeve of the second ... SLN Base
George Zalzal and Matthew Gorham,
Editors

June 2015
Function Preservation in Laryngeal Cancer
Babak Sadoughi, Editor

August 2015
Medical and Surgical Complications in the
Treatment of Chronic Rhinosinusitis
James A. Stankiewicz, Editor

RECENT ISSUES

December 2014
...
Orlo Driscoll and Brad Hall, Editors

October 2014
Common ENT Disorders in Children
Charles Bower and Gresham Richter,
Editors

August 2014
Thyroid Cancer: Current Diagnosis
Management, and Reconstruction
Robert L. Witt, Editor

June 2014
Robotic Surgery in Otolaryngology
Neil D. Gross and Eric Holsinger, Editors

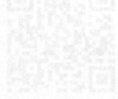

Preface

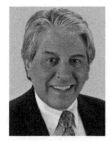
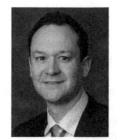

John Maddalozzo, MD   Jeffrey C. Rastatter, MD
Editors

The preface of this issue consists of statements by 3 distinct physicians at various stages of their careers, demonstrating where we come from, where we are, and where we are going.

> *If I can see farther, it is because I stand on the shoulders of giants.*
> —Sir Isaac Newton

The subspecialty of Pediatric Otolaryngology Head and Neck surgery continues to change and evolve. The origin of this subspecialty can be traced to the studies and advancements made by Chevalier Jackson, MD (November 4, 1865 to August 16, 1958) in the early and middle portions of the twentieth century. His work primarily concerned pediatric bronchoesophagology and attracted students who devoted their practice and research to advance the techniques he pioneered. New standards of care began to emerge, which led to the establishment of societies and university-based fellowship programs devoted to studying, describing, and treating otolaryngology diseases of children.

As pediatric care became concentrated at major pediatric referral centers, practitioners recognized that there were many congenital lesions as well as benign and malignant tumors of the head and neck region that were unique to the pediatric population. This led to a renewed interest and investigation into the anatomic features, physiology, and treatment of these unique pediatric disorders, contributing to better patient outcomes. Having devoted my professional career to the study and care of children with head and neck masses, I am pleased that there is continued interest in this subspecialty. This volume was compiled as a testament to past and present efforts and to provide a framework that encourages others to make advancements in the development of pediatric otolaryngology and head and neck mass surgery.

Otolaryngol Clin N Am 48 (2015) xv–xvii
http://dx.doi.org/10.1016/j.otc.2014.10.001
0030-6665/15/$ – see front matter © 2015 Elsevier Inc. All rights reserved.

oto.theclinics.com

John Maddalozzo, MD
Division of Otolaryngology–Head & Neck Surgery
Ann & Robert H. Lurie Children's Hospital of Chicago
Northwestern University Feinberg School of Medicine
225 East Chicago Avenue
Box #25
Chicago, IL 60611, USA

E-mail address:
JPMaddal@luriechildrens.org (J. Maddalozzo)

Pediatric otolaryngology head and neck surgery certainly has a rich and well-established history. The field has proven to be dynamic and progressive as major advancements and contributions have been made over a wide range of pathologies and clinical situations. Regarding management of pediatric head and neck lesions specifically, many of the foremost leaders of this discipline are represented as authors in this collection of articles. As a coeditor of this volume, I have truly enjoyed working with each author.

Regarding my own history, a complete list of otolaryngologists that have contributed to my passion for treating patients with pediatric head and neck lesions would be long indeed. Of particular significance, my years in residency training, learning from Dr David Schuller, a true giant and pioneer in the field of head and neck surgery, gave me the necessary foundation of knowledge and skill. As hard-working, caring, and passionate as they come, Dr Schuller will always be a role model to me. In my pediatric otolaryngology fellowship training, working with Dr John Maddalozzo provided a breadth of experience and refinement of knowledge specific to the management of the unique and challenging aspects of pediatric head and neck lesions. Over the last several years, management of pediatric head and neck lesions has become a primary focus of my tertiary practice. Through patient care, research, and education, I hope to continue to contribute to and advance the field of pediatric head and neck surgery for the benefit of our patients and the next generation of surgeons.

Jeffrey C. Rastatter, MD
Division of Pediatric Otolaryngology
Ann & Robert H. Lurie Children's Hospital of Chicago
225 East Chicago Avenue
Box 25
Chicago, IL 60611, USA

Department of Otolaryngology–Head and Neck Surgery
Northwestern University Feinberg School of Medicine
NMH/Galter Room 15-200
675 N Saint Clair
Chicago, IL 60611, USA

E-mail address:
JRastatter@luriechildrens.org (J.C. Rastatter)

Being chosen to contribute to the preface of this volume has been a humbling experience. Looking through the index, one can see the contributions of so many well-known clinicians in our field who share a passion for the care of the pediatric patient with head and neck pathology. When considering the Venn diagram of specialties in our field, pediatric head and neck surgery will represent a place of great curiosity and inquiry in my practice, nestled firmly in the principles of head and neck surgery with a keen focus on the unique problems presenting in the pediatric population. I draw equally on my experiences working with leaders in the fields of both Pediatric Otolaryngology and Head and Neck Surgery when addressing a pediatric head and neck patient. While I hope to contribute to this field in a meaningful way for years to come, any further vision I will have gained is not by standing on the shoulders of these giants but by working with them side by side and learning the technical and clinical considerations so critical to the care of this unique patient population. In this volume is the shared wisdom of many of these experts and the rising generation of leaders in the field, compiled with an eye to providing a thoughtful, systematic approach to the pediatric head and neck.

Patrick C. Walz, MD
Department of Pediatric Otolaryngology
Ann and Robert H. Lurie Children's Hospital of Chicago
225 E. Chicago Avenue
Box 23
Chicago, IL 60611-2991, USA

Department of Otolaryngology–Head and Neck Surgery
The Ohio State University
9000 Olentangy River Road
Suite 4000
Columbus, OH 43212, USA

E-mail address:
pcwalzmd@gmail.com (P.C. Walz)

Branchial Cleft Anomalies and Thymic Cysts

J. Drew Prosser, MD, Charles M. Myer III, MD*

KEYWORDS

- Branchial cleft cyst • Branchial cleft anomaly • Pediatric neck mass
- Branchial remnant • Thymic cyst

KEY POINTS

- Thorough knowledge of the embryology of branchial arch derivatives is essential for accurate diagnosis and surgical management of these anomalies.
- A history of preauricular infections and otorrhea with a normal tympanic membrane should raise suspicion of a first branchial arch anomaly.
- Always consider the diagnosis of a cystic metastasis in the differential of a presumed branchial cleft anomaly in an adult.
- CT scan with contrast, MRI, fistulograms, and ultrasound have all been used to aid in the diagnosis of congenital neck masses and predict the intraoperative findings before surgical excision.
- When managing first arch anomalies, be prepared to identify the facial nerve and perform a superficial or total parotidectomy (ie, informed consent, adequate sterile preparation, nerve monitoring, parotid instruments).
- Direct laryngoscopy and attention to the pyriform sinus with palpation on the ipsilateral neck can aid in pre-excision diagnosis of a third or fourth branchial cleft fistula.

INTRODUCTION

Branchial or pharyngeal cleft anomalies are an important diagnostic consideration in pediatric neck pathology. They represent the most common congenital lateral neck mass, and are second only to thyroglossal duct cysts when all cervical sites are included.[1] These anomalies can occur as a cyst (epithelial-lined structure that lacks a connection to the skin or pharynx), a sinus (connecting either the skin or pharynx to a blind pouch in the neck), or a fistula (an open tract connecting the skin and pharynx).

Disclosures: None.
Department of Pediatric Otolaryngology, Cincinnati Children's Hospital Medical Center, 3333 Burnet Avenue, Cincinnati, OH 45229, USA
* Corresponding author. 3333 Burnet Avenue, MLC 2018, Cincinnati, OH 45229.
E-mail address: charles.myer@cchmc.org

Otolaryngol Clin N Am 48 (2015) 1–14
http://dx.doi.org/10.1016/j.otc.2014.09.002
0030-6665/15/$ – see front matter © 2015 Elsevier Inc. All rights reserved.

oto.theclinics.com

Abbreviations	
BCA	Branchial cleft anomalies
CT	Computed tomography
MRI	Magnetic resonance imaging
SCM	Sternocleidomastoid muscle

The term branchial is derived from the Greek term "branchia," meaning gills. This terminology stems from the transient structures that appear from the fourth to the seventh week of gestation on the lateral aspects of the developing fetus. They are thought to be phylogenetically related to gill slits in amphibians. The branchial or pharyngeal apparatus is composed of mesodermal arches that appear on the superior-lateral aspects of the developing fetus. These arches are separated by external clefts or grooves (found on the epithelial surface between each arch and, with the exception of the first cleft, obliterate during normal development) and internal pouches (endodermal-derived elements). Each of these numbered arches develops into an associated nerve, blood vessel, and muscle group (**Table 1**). Aberrant development of these structures or incomplete obliteration of the clefts and grooves that divide them can lead to a variety of different anomalies. Here we present an overview of these anomalies and discuss their cause, presentation, and treatment.

RELEVANT ANATOMY AND PATHOPHYSIOLOGY

As with any congenital condition, a complete understanding of the normal developmental process is critical to understanding the pathology that results when this process is interrupted in some way. During fetal development, six paired outpouchings (arches) originate on the ventrolateral aspect of the developing embryonic head and join in the midline. Each arch is separated externally by grooves or clefts, which are lined with ectodermal tissue. The internal surface of the arches is separated by pouches, which are lined by endodermal tissue. The individual arches themselves are composed of mesodermal tissue, which develops into an artery, nerve, muscular, and cartilageous elements (see **Table 1**). As the fetus matures, these elements form well-defined anatomic structures that are present at birth.

Initially during development the endodermal and ectodermal linings come into close contact, further separating the arches. As the fetus matures, most of the external cleft and internal pouches are obliterated as the adjacent arches subsequently fuse (see **Table 1**). Branchial cleft anomalies (BCAs) result from incomplete obliteration of the associated cleft or pouch during this process. The resulting cyst, sinus, or fistula is based on the specific arch and degree of obliteration that is completed. This embryologic basis means that each anomaly courses inferior to the anatomic derivatives of its associated arch and superior to all derivatives of the next arch (see **Table 1**). This knowledge allows the surgeon to identify correctly the associated arch and predict its tract intraoperatively. Depending on the arch of origin, these anomalies can present as a mass or draining tract anywhere from the preauricular skin down to the clavicle with the external opening at the anterior border of the sternocleidomastoid muscle (SCM).

CLINICAL PRESENTATION AND EXAMINATION

Many symptoms of BCA are nonspecific, including neck swelling, recurrent infections, and drainage. Because of the nonspecific nature of many of these complaints, most

Table 1
Branchial cleft development

Arch	Skeletal	Nerve	Muscles	Artery	Pouch	Cleft
First (mandibular arch)	Meckel cartilage Malleus Incus Portion of the mandible	Trigeminal (V)	Muscles of mastication Tensor tympani Tensor palatini Mylohyoid Anterior belly of digastric	Maxillary	Eustachian tube Middle ear	External auditory canal
Second (hyoid arch)	Reichert cartilage Stapes Styloid process Hyoid bone-lesser horn, upper half of body	Facial (VII)	Muscles of facial expression Stapedius Stylohyoid Posterior belly of digastric	Stapedial (normally obliterates)	Lining (crypts) of palatine tonsils	Obliterates
Third	Hyoid bone-greater horn, lower half of body	Glossopharyngeal (IX)	Stylopharyngeus	Common/internal carotid	Inferior parathyroid gland Thymus	Obliterates
Fourth	Thyroid cartilage Epiglottic cartilage	Vagus (X) Superior laryngeal nerve	Cricothyroid All muscles of pharynx (except stylopharyngeus) All muscles of soft palate (except tensor palatini)	Aortic arch and subclavian	Superior parathyroid gland C-cells of Thyroid	Obliterates
Fifth arch is transient and no structures are derived from this arch in mammals						
Sixth	Cricoid cartilage Arytenoid complex	Vagus (X) Recurrent laryngeal nerve	Intrinsic muscles of the larynx except the cricothyroid	Pulmonary arteries and ductus arteriosis	—	Obliterates

patients present initially to their primary care physician or pediatrician. Once the diagnosis is suspected, the surgeon is consulted. Only a small minority of these are discovered incidentally, either by physical examination or during imaging for a nonrelated complaint. The clinical presentation of each lesion ultimately depends on the arch involved and the exact anomaly present.

Most patients with a cyst (no connection to the external skin or pharynx) present with a firm, nontender mass, usually in the anterior cervical triangle anywhere from the preauricular region to the supraclavicular fossa. If the cyst is large, dysphagia, dyspnea, and stridor can be present. Infection or hemorrhage into a cyst can lead to an abrupt increase in size, worsening pain, or abscess formation. When a sinus connecting to the pharynx is present, these tend to present with recurrent infections. A connection to the skin can present with infections, drainage, or an external skin pit. A fistula usually presents with a draining skin pit.

Although BCAs can present at any age, most cases are diagnosed in early childhood. A 10-year review of pediatric BCAs showed that the average age of presentation was younger than 5 years with fistulas presenting at the youngest age. Sinuses and cysts tended to present at an older age. Second arch anomalies were the most common followed by first arch anomalies.[2] Overall there is no predilection for sex (male or female) or side (left or right); however, complete second branchial cleft fistulas have recently been shown to be more common on the right, whereas third arch anomalies tend to affect the left.[3] Most occur spontaneously; however, a minority is associated with a syndrome (most commonly branchio-oto-renal syndrome, which often presents with bilateral BCA, bilateral preauricular pits, and renal anomalies).

First Branchial Cleft Anomalies

Periauricular pits, sinuses, and tags are the most common first branchial arch anomalies.[4] These lesions result from aberrant development of the first three hillocks of His, which form from the dorsal aspect of the first branchial arch and contribute to formation of the auricle. They do not involve the first branchial cleft and therefore are not true BCAs; however, it is important to know and recognize the distinction between these two conditions because preauricular pits are a common incidental finding in pediatric patients and often do not require surgical management. Preauricular pits and tags usually occur in the preauricular skin anterior to the tragus or the ascending rim of the helix. Although preauricular tags mostly present only cosmetic concerns, preauricular sinuses can have a history of drainage at the site of a skin pit. Recurrent infection with cellulitis and abscess formation also occurs, although most are asymptomatic. Physical examination should pay particular attention to the site of the lesion or skin opening and the presence of any signs of infection (erythema, tenderness, fluctuance, or induration of surrounding structures). The ear canal should be examined carefully to ensure that there are no signs of connection or duplication, which would represent a true first cleft anomaly. If the patient tolerates, gentle probing of the tract can give the surgeon valuable information about the extent of the anomaly.

First BCAs, which exclude pits and tags, are rare and account for less than 20% of all BCAs.[2,5] The epithelial component of these anomalies is found above the hyoid bone with a tract coursing through the parotid gland. Because the gland and facial nerve are developing at the same time as the tract is obliterating, the relationship of the tract to the facial nerve is variable in these anomalies. This lesion can course either superficial or deep to the main trunk or even travel between nerve branches.[6] If an internal communication is present, the opening courses into the external auditory canal or middle ear cleft.

Because of their location, first branchial cleft remnants can present with recurrent preauricular or upper neck swelling. If they rupture, a draining sinus often results. One should be suspicious of a first branchial anomaly when a child presents with recurrent otorrhea without evidence of middle ear disease or significant canal inflammation. The cysts may occur in the parotid gland itself thus leading to the misdiagnosis of salivary pathology.[7]

Several authors have attempted to classify first BCAs; however, the most widely used scheme was published by Work in 1972. He proposed a system of dividing first branchial anomalies according to their embryologic derivative.[8] Type I anomalies consisted only of ectodermal elements. In contradistinction type II anomalies consisted of ectodermal and mesodermal elements. This method adds a histologic component to the traditional anatomic classification. Several authors have proposed revisions of Work's classification. Belenky and Medina[9] proposed a modification where a type 1 anomaly is a preauricular cyst or sinus, which courses lateral or superior to the facial nerve and terminates without an opening in the external auditory canal. A type II anomaly can be a cyst, sinus, or fistula where the tract starts near the angle of the mandible and tracts superior medially to join or open into the cartilaginous external auditory canal. This tract can have a variable relationship to the facial nerve. This classification is purely anatomic and removes the histologic basis and is preferred by some authors.

However one classifies the anomaly, the relationship of the lesion or tract to the facial nerve is a critically important one and there is not currently an accurate way for the clinician to determine this relationship before surgery. Given this, if a surgeon is not prepared or capable of identifying, preserving, and protecting the facial nerve during surgery, then no attempt should be made at removal of first BCAs.

Second Branchial Cleft Anomalies

Most (70%–90%) BCAs originate from the second cleft.[2,10] The skin opening of a second BCA is lower in the neck at the anterior border of SCM. Clinically, these anomalies have much in common with some third arch anomalies; however, the diagnosis is made clear during surgical excision. The tract of the second cleft anomaly starts in the tonsillar fossa, courses inferior-laterally, and travels superior-lateral to the glossopharyngeal and hypoglossal nerves. The tract courses between the internal and external carotid arteries and terminates at a skin opening anterior to the SCM. Cleft anomalies can present anywhere along this tract.

Cysts are the most common second BCA, followed by sinuses and then fistulas. Second branchial cleft cysts present most commonly with a cystic neck mass located deep to the SCM. When the anomaly involves a tract (ie, sinus or fistula), the most common presenting complaint is an external skin opening with drainage, followed by recurrent infections. Abscess formation can also occur, and in patients with a history of infection, they tend to be recurrent in nature.

Third Branchial Cleft Anomalies

Third BCAs are rare but can have many similarities with second arch anomalies. Cysts again present with a mass deep to the SCM, as with second arch anomalies. The skin opening again is low in the lateral neck anterior to the SCM. These tend to occur on the left side of the neck. The theoretic tract of a third BCA originates in the apex of the piriform sinus, pierces the thyrohyoid membrane, and travels inferior and posterior to the glossopharyngeal nerve and superior to the hypoglossal nerve. The tract courses posterior to the internal carotid artery and exits the skin just anterior to the SCM.

A key clinical piece of information that can lead to suspicion of a third arch anomaly is the close relation of these arch elements to the thyroid gland. Inflammation of these anomalies can often lead to recurrent bouts of thyroiditis. Furthermore, an abscess in the neck located within or surrounding the thyroid gland should raise suspicion of a third arch anomaly.[11] Although not always typical in second branchial cleft sinuses, a neck abscess is typical of a third branchial cleft sinus. The connection to the dependent pyriform sinus leads to frequent contamination by oropharyngeal secretions in third branchial cleft sinuses, whereas the lateral location of the tonsillar crypts without dependent drainage makes this rarer in second cleft anomalies.

Cervical Thymic Anomalies

Cervical thymic anomalies are themselves branchial arch anomalies because of their embryologic derivative from the third arch (see **Table 1**). Although ectopic cervical thymic tissue can be seen anywhere along the course of the thymic descent, this condition is exceedingly rare. Cervical thymic cysts are more common than ectopic thymic tissue but remain a rare presentation of congenital neck lesions.[12] A review of 20 cases at Cincinnati Children's Hospital revealed the most common presentation of cervical thymic anomalies is a mass with associated compressive symptoms.[13] There was a predilection for these anomalies on the left side; however, midline and right-sided anomalies were seen. Most patients were male with age ranges from 1 to 16 years. An association with lymphoma or its treatment has been suggested but this condition is so rare that finding consistent associations can be difficult.[14]

Fourth Branchial Cleft Anomalies

Fourth BCAs are without question the rarest with few having been described in the literature. These cysts and sinuses present with recurrent lower neck or upper chest infections. Thyroiditis also can be seen and these patients have frequently been misdiagnosed and had inappropriate surgical interventions. Although cysts and sinuses have been reported, a fourth branchial cleft fistula is thought to have never occurred because of the long tortuous course that this anomaly would have to take from the pyriform sinus to the skin. The theoretic path of this tract originates in the pyriform sinus and courses inferiorly, deep to the superior laryngeal nerve and superficial to the recurrent laryngeal nerve and tracts inferiorly to wrap around the aortic arch on the left and subclavian artery on the right, then ascends superiorly, posterior to the carotid artery and attaches to the skin low in the neck anterior to the SCM.

DIAGNOSTIC PROCEDURES

Although the diagnosis can be suspected on clinical history and physical examination alone, the true diagnosis of a BCA comes from surgical excision and pathologic examination. Various imaging techniques have been used to aid in preoperative localization of the lesion and the relation to critical neck structures. These can be particularly helpful in recurrent lesions, or those with a history of multiple infections who have previously undergone surgical drainage. However, imaging should not be used for diagnosis alone. The choice of imaging modality varies by treatment center based on the risks and benefits of each modality described next.

Computed Tomography Scan

Computed tomography (CT) scanning with intravenous contrast is probably the most widely used imaging modality when evaluating cervical masses. When clinical history is classic, and no prior surgery has been performed, often no imaging is ordered. When the history is equivocal or if there is a question of abscess formation or a significant inflammatory component, a CT scan can help to define the extent of the lesion preoperatively, guide the timing of surgical intervention, and aid in preoperative planning for complete excision. CT characteristics of BCAs tend to show a well-circumscribed lesion with thin walls and central mucous attenuation (10–25 HU). When infected the cyst wall or tract tends to become thickened and irregular, and enhancing with intravenous contrast. Usually, only when the lesion is infected and has inflamed walls is the tract visible. When the tract is visible, the most reliable predictor in identifying the affected arch is its relationship to the cervical vasculature.[15] The main drawback of this modality is the radiation exposure and occasional need for sedation. The relatively low cost and ease of obtaining make it the primary choice of some centers.

MRI

MRI scans show a cystic lesion with low to intermediate T1-weighted and high T2-weighted signal intensity. With chronic infection, high T1-weighted signal can be seen and is related to a change in the protein content of the mucous. MRIs can be beneficial in parotid masses and may be the primary imaging choice depending on the suspected pathology. They should be ordered with contrast to aid in identification of the cyst tract and its relationship to the facial nerve.[15] The main drawback of this modality is the cost and need for sedation in most children. The excellent soft tissue detail and lack of radiation exposure make it the primary choice of some centers.

Ultrasound

There has been a recent push toward ultrasound as an imaging modality in the pediatric population. This has the benefit of a rapid, low-cost imaging study that avoids radiation exposure. The drawbacks are that it is operator dependent and generally gives less anatomic detail than CT or MRI. Findings on ultrasound usually demonstrate a round mass with uniform low echogenicity and a lack of internal septations with no acoustic enhancement or enlargement.[16] Ultrasound can be useful in determining the relationship of the lesion to the cervical vasculature and aid in needle decompression in the infected cyst where one is avoiding a formal incision and drainage. Ultrasound may also be beneficial for third or fourth arch anomalies that pass close to or go through the thyroid gland. Tsai and coworkers[17] recently reported the prenatal diagnosis of a branchial cleft cyst via three-dimensional ultrasound that caused tracheal deviation and resulted in early surgical excision.

Barium Esophagram

When recurrent neck infections or fistulas are noted, a barium esophagram can help identify an opening in the hypopharynx that tracks into the neck. This study also can be combined with a noncontrast CT scan to show the relationship of the tract to critical structures.[11] This modality can be greatly beneficial but should not supplant direct visualization of the opening via endoscopy. Furthermore, the insertion of a catheter at the time of endoscopy can aid in identification of the sinus tract during open surgical management and allow for complete excision of the tract.

SURGICAL TECHNIQUE

Surgery is performed in these cases for a variety of reasons but the most frequent are a history of recurrent infections, desire for improved cosmesis, a mass with recent increase in size, or an unknown lesion in need of a histopathologic diagnosis. The underlying surgical principle in diagnosing and treating all BCAs is complete surgical excision of the cyst or sinus tract, in addition to any previously dissected tissues, which may harbor epithelial components.

Surgical excision of an acutely infected branchial cleft cyst or tract increases the technical difficulty and leads to higher recurrence rates and complications.[18] Local edema and inflammation leads to obscuring of tissue planes and purulent contents under pressure can predispose to intraoperative cyst rupture. When an infected cyst, sinus, or fistula is present, appropriate antibiotics should be started and continued for at least 10 days if clinically improving. If the patient fails to improve, needle aspiration, using ultrasound guidance if needed, can be used to identify the organism and guide antibiotic therapy. If this is done, therapy should consist initially of intravenous antibiotics until cultures and sensitivities return, then allowing for prolonged oral antibiotics followed by surgical excision when the infection has resolved. Every reasonable attempt should be made to avoid incision and drainage because this can make the definitive surgical treatment more difficult. If incision and drainage is required, when definitive treatment is undertaken, the scar tissue should be excised with the specimen.

Preauriclar Pits and Cysts and Sinuses

Excision of preauricular cysts and sinuses is performed usually for a history of recurrent infections. The tract is first cannulated with a lacrimal duct probe before injection of local anesthetic because the local injection can make cannulation of the sinus tract more difficult. A vertical elliptical incision is placed in a preauricular skin crease and surrounds the preauricular skin opening. Any scar tissue from previous surgery should be excised with the sinus tract. Blunt and sharp dissection is used to delineate the tract, taking care not to violate the wall. These generally track down to the anterior helical or tragal cartilage rim. If scaring is present, a margin of cartilage can be removed to ensure complete excision. Every attempt should be made to excise the entire cyst and tract down to the temporalis fascia if required. These preauricular cysts and sinuses are not typically associated with the facial nerve and surface landmarks for nerve anatomy should be used to ensure dissection is away from the nerve.

First Branchial Cleft Anomalies

First branchial cleft cysts, sinuses, and fistulas are excised in a manner similar to parotid surgery. If electrophysiologic monitoring is used, the surgeon should communicate this to the anesthesia team to ensure no muscle relaxants are administered. The incision should be performed in the preauricular skin fold and extend around the lobule into either the hairline for a modified facelift approach or curve anteriorly into a cervical skin crease at least 2 cm below the angle of the mandible. Any previous incision and drainage incisions should be incorporated and removed with the specimen. The skin flaps are elevated over the parotid and SCM, preserving the greater auricular nerve if possible.

Next, the parotid is freed from the SCM posteriorly and the external auditory canal anteriorly. The posterior belly of the digastric is identified and the facial nerve trunk identified as it exits the stylomastoid foramen. The nerve is traced anteriorly to the pes aneserinus and, at this point, depending on the relationship of the cyst to the main truck, dissection of the anomaly can proceed. Removal of either a portion or the entire superficial lobe of the parotid gland may be required to excise the anomaly totally (**Fig. 1**). If intraoperatively or on preoperative imaging the tract does not course deep to the parotid fascia, identification of the nerve may not be required.

The tract is dissected to the external auditory canal where a segment of canal cartilage may need to be excised to ensure complete resection of the tract. This area can

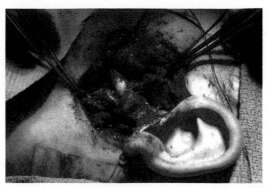

Fig. 1. Intraoperative view of a first branchial cleft cyst (Work type II). DeBakey forceps are seen retracting the residual superficial parotid lobe. The anomaly can be seen coursing deep to the upper branch of the facial nerve, which has been traced and preserved. A portion of the superficial parotid has been removed such that the full extent of the cyst can be identified and safely but completely resected.

be left to heal by secondary intention or reconstructed as necessary. The incision should be closed in layers using a drain. Postoperatively, antibiotics should be used while the drain is in place and facial nerve function should be assessed as soon as the patient is awake.

Second and Third Branchial Cleft Anomalies

Second and third BCAs can have many things in common during presentation, and in the absence of a history of thyroiditis the distinction is not clear until surgical excision is performed. For cysts with no apparent connection to the skin, the incision should be placed on the ipsilateral side of the neck in a relaxed skin tension line, realizing that if the cyst is in fact connected to a tract, this tract courses either superiorly toward the tonsillar fossa or medially toward the pyriform sinus. Given this, it is often advisable to choose an incision near the superior aspect of the cyst if it does not violate a zone 2 cm from the angle of the mandible. Previous scars should be incorporated.

Subplatysmal flaps are raised superiorly to the submandibular gland, posteriorly to the posterior border of the SCM, inferiorly to the clavicle, and medially to the strap muscles. The fascia of the SCM is divided at the anterior border and the muscle is retracted, exposing the cyst. The cyst is then freed from surrounding critical structures and any tracts should be identified and traced. Pay careful attention to the relationship of the cyst to the carotid artery. If the tract is traced to the pharynx, this internal opening may be removed and then closed in a layered fashion. Skin closure is performed in a layered fashion over a drain. Antibiotics are continued while the drain is in place.

Fistulas or sinuses with an external skin opening may be cannulated with a lacrimal duct probe or angiocatheter before incision to define the extent of the tract. Preincision direct laryngoscopy with careful inspection of the ipsilateral pyriform and tonsillar fossa while palpating the neck can identify the pharyngeal opening and facilitate cannulation of the tract from the pharyngeal side. Complete excision may require "stair stepping" incisions to allow for excision of the entire tract. Tracts that course close to or through the thyroid gland may need to be managed with a hemithyroidectomy with identification and preservation of the recurrent laryngeal nerve.

Cervical Thymic Anomalies

Because of the rare nature of these anomalies, frequently a separate diagnosis is suspected (ie, neoplasm, adenopathy, a separate branchial anomaly, or lymphatic malformation). These anomalies can be found anywhere along the tract of descent of the thymus and can commonly be associated with other third arch derivatives, such as the parathyroid glands. These cysts can become quite large and involve the mediastinum, splay the great vessels, and extend superiorly to involve the tracheoesophageal groove and retropharyngeal space (**Figs. 2–4**). Most are found deep in the lower neck and are associated with the carotid sheath. The pathologic hallmark is thymic parenchyma with lymphoid tissue and Hassall corpuscles found within the cyst wall. Complete excision is curative and complications and recurrence rates are low.[13]

Endoscopic Treatment

For third or fourth cleft sinuses where there is no skin opening but only an opening in the pyriform sinus (**Fig. 5**), some authors have advocated for a purely endoscopic approach to these lesions.[19] Chen and colleagues[19] reported nine patients diagnosed with pyriform fossa sinus tracts treated with laryngoscopy and endoscopic electrocauterization of the sinus tract. In this study, 78% of patients had no recurrences, whereas 22% had recurrent infections and underwent excision with a left hemithyroidectomy. Trichloroacetic acid also has been used for endoscopic chemical cauterization.[20] Others have used the endoscope to facilitate open resection of these lesions with some using a retroauricular incision with robotic technology aiding in resection.[21] This is not widespread.

Controversies

There is controversy surrounding the entity of "branchiogenic carcinoma," which is carcinoma arising within a branchial cleft cyst.[22] This controversy centers on whether this is a true occurrence or represents a cystic lymph node metastasis to cervical nodes from tonsillar fossa, base of tongue, or unknown primary squamous cell carcinomas. Full discussion of this controversy is beyond the scope of this article except to

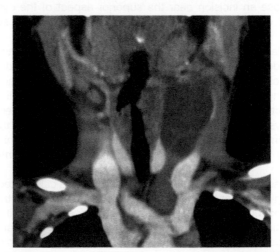

Fig. 2. Coronal CT scan of the neck with contrast showing a large cystic structure closely associated with the great vessels, extending down into the mediastinum and deviating the airway to the right.

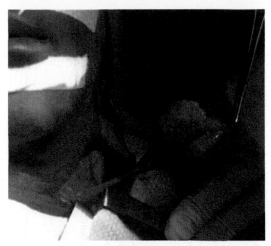

Fig. 3. Intraoperative view of a cervical thymic anomaly as it is excised off of the carotid sheath and associated vascular structures.

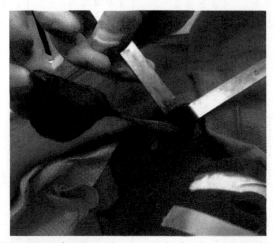

Fig. 4. Intraoperative view showing the cervical thymic cyst tracking deep into the mediastinum.

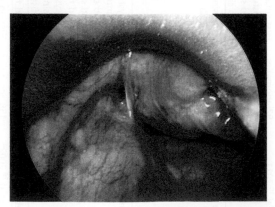

Fig. 5. Endoscopic view of the left pyriform fossa showing a tract positioned at the deep portion of the fossa. The esophageal introitus can be seen posteriorly with the arytenoids at the upper right of the view. This anomaly was treated endoscopically with electrocauterization of the sinus tract.

Table 2
Recent literature on branchial cleft anomalies

Author, Year	Numbers	Anomalies (Number)	Recurrence Rates	Complications
Cheng Elden,[18] 2012	85 anomalies	Second cysts (20) Second sinus (29) Second sinus (36)	One reported in fistula (2.8%)	None reported
Maddalozzo et al,[3] 2012	31 anomalies	Second fistula (31)	None reported	None reported
Bajaj et al,[10] 2011	92 anomalies	First sinus (12) First fistula (3) Second sinus/fistula (74) Fourth sinus (3)	None reported	One temporary marginal nerve weakness (first cleft) One incomplete excision (second sinus/fistula)
Nicoucar et al,[24] 2010[a]	202 anomalies	Third sinus/cyst/fistula (202)	For those treated with incision (I) and drainage (D) (94% initial recurrence) For the open surgical resection (15% recurrence) Endoscopic treatment (18% recurrence)	Three vocal cord paralysis, one vocal cord paresis, three salivary fistulas, one facial nerve paralysis, one Horner syndrome, one patient with IX/X/XI cranial nerve paralysis
Schroeder et al,[2] 2007	74 anomalies	First cyst (7) First sinus (6) Second cyst (14) Second sinus (23) Second fistula (14) Third cyst (1) Third sinus (2) Third fistula (1)	6% overall	Five wound infections One temporary XII nerve paresis One seroma Three hypertrophic scars One keloid
Rattan et al,[25] 2006	63 anomalies	Second fistula (63)	3%	None reported
D'Souza et al,[26] 2002[a]	158 anomalies	First sinus (67) First fistula (72) Unspecified (19)	8%	Twenty-three facial nerve palsy Three facial nerve paralysis Eight postoperative infections One tympanic membrane (TM) perforation One external auditory canal stenosis One keloid

[a] Denotes review article that reports data published before the referenced article.

mention that, in an adult patient with a cystic neck mass, every attempt should be made to rule out carcinoma as the cause. Should carcinoma be identified in the cystic mass, attention should be paid to the tonsillar fossa and base of tongue as potential primary sites.

Some controversy exists surrounding the identification of third and fourth branchial cleft sinuses. Some authors prefer the classification of pyriform sinus tracts and believe that these anomalies are more consistent with a remnant of the thymopharyngeal duct, which is formed as the thymus descends into the anterior mediastimum.[23] Others believe this terminology simply serves to broadly classify third and fourth cleft sinus tracts that have not been fully identified based on their relation to the superior laryngeal nerve. If surgical excision is performed, the exact cleft or origin often can be identified.

CLINICAL OUTCOMES IN THE LITERATURE

With adequate surgical excision of these anomalies, recurrence rates are low. A history of recurrent infections or previous surgery leads to higher rates of recurrence and complications. **Table 2** summarizes the recent literature, published since 2000, which reports the outcomes of 30 or more patients diagnosed with BCAs. The number and types of anomalies studied and any complications are included.

SUMMARY

BCAs represent varied clinical pathology that can present in children and adults. In many cases, a high index of suspicion is necessary for appropriate diagnosis and treatment. Although the mainstay of treatment is complete surgical excision, in some sinus tracts that open into the pyriform fossa, endoscopic cauterization may provide relief from symptoms and obliviate the need for surgical excision. Overall, complications and recurrence rates are low, but a sound understanding of the embryologic basis of the anomaly and experience in open head and neck surgery is critical to safe surgical excision.

REFERENCES

1. LaRiviere CA, Waldhausen JH. Congenital cervical cysts, sinuses, and fistulae in pediatric surgery. Surg Clin North Am 2012;92(3):583–97.
2. Schroeder JW Jr, Mohyuddin N, Maddalozzo J. Branchial anomalies in the pediatric population. Otolaryngol Head Neck Surg 2007;137(2):289–95.
3. Maddalozzo J, Rastatter JC, Dreyfuss HF, et al. The second branchial cleft fistula. Int J Pediatr Otorhinolaryngol 2012;76(7):1042–5.
4. Nofsinger YC, Tom LW, LaRossa D, et al. Periauricular cysts and sinuses. Laryngoscope 1997;107:883–7.
5. Olsen KD, Maragos NE, Weiland LH. First branchial cleft anomalies. Laryngoscope 1980;90:423–36.
6. Solares CA, Chan J, Koltai PJ. Anatomical variations of the facial nerve in first branchial cleft anomalies. Arch Otolaryngol Head Neck Surg 2003;129(3):351–5.
7. Triglia JM, Nicollas R, Ducroz V, et al. First branchial cleft anomalies. A study of 39 cases and a review of the literature. Arch Otolaryngol Head Neck Surg 1998;124: 291–3.
8. Work WP. Newer concepts of first branchial cleft anomalies. Laryngoscope 1972; 82:1581–93.

9. Belenky WM, Medina JE. First branchial cleft cyst anomalies. Laryngoscope 1980;90:28–39.
10. Bajaj Y, Ifeacho S, Tweedie D, et al. Branchial anomalies in children. Int J Pediatr Otorhinolaryngol 2011;75(8):1020–3.
11. Stone ME, Thompson Link D, Egelhoff JC, et al. A new role for computed tomography in the diagnosis and treatment of pyriform sinus fistula. Am J Otolaryngol 2000;21:323–5.
12. Khariwala SS, Nicollas R, Triglia JM, et al. Cervical presentations of thymic anomalies in children. Int J Pediatr Otorhinolaryngol 2004;68(7):909–14.
13. Statham MM, Mehta D, Willging JP. Cervical thymic remnants in children. Int J Pediatr Otorhinolaryngol 2008;72(12):1807–13.
14. Lewis CR, Manoharan A. Benign thymic cysts in Hodgkin's disease: report of a case and review of published cases. Thorax 1987;42:633–4.
15. Som PM, Smoker WRK, Curtin HD, et al. Congenital lesions of the neck. In: Som PM, Curtin HD, editors. Head and neck imaging. 5th edition. St Louis, MO: Elsevier and Mosby publishers; 2011. p. 2235–52.
16. Reynolds JH, Wolinski AP. Sonographic appearance of branchial cysts. Clin Radiol 1993;48:109–10.
17. Tsai PY, Chang CH, Chang FM. Prenatal imaging of the fetal branchial cleft cyst by three-dimensional ultrasound. Prenat Diagn 2003;23:599–610.
18. Cheng J, Elden L. Management of pediatric second branchial fistulae: is tonsillectomy necessary? Int J Pediatr Otorhinolaryngol 2012;76(11):1601–3.
19. Chen EY, Inglis AF, Ou H, et al. Endoscopic electrocauterization of pyriform fossa sinus tracts as definitive treatment. Int J Pediatr Otorhinolaryngol 2009;73(8):1151–6.
20. Kim KH, Sung MW, Koh TY, et al. Pyriform sinus fistula: management with chemocauterization of the internal opening. Ann Otol Rhinol Laryngol 2000;109(5):452–6.
21. Park YM, Byeon HK, Chung HP, et al. Robotic resection of benign neck masses via a retroauricular approach. J Laparoendosc Adv Surg Tech A 2013;23(7):578–83.
22. Singh B, Balwally AN, Sundaram K, et al. Branchial cleft cyst carcinoma: myth or reality? Ann Otol Rhinol Laryngol 1998;107:519–24.
23. James A, Stewart C, Warrick P, et al. Branchial sinus of the piriform fossa: reappraisal of third and fourth branchial anomalies. Laryngoscope 2007;117(11):1920–4.
24. Nicoucar K, Giger R, Jaecklin T, et al. Management of congenital third branchial arch anomalies: a systematic review. Otolaryngol Head Neck Surg 2010;142(1):21–8.
25. Rattan KN, Rattan S, Parihar D, et al. Second branchial cleft fistula: is fistulogram necessary for complete excision. Int J Pediatr Otorhinolaryngol 2006;70(6):1027–30.
26. D'Souza AR, Uppal HS, De R, et al. Updating concepts of first branchial cleft defects: a literature review. Int J Pediatr Otorhinolaryngol 2002;62(2):103–9.

Thyroglossal Duct Cyst and Ectopic Thyroid

Surgical Management

Karin P.Q. Oomen, MD, PhD[a,b], Vikash K. Modi, MD[c],
John Maddalozzo, MD[d],*

KEYWORDS

- Surgical management • Thyroglossal duct cyst • Ectopic thyroid • Carcinomas

KEY POINTS

- Thyroglossal duct cyst carcinomas.
- Posterior Hyoid Space.

INTRODUCTION

The thyroglossal duct cyst (TGDC) is the most common congenital malformation in the neck, accounting for 70% of all congenital neck lesions.[1] Although TGDCs may occur at any age, most are detected in the first 2 decades of life.[2] A previous histopathologic study of adult larynges showed TGDCs to be present in 7% of the population.[3] TGDCs occur as a result of failure of the thyroglossal duct to obliterate during embryonic development. During the fourth week of fetal development, epithelium located in the floor of the pharynx (an area that later becomes the foramen cecum of the tongue) invaginates to form the thyroglossal duct. This duct then extends in a fingerlike fashion to a terminus in the lower midline neck, where its distal end becomes bilobed and further differentiates into the thyroid gland. Thyroid development is completed at the eighth week of gestation, after which the thyroglossal duct involutes between the eighth and 10th week. A TGDC may occur if viable epithelium persists anywhere

[a] Department of Otolaryngology-Head & Neck Surgery, Wilhelmina Children's Hospital, University Medical Center Utrecht, Heidelberglaan 100, Utrecht 3584 CX, The Netherlands; [b] Pediatric Otolaryngology-Head & Neck Surgery, Wilhelmina Children's Hospital, University Medical Center Utrecht, Heidelberglaan 100, Utrecht 3584 CX, The Netherlands; [c] Pediatric Otolaryngology-Head & Neck Surgery, Department of Otolaryngology-Head & Neck Surgery, Weill Cornell Medical College, 428 East 72nd Street, Suite 100, New York, NY 10021, USA; [d] Division of Otolaryngology-Head & Neck Surgery, Ann & Robert H. Lurie Children's Hospital of Chicago, Northwestern University Feinberg School of Medicine, 225 East Chicago Avenue, Box #25, Chicago, IL 60611, USA
* Corresponding author.
E-mail address: JPMaddal@luriechildrens.org

Otolaryngol Clin N Am 48 (2015) 15–27
http://dx.doi.org/10.1016/j.otc.2014.09.003
0030-6665/15/$ – see front matter © 2015 Elsevier Inc. All rights reserved.

along the course of the thyroglossal duct. As a consequence, the cyst can form any-where from the level of the foramen cecum to the thyroid.[4–6] During its descent, the thyroglossal duct passes close to the hyoid bone, which is concomitantly undergoing anterior fusion. Consequently, the 2 structures assume a close anatomic relationship. In a previous histopathologic study of TGDCs,[3] most cyst tracts were noted to be ventral and closely adherent to the hyoid bone. A more recent study[7] reported that the tract may be found posterior to the hyoid in approximately 30% of cases, which has important implications in treatment. The tract has never been reported to lie within the bone itself.

TGDCs normally present as indolent, asymptomatic soft masses, which move up-ward on tongue protrusion and swallowing.[8,9] However, restricted movement of the cyst does not rule out diagnosis.[10] According to Shah and colleagues,[8] locations of TGDCs are classified into 4 subdivisions: (1) intralingual, (2) suprahyoid or submental, (3) thyrohyoid, and (4) suprasternal. TGDCs usually appear as midline cervical masses located just above or below the hyoid bone, but approximately one-third may present submentally or in lower cervical levels. Less than 1% are located off the midline.[4–6] Most TGDCs are asymptomatic; however, the lingual subtype may cause laryngeal stridor, respiratory obstruction, and dysphagia.[8,11,12] TGDCs may show similarities to dermoid cysts, lymphadenopathy, lymphatic malformations, ectopic thyroid gland, branchial cleft cysts, hemangiomas, lipomas, and sebaceous cysts.[9,13] Thyroglossal duct carcinomas occur in less than 1% of TGDCs.[14,15]

The epithelial lining of a TGDC ranges from squamous epithelium to pseudostrati-fied ciliated columnar epithelium. Salivary gland tissue or thyroid gland tissue may be seen in the wall of the cyst.[7] The cyst fluid can be described as mucoid, gelatinous, or purulent yellowish-white to dark brown, and may contain cholesterol.[16] Sono-graphic studies have shown that stratified squamous epithelium tends to line cysts located near the foramen cecum, whereas thyroidal acinar epithelium tends to line cysts located more proximal to the thyroid gland.[17]

Radiologic criteria for diagnosing TGDCs are usually based on the presence of duct-ular or cystic structures.[18]

TREATMENT GOALS AND PLANNED OUTCOMES

Surgical extirpation of TGDCs is recommended, because of the likelihood of recurrent infections and the rare possibility of malignancy. Surgical management requires a thorough understanding of the embryogenesis of the thyroid gland and of the hyoid bone. The main aim of surgical treatment is the complete removal of the cyst and the duct. Historically, TGDCs were treated by simple excision or incision and drainage, which resulted in recurrence rates of greater than 50%.[19]

Surgical approaches to the TGDC have been developed primarily to avoid compli-cations associated with chronic infection, usually resulting in a cutaneous fistula. Schlange[20] in 1893 was the first to propose excision of the TGDC, along with the cen-tral portion of the hyoid bone based on embryologic procedures. This technique was later refined in 1920 by Sistrunk,[21] who included not only resection of the central hyoid but also a cuff of lingual musculature oriented toward the foramen cecum. The Sis-trunk procedure is now recognized as the most efficacious surgical treatment of TGDCs, because of its low rate of recurrence.[2] Nevertheless, recurrence remains a frequent complication in the treatment of TGDCs, even when the Sistrunk procedure is adhered to.[22–24] Several investigators have proposed variants of the Sistrunk proce-dure in an attempt to further reduce these recurrence rates.[8,22–27] These variants consist of different types of wider dissections, which include more tongue base tissue, an extension to the infrahyoid space including strap muscles, or an en bloc central neck dissection. However, none of them has been proved to significantly improve the outcome. Several other investigators have focused on different factors related to TGDC recurrence. Perkins and colleagues[22] reported results of the Sistrunk procedure for 231 patients, based on 23 years' experience. These investigators reported that TGDC recurrence was related to incorrect initial diagnosis in 50% of cases, previous infection in 15% of cases, TGDC presentation in unusual locations (ie, lateral neck or base of tongue) in 15% of cases, and lack of removal of tongue base muscle tissue and relative inexperience of the surgeon, both in 2% of cases. These factors identified to be related to TGDC recurrence are in agreement with those found in previous studies.[19,28] It is our opinion that performing the wrong operation secondary to an error in diagnosis does not represent recurrence. Preoperative infection is a common TGDC complication affecting surgical outcome, with rates ranging from 10% to 70%.[3,28] Traditional management has been to avoid incision and drainage and to rely on antibiotics and possible needle aspiration for refractory cases. The reason for this approach has been that incision and drainage create scarring and obscure natural tissue planes, making dissection difficult and decreasing the likelihood of successful surgical extirpation. Previous studies have reported the rate of recurrence after Sistrunk procedure to be higher when a previous incision and drainage had been required than when they were not.[28,29] However, a more recent study contradicts this finding, showing that incision and drainage of previous infections were not associated with an increased risk of recurrence when compared with treatment with antibiotics alone.[30]

Marianowski and colleagues[28] reported age to be a factor of importance; an age older than 2 years at time of surgery was in their study correlated to a significantly lower TGDC recurrence rate. However, this finding is contradicted by Shah and colleagues,[8] who found TGDC recurrence to be independent of age at presentation.

In 2010, Maddalozzo and colleagues[31] defined a previously undescribed anatomic area, the posterior hyoid space (PHS), which plays an important role in TGDC surgery and minimizes the risk of recurrence. The investigators ascribe the recurrence of TGDCs to incomplete resection of (1) the suprahyoid ductules, which are microscopic, or (2) infrahyoid and perihyoid tissue. The PHS is demarcated caudally by the inferior rim of the hyoid, cranially by the superior rim of the hyoid and thyrohyoid membrane, ventrally by the posterior surface of the hyoid, and dorsally by the thyrohyoid membrane (**Figs. 1–4**). Identification of the PHS allows surgeons to accurately assess the dimensions of the hyoid in both its inferior to superior aspect, as well as the anterior to posterior. This assessment facilitates complete resection of the hyoid and unroofing of the PHS, allowing evacuation of abnormal tissue from this area. These investigators reported that understanding and applying the anatomic concept of the PHS can prevent inadequate cyst resection in the area of the hyoid, reporting a recurrence rate of less than 2%.

PREOPERATIVE PLANNING AND PREPARATION

Although clinical examination is often sufficient,[32] most surgeons request preoperative imaging in diagnosing a TGDC. The purpose of imaging is to primarily identify a normal thyroid gland and to rule out ectopic thyroid tissue, which may represent the patient's only functioning thyroid.[13,33,34] Secondarily, it is used to appreciate the characteristics of the cyst. The role of computed tomography (CT) and MRI have been previously well established.[35,36] However, high-resolution ultrasonography (US) remains the ideal initial investigation of choice in diagnosing TGDCs.[37] This option is particularly

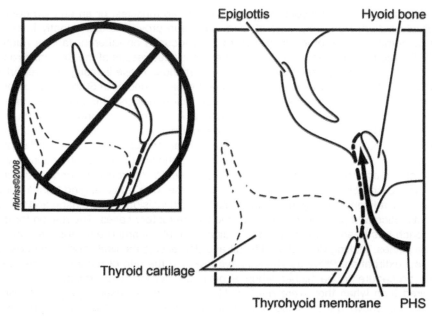

Fig. 1. PHS, sagittal view.

applicable to children, because US does not involve ionizing radiation, does not usually require sedation, is readily available, and in most cases, provides the necessary preoperative information. Echographic patterns for TGDCs in children range from anechoic to heterogeneous. Uncomplicated TGDCs tend to be anechoic, whereas a pseudosolid echo pattern most likely represents cholesterol crystals, proteinaceous

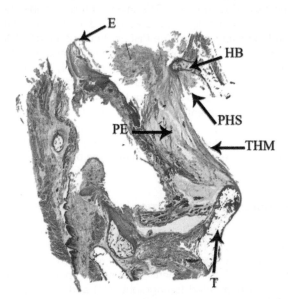

Fig. 2. Histologic sagittal section showing relationship of thyroid cartilage (T), thyrohyoid membrane (THM), pre-epiglottic space (PE), PHS, hyoid bone (HB), and epiglottis (E).

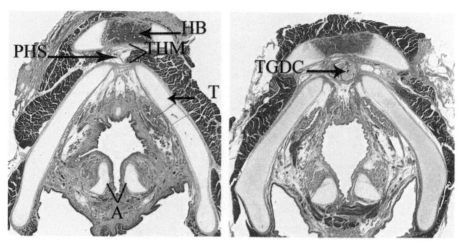

Fig. 3. Histologic cornal section showing relationship of thyroid cartilage (T), thyrohyoid membrane (THM), PHS, and hyoid bone (HB).

fluid content, or keratin.[37–39] Evidence of thick walls and internal septae indicates inflammation.[13] Although US is the most common preoperative diagnostic technique used for pediatric TGDCs, the literature[9] suggests that CT is used more often in adults. Typically, TGDCs are visualized on CT as well-circumscribed lesions, with homogeneous fluid attenuation surrounded by a thin enhancing rim. However, an increased density may be observed, as in US, caused by cholesterol crystals, fluid-containing proteins, and keratin.[37–39] The use of MRI for TGDCs is largely reserved for recurrences. Although MRI has the benefit of not involving any radiation, it often does require sedation in children.[39] Lingual TGDCs (**Fig. 5**), which present superior

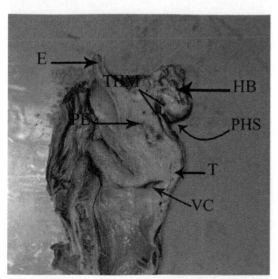

Fig. 4. Gross cadaveric sagittal section showing relationship of vocal cord (VC), thyroid cartilage (T), thyrohyoid membrane (THM), pre-epiglottic space (PE), PHS, hyoid bone (HB), and epiglottis (E).

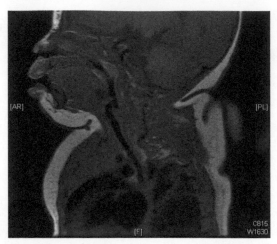

Fig. 5. Sagittal MRI T1 of intralingual TGDC.

to the hyoid bone, require the aid of other diagnostic modalities, such as flexible fiber-optic laryngoscopy (**Fig. 6**), direct laryngoscopy (**Fig. 7**), or three-dimensional CT imaging for diagnosis.[12] Fine-needle aspiration biopsy has also been used to confirm TGDC diagnosis as well as to determine the composition of the cyst fluid.[37] Fine-needle aspiration biopsy can also, to a limited degree, confirm malignancy, although the rate of true-positive results is only 53%.[15,17] A recent study by Lee and colleagues[40] concluded that fine-needle aspiration is not routinely necessary for diagnosing TGDC in children, especially given the concerns about possible injury, low sensitivity, and low positive predictive value.

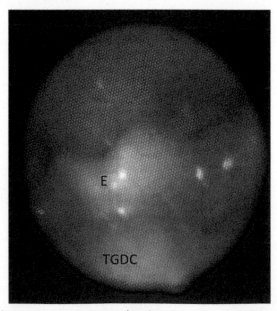

Fig. 6. Flexible fiber-optic laryngoscopy showing intralingual TGDC relationship to the epiglottis (E).

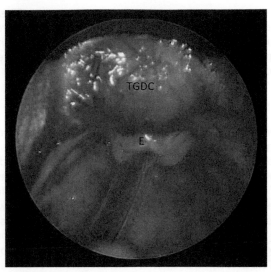

Fig. 7. Direct laryngoscopy showing intralingual TGDC relationship to the epiglottis (E).

PROCEDURAL APPROACH

A horizontal incision approximately 4 cm long is made in a skin crease inferior to the lesion and carried through subcutaneous tissue and platysma. Superior and inferior myocutaneous flaps are developed. Superiorly, the flap is elevated adequately to expose the hyoid bone and inferior portion of the submental triangle of the neck. Inferiorly, the flap is extended to expose the thyroid cartilage. The strap muscles are divided along their median raphe, and dissection is extended to the level of the thyroid cartilage. The alae of the thyroid cartilage are exposed, and the notch of the thyroid cartilage is identified. The thyrohyoid membrane is used as a conduit to identify the posterior aspect of the hyoid bone and the space between the bone and membrane (PHS) (**Fig. 8**). The height of the hyoid can be seen after these steps. The hyoid is grasped with an Allis clamp or elevated with a tracheal hook, and the hyoid can

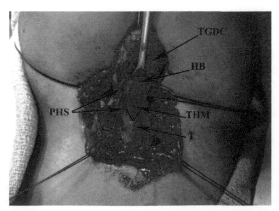

Fig. 8. Intraoperative photograph showing relationship of thyroid cartilage (T), thyrohyoid membrane (THM), PHS, and hyoid bone (HB) to the TGDC.

then be transected medial to the tendon of the digastric muscle. Dissection continues superiorly to include the cyst tract and a core of lingual musculature to the approximate level of lingual mucosa, where the specimen is transected. The tongue defect and surgical stump are then oversewn with dyed monofilament suture, and the wound is drained before closure.[2,31]

POTENTIAL COMPLICATIONS AND THEIR MANAGEMENT

Recurrence remains the most commonly encountered complication of the Sistrunk procedure.[19] Current literature indicates that the recurrence rates of TGDCs may vary from 5.2% to 33% using the Sistrunk procedure or some modification, but are usually on the lower end of this range.[9,32,41] A recent systematic review of 16 retrospective studies[42] concluded that about 1 in 10 children operated for TGDC experience a recurrence; however, not all studies concerned the Sistrunk procedure, and the investigators concluded that adhering to this procedure at least reduces recurrence rates. They also identified recurrent infection as a risk factor for recurrence. Hewitt and colleagues[27] suggested modifications to the Sistrunk procedure for the management of TGDC recurrences. These investigators recommend approaching the recurrence in the following steps: excision of previous skin incision, including fistula (if present); elevation of superior and inferior skin flaps; dissection of the lesion with a cuff of normal tissue (0.5 cm) and any granulation tissue, maintaining hemostasis; thyroid isthmus removal (may be required for inferior dissections); identification of the hypoglossal nerve in superior dissections as it enters the genioglossus muscle; removal of a 1-cm core of tissue around the foramen cecum, with or without mucosa resection; clamping and transection of the base of the tongue around the foramen cecum within 1 cm; and confirmation of the absence of epithelial tissue by taking a frozen section sample of tongue tissue deep to transection site. Although recurrence of TGDCs has classically been attributed to incomplete resection, as described earlier, Bakar and colleagues[43] suggested that in a subset of patients, the postoperative drainage may represent a salivary fistula and not always a residual, actively secreting thyroglossal duct remnant. This theory was supported by an immunohistochemical analysis of the investigators' own patient population with postoperative drainage, noting a higher incidence of salivary tissue within the resection specimen (66% vs 14% of specimens without postoperative drainage). This wide disparity suggests that the presence of salivary tissue within the resection specimen may be a risk factor for the occurrence of postoperative drainage. However, the sample size in this study is small, and the investigators agree that these findings need to be confirmed in larger studies.

In 2001, Maddalozzo and colleagues[2] retrospectively reviewed their experience with the Sistrunk procedure and its associated surgical complications. They reported a 29% incidence of minor wound-related complications associated with the Sistrunk procedure, including seroma, local wound infection, stitch abscess, and wound dehiscence. There were no recurrences or major complications in their cohort of 35 pediatric patients.

Complications defined as major complications of TGDC surgery include abscess or hematoma requiring surgical drainage, the need for a blood transfusion, violation of the airway or tracheotomy, (hypoglossal) nerve paralysis, hypothyroidism, and death.[2] Some of these complications may be avoided by careful preoperative planning and intraoperative dissection. Neurovascular complications can be avoided by transecting the hyoid at the level of the lesser cornu medial to the anterior belly of the digastric, thus avoiding the nerve and the lingual artery and vein. Placement of a drain also avoids hematoma formation. Identification of the thyroid gland with preoperative US precludes the possibility of excision of solitary ectopic thyroid tissue and resultant hypothyroidism.

Laryngotracheal injury is a highly uncommon but dreaded major complication of TGDC excision. A retrospective analysis by Wootten and colleagues[44] reported on 4 cases of TGDC excision using the Sistrunk procedure in which the airway was significantly injured. In all of the cases, the thyroid cartilage was mistaken for the hyoid, resulting in a pattern of injury that involved resection of the anterior thyroid cartilage with the anterior vocal folds and commissure. One of the factors identified to play a role in this misidentification is that in young patients, the ossified hyoid bone may override the top of the thyroid cartilage. The investigators recommend that as soon as airway injury is suspected, a safe, secure airway must be established first, before performing a direct laryngoscopy and bronchoscopy to determine the nature of the injury. Subsequently, laryngotracheal reconstruction needs to be performed with placement of a (preferably costal) cartilage graft. The investigators advocate for performing tracheotomy at the time of repair. All of their patients could be decannulated afterward. These recommendations are confirmed by Maddalozzo and colleagues,[2] who suggest that if the thyroid cartilage is violated, surgical repair with concomitant tracheotomy is required. If entry into the airway is minor (eg, tracheal puncture), the investigators recommend placement of a drain to prevent subcutaneous emphysema and allowing the wound to heal by secondary intention. Inadvertent entry into the airway can be avoided by intraoperatively identifying the notch of the thyroid cartilage and the thyrohyoid membrane. This maneuver not only allows the surgeon to avoid an erroneous transection of these structures, but identification of the membrane also provides a surgical conduit to identify the hyoid bone and the PHS.[31]

Intraoperative hemorrhage or hypoglossal nerve injury, or both, may occur if the hyoid is divided too laterally or if subsequent dissection is too aggressive in a superior lateral direction. This type of neurovascular injury would be the consequence of disrupting the contents of the Lesser triangle. This inverted triangle is a subanatomical unit of the submandibular triangle and is bounded by the tendon of the digastric and the hypoglossal nerve. Within this triangle, lying deep to the mylohyoid muscle, traverse the lingual artery and vein.[45] Injury to these structures can be avoided by transecting the hyoid at the level of the lesser cornu and by maintaining subsequent dissection medial to the anterior belly of the digastric, confined to the submental triangle of the neck.

MANAGEMENT OF THYROGLOSSAL DUCT CYST CARCINOMAS

Most TGDC carcinomas are well-differentiated papillary thyroid carcinomas, which are usually diagnosed after initial surgery for what is believed to be a normal TGDC. No clear consensus exists regarding further management after adequate excision of the cyst. Although there are proponents of aggressive therapy in this setting, many believe that such a regimen condemns the patient to lifelong sequelae associated with total thyroidectomy, radioactive iodine therapy, and hormone replacement therapy. A retrospective pooled analysis of 62 cases in the literature by Patel and colleagues[46] reported that the Sistrunk procedure is adequate for most patients with TGDC carcinomas in the presence of a clinically and radiologically normal thyroid gland. The addition of total thyroidectomy did not have a significant impact on outcome. Furthermore, routine elective nodal dissection is not recommended. However, the investigators concluded that high-risk patients (those older than 45 years, tumor >4 cm in diameter, soft tissue extension, presence of distant metastases), as well as those with clinically or radiologically abnormal regional nodes, require more aggressive management, including total thyroidectomy and radioactive iodine therapy.

ECTOPIC THYROID

Ectopic thyroid tissue is a rare midline congenital anomaly resulting from the lack of normal caudal migration of the thyroid gland.

Although approximately 90% of ectopic thyroid tissue occurs in the tongue, it has also been reported between the geniohyoid and mylohyoid muscles (sublingual thyroid), above the hyoid bone (prelaryngeal thyroid) and in other rare sites such as the mediastinum, precardial sac, heart, breast, pharynx, esophagus, trachea, lung, duodenum, mesentery of the small intestine, and adrenal gland.[47,48] Dual ectopic thyroid has been described,[49,50] even with the thyroid gland in a normal location.[51]

Ectopic thyroid tissue occurs more frequently in females (with a male/female ratio of 4:1), is seen in any age, is more frequently detected in the second decade of life, and its clinical incidence varies between 1:3000 and 1:10,000.[49] Moreover, in approximately 75% of cases, the lingual thyroid represents the only functional thyroid tissue.[48] Differential diagnosis includes lymphatic malformation, minor salivary gland tumors, midline branchial cysts, TGDCs, epidermal and sebaceous cysts, angioma, adenoma, fibroma, and lipoma.[50,52]

Diagnosis of ectopic thyroid can be made through physical examination, US, CT, and MRI, but most importantly, the use of a thyroid scan with technetium 99m sodium. CT and MRI enable estimation of gland size and position, but a thyroid scan may also show whether other sites of thyroid tissue localizations exist and may show radionuclide activity at the normal position of the thyroid in the neck. The choice of treatment of patients with ectopic thyroid tissue depends on several factors: size of the lesion, presence of local symptoms, age of the patient, state of the thyroid gland, and presence of complications, such as ulceration, hemorrhage, cystic degeneration, or malignancy.[52,53]

No treatment is required when the lingual thyroid is asymptomatic and the patient is in an euthyroid state; however, the patient should be followed to avoid the development of complications. Malignant transformation has been described,[54–57] and for this reason, some investigators advocate complete surgical removal of the gland as appropriate treatment.[55–57] For patients with absent or mild clinical symptoms and increased thyroid-stimulating hormone concentration, substitutive therapy with thyroid hormone may be successful, producing a slow reduction of the mass. Ablative radioiodine therapy is an alternative approach recommended in patients who are symptomatic and deemed unfit for surgery. Because ectopic thyroid tissue is often hypoactive and the dose of radioiodine required is generally high, this treatment should be avoided in children and young adults, because the systemic doses required have potentially damaging effects on the gonads or other organs.[58–60]

Surgical treatment should be considered if suppressive therapy has failed or to provide relief of symptoms.[48,55] Respiratory distress, difficulty swallowing, obstructive symptoms, recurrent hemorrhage, and increase in size are all indications for biopsy and surgical management. Surgical excision can be performed transorally or externally via a median or lateral pharyngotomy.[55] The transoral approach seems to avoid injury to the deep neck structures, with subsequent complications (such as injury of the lingual nerve, fistula formation, deep cervical infection, and visible scar). A transoral approach should be considered as treatment of a small mass, whereas external approaches with temporary tracheotomy can allow for better control of bleeding and are recommended for bulky masses. For the transoral approach, cold instruments with monopolar coagulation and laser CO_2 or laser diode have been used.[61]

The possibility that the ectopic thyroid tissue could be the only functioning tissue must always be considered; in those cases, transplantation of the excised ectopic tissue is usually recommended in order to avoid permanent hypothyroidism. Transplantation is not necessary in cases of partial surgical eradication, may be necessary to preserve euthyroid state and avoid recurrence of the mass.[62]

REFERENCES

1. Santiago W, Rybak LP, Bass RM. Thyroglossal duct cyst of the tongue. J Otolaryngol 1985;14:261–4.
2. Maddalozzo J, Venkatesan TK, Gupta P. Complications associated with the Sistrunk procedure. Laryngoscope 2001;111:119–23.
3. Ellis PD, van Nostrand AW. The applied anatomy of thyroglossal tract remnants. Laryngoscope 1977;87:765–70.
4. Guarisco JL. Congenital head and neck masses in infants and children, I. Ear Nose Throat J 1991;70:40–7.
5. Guarisco JL. Congenital head and neck masses in infants and children, II. Ear Nose Throat J 1991;70:75–82.
6. Maddalozzo J. Head and neck masses in children. Child Doctor 1995;12:9–17.
7. Chandra RK, Maddalozzo J, Kavark P. Histological characterization of the thyroglossal duct tract: implications for surgical management. Laryngoscope 2001; 111:1002–5.
8. Shah R, Gow K, Sobol SE. Outcome of thyroglossal duct cyst excision is independent of presenting age or symptomatology. Int J Pediatr Otorhinolaryngol 2007; 71:1731–5.
9. Lin ST, Tseng FY, Hsu CJ, et al. Thyroglossal duct cyst: a comparison between children and adults. Am J Otolaryngol 2008;29:83–7.
10. Prasad KC, Dannana NK, Prasad SC. Thyroglossal duct cyst: an unusual presentation. Ear Nose Throat J 2006;85:454–6.
11. Fu J, Xue X, Chen L, et al. Lingual thyroglossal duct cyst in newborns: previously misdiagnosed as laryngomalacia. Int J Pediatr Otorhinolaryngol 2008;72: 327–32.
12. Bai W, Ji W, Wang L, et al. Diagnosis and treatment of lingual thyroglossal duct cyst in newborns. Pediatr Int 2009;51:552–4.
13. Kutuya N, Kurosaki Y. Sonographic assessment of thyroglossal duct cysts in children. J Ultrasound Med 2008;27:1211–9.
14. Motamed M, McGlashan JA. Thyroglossal duct carcinoma. Curr Opin Otolaryngol Head Neck Surg 2004;12:106–9.
15. Torcivia A, Polliand C, Ziol M, et al. Papillary carcinoma of the thyroglossal duct cyst: report of two cases. Rom J Morphol Embryol 2010;51:775–7.
16. Allard RH. The thyroglossal cyst. Head Neck Surg 1982;5:134–46.
17. Ahuja AT, King AD, King W, et al. Thyroglossal duct cysts: sonographic appearances in adults. AJNR Am J Neuroradiol 1999;20:579–82.
18. Lee DH, Jung SH, Yoon TM, et al. Computed tomographic evaluation of thyroglossal duct cysts in children under 11 years of age. Chonnam Med J 2012;48: 179–82.
19. Pelausa ME, Forte V. Sistrunk revisited: a 10-year review of revision thyroglossal duct surgery at Toronto's Hospital for Sick Children. J Otolaryngol 1989;18: 325–33.

20. Schlange H. Ueber die Fistula Colli Congenita. Arch Klin Chir 1893;46:390–2 [in German].
21. Sistrunk WE. The surgical treatment of cysts of the thyroglossal tract. Ann Surg 1920;71:121–2.
22. Perkins JA, Inglis AF, Sie KC, et al. Recurrent thyroglossal duct cysts: a 23-year experience and a new method for management. Ann Otol Rhinol Laryngol 2006; 115:850–6.
23. Narayana MS, Arcot R. Thyroglossal duct cyst–more than just an embryological remnant. Indian J Surg 2011;72:28–31.
24. Ahmed J, Leong A, Jonas N, et al. The extended Sistrunk procedure for the management of thyroglossal duct cysts in children: how we do it. Clin Otolaryngol 2011;36:271–5.
25. Kim MK, Pawel BR, Isaacson G. Central neck dissection for the treatment of recurrent thyroglossal duct cysts in childhood. Otolaryngol Head Neck Surg 1999;121:543–7.
26. Patel NN, Hartley BE, Howard DJ. Management of thyroglossal tract disease after failed Sistrunk's procedure. J Laryngol Otol 2003;117:710–2.
27. Hewitt K, Pysher T, Park A. Management of thyroglossal duct cysts after failed Sistrunk procedure. Laryngoscope 2007;117:756–8.
28. Marianowski R, AitAmer JL, Morisseau-Durand MP, et al. Risk factors for thyroglossal duct remnants after Sistrunk procedure in a pediatric population. Int J Pediatr Otorhinolaryngol 2003;67:19–23.
29. Athow AC, Fagg NL, Drake DP. Management of thyroglossal cysts in children. Br J Surg 1989;76:811–4.
30. Simon LM, Magit AE. Impact of incision and drainage of infected thyroglossal duct cyst on recurrence after Sistrunk procedure. Arch Otolaryngol Head Neck Surg 2012;138:20–4.
31. Maddalozzo J, Alderfer J, Modi V. Posterior hyoid space as related to excision of the thyroglossal duct cyst. Laryngoscope 2010;120:1773–8.
32. Davenport M. Lumps and swellings of the head and neck. BMJ 1996;312:368–71.
33. Gupta P, Maddalozzo J. Preoperative sonography in presumed thyroglossal duct cysts. Arch Otolaryngol Head Neck Surg 2001;127:200–2.
34. Tanphaichitr A, Bhushan B, Maddalozzo J, et al. Ultrasonography in the treatment of a pediatric midline neck mass. Arch Otolaryngol Head Neck Surg 2012;138:823–7.
35. Weissman JL. Nonnodal masses of the neck. In: Som PM, Curtin HD, editors. Head and neck imaging. 3rd edition. St Louis (MO): Mosby Year Book; 1996. p. 794–822.
36. Harnsberger RH. Handbook of head and neck imaging. 2nd edition. St Louis (MO): Mosby Year Book; 1995. p. 199–223.
37. Ahuja AT, King AD, Metreweli C. Sonographic evaluation of thyroglossal duct cysts in children. Clin Radiol 2000;55:770–4.
38. Ahuja AT, Wong KT, King AD, et al. Imaging for thyroglossal duct cyst: the bare essentials. Clin Radiol 2005;60:141–8.
39. Yang YJ, Haghir S, Wanamaker JR, et al. Diagnosis of papillary carcinoma in a thyroglossal duct cyst by fine-needle aspiration biopsy. Arch Pathol Lab Med 2000;124:139–42.
40. Lee DH, Yoon TM, Lee JK, et al. Is fine needle aspiration cytology appropriate for preoperatively diagnosing thyroglossal duct cysts in children under the age of 10 years? Int J Pediatr Otorhinolaryngol 2012;76:480–2.
41. Swaid AI, Al-Ammar AY. Management of thyroglossal duct cyst. Open Otorhinolaryngol J 2008;2:26–8.

42. Galluzzi F, Pignataro L, Gaini RM, et al. Risk of recurrence in children operated for thyroglossal duct cysts; a systematic review. J Pediatr Surg 2013;48:221–7.
43. Bakar SA, Martinez-Alvernia EA, Mankarious LA. Drainage post-thyroglossal duct remnant surgery: possible source and analysis. Otolaryngol Head Neck Surg 2009;140:343–7.
44. Wootten CT, Goudy SL, Rutter MJ, et al. Airway injury complicating excision of thyroglossal duct cysts. Int J Pediatr Otorhinolaryngol 2009;73:797–801.
45. Tenta LT, Keyes GR. The viscerovertebral angle: the surgical avenue of the neck. Clin Plast Surg 1985;12:313–22.
46. Patel SG, Escrig M, Shaha AR, et al. Management of well-differentiated thyroid carcinoma presenting within a thyroglossal duct cyst. J Surg Oncol 2002;79: 134–9.
47. Thomas G, Hoilat R, Daniels JS, et al. Ectopic lingual thyroid: a case report. Int J Oral Maxillofac Surg 2003;32:219–21.
48. Turgut S, Murat Ozacan K, Celikkanat S, et al. Diagnosis and treatment of lingual thyroid: a review. Rev Laryngol Otol Rhinol (Bord) 1997;118:189–92.
49. Ulug T, Ulubil SA, Alagol F. Dual ectopic thyroid: report of a case. J Laryngol Otol 2003;117:574–6.
50. Hazarika P, Siddiqui SA, Pujary K, et al. Dual ectopic thyroid: a report of two cases. J Laryngol Otol 1998;112:393–5.
51. Huang TS, Chen HY. Dual thyroid ectopia with a normally located pretracheal thyroid gland: case report and literature review. Head Neck 2007;29:885–8.
52. Benedetto V. Ectopic thyroid gland in the submandibular region simulating a thyroglossal duct cyst: a case report. J Pediatr Surg 1997;32:1745–6.
53. Williams JD, Scalafani AP, Slupchinskij O, et al. Evaluation and management of the lingual thyroid gland. Ann Otol Rhinol Laryngol 1996;105:312–6.
54. Paludetti G, Galli J, Almadori G, et al. Ectopic lingual thyroid. Acta Otorhinolaryngol Ital 1991;11(2):117–33.
55. Shah BC, Ravichand CS, Juluri S, et al. Ectopic thyroid cancer. Ann Thorac Cardiovasc Surg 2007;13:122–4.
56. Perez JS, Munoz M, Naval L, et al. Papillary carcinoma arising in lingual thyroid. J Craniomaxillofac Surg 2003;31:179–82.
57. Falvo L, Berni A, Catania A, et al. Sclerosing papillary carcinoma arising in a lingual thyroid: report of a case. Surg Today 2005;35:304–8.
58. Danner C, Bodenner D, Breay R. Lingual thyroid: iodine 131: a viable treatment modality revisited. Am J Otolaryngol 2001;22:276–81.
59. Alderson DJ, Lannigan FJ. Lingual thyroid presenting after previous thyroglossal cyst excision. J Laryngol Otol 1994;108:341–3.
60. Weider DJ, Parker W. Lingual thyroid: review, case reports, and therapeutic guidelines. Ann Otol Rhinol Laryngol 1977;86:841–8.
61. Hafidh MA, Sheahan P, Khan NA, et al. Role of CO2 laser in the management of obstructive ectopic lingual thyroids. J Laryngol Otol 2004;118:807–9.
62. Toso A, Colombani F, Averono G, et al. Lingual thyroid causing dysphagia and dyspnea. Case reports and review of the literature. Acta Otorhinolaryngol Ital 2009;29:213–7.

Head and Neck Vascular Lesions

Stephen R. Hoff, MD[a,b,]*, Jeffrey C. Rastatter, MD[a,b], Gresham T. Richter, MD[c]

KEYWORDS

- Infantile hemangioma • Venous malformation • Lymphatic malformation
- Arteriovenous malformation

KEY POINTS

- Vascular malformations represent a complex and highly variable group of head and neck masses, for which correct diagnosis is of the utmost importance.
- A thorough history and examination can usually lead to diagnosis, which is confirmed with imaging.
- The decision-making process of whether and when to treat these lesions requires expertise across multiple disciplines, and will be dually rewarding and frustrating.
- Using these guidelines, the clinician can set a realistic expectation and plan for each individual patient.

INTRODUCTION

Vascular anomalies represent a broad range of vascular malformations and tumors, which predominantly occur in the head and neck and are seen in approximately 4.5% of children.[1–6] Due to the wide variety of different presentations, growth behavior, and available treatments, which depend on the lesion, accurate diagnosis is of utmost importance. Proper diagnosis will aid in patient and family counseling and expectations, and it is helpful if they understand from the beginning that treatment will tend to be long-term. Using hemangioma as a blanket diagnosis to include vascular malformations (venous, lymphatic, and arteriovenous), with the incorrect

Funding Sources: None.
Conflict of Interest: None.
[a] Department of Otolaryngology–Head and Neck Surgery, Northwestern University Feinberg School of Medicine, 675 N St Clair St, Chicago, IL 60611, USA; [b] Division of Pediatric Otolaryngology–Head and Neck Surgery, Ann & Robert H. Lurie Children's Hospital of Chicago, 225 East Chicago Avenue, Box 25, Chicago, IL 60611, USA; [c] Department of Otolaryngology–Head and Neck Surgery, University of Arkansas for Medical Sciences, 4301 W Markham St, Little Rock, AR 72205, USA
* Corresponding author. Division of Pediatric Otolaryngology, Ann & Robert H. Lurie Children's Hospital of Chicago, 225 East Chicago Avenue, Box 25, Chicago, IL 60611.
E-mail address: stephen.hoff@northwestern.edu

implication that the lesion will regress over time, will lead to unrealistic expectations and increased the chance of complications from the lesion.

Vascular anomalies are divided into vascular tumors and vascular malformations, according to the International Society for the Study of Vascular Anomalies classification system, which is based on the work of Mulliken and Glowacki[1] in 1982 (**Table 1**). This is an important distinction because malformations and tumors show different growth characteristics. Infantile hemangioma (IH) is the most common and is considered a benign vascular tumor. IH will rapidly enlarge, then slowly regress over time, but many will still need treatment.

Vascular malformations are relatively uncommon, rarely regress, and will continue to enlarge and cause increased complications over time.[2,7–9] This includes venous malformation (VM), lymphatic malformation (LM), and arteriovenous malformation (AVM). The paradigm is shifting toward early treatment of vascular malformations when the lesion is smaller and there has been less distortion or invasion of local tissues.

Vascular anomalies represent an opportunity for collaboration in conjunction with a multidisciplinary vascular anomalies team. The authors encourage an active and frequent dialogue between otolaryngology, dermatology, interventional radiology, plastic surgery, hematology-oncology, pediatric surgery, orthopedic surgery, physical therapy, psychology, and social work. This article discusses the spectrum of common vascular anomalies, with a focus on IH as well as VMs, LMs, and AVMs.

INFANTILE HEMANGIOMAS
Diagnosis

IHs are true benign tumors of infancy and are the most common vascular anomaly. IHs are seen in approximately 4% to 10% of infants, usually before the age of 1 year, and 60% of these will present in the head and neck.[10–12] IHs are more common in whites, low-birth weight infants, and multiple gestations (2–3:1 girl/boy ratio).[2]

Histologically, IHs are composed of proliferating immature endothelial cells and disorganized vessels. The exact pathway is not fully understood, but IHs derive from endothelial stem cells with abnormal angiogenesis and vasculogenesis. Current areas of study have implicated the vascular endothelial growth factor (VEGF) and adrenergic receptor pathway, which may be the mechanism by which propranolol can shrink these tumors.[12] GLUT-1 has been identified as a specific marker for IH,

Table 1
Vascular anomaly classification based on International Society for the Study of Vascular Anomalies guidelines

Vascular Anomalies	
Vascular Tumors	**Vascular Malformations**
Hemangioma	High-flow
Infantile	Arteriovenous
Congenital (RICH or NICH)	Mixed Arterial
KHE	Low-flow
Tufted angioma	Venous
Pyogenic granuloma	Lymphatic
Other rare vascular tumors	Capillary or venular

Abbreviations: KHE, kaposiform hemangioendothelioma; NICH, noninvoluting congenital hemangioma; RICH, rapidly involuting congenital hemangioma.

with 97% of IH testing positive for GLUT-1.[13,14] Interestingly, GLUT-1 is only otherwise seen in placental tissue and endothelial cells at the blood-brain barrier. The specificity of GLUT-1 for IH has an important role in management. If a lesion is not behaving as an IH should and is suspected to be another type of vascular lesion (or is not responding to propranolol; see later discussion), a biopsy should be performed with GLUT-1 as a marker. Tumors that are GLUT-1 negative should not be expected to follow the typical proliferation-involution cycle of IH.

IHs can be classified as unifocal, segmental, or multifocal if multiple sites are involved. More than 5 cutaneous IHs necessitates an ultrasound or MRI to investigate for liver hemangiomas, which may bleed and be life-threatening.[15] Segmental IH will present along the dermatome of a cranial nerve, usually trigeminal distribution, and may have the classic beard distribution. Patients with segmental facial hemangiomas should be evaluated for posterior fossa, hemangioma, arterial lesions, cardiac abnormalities, eye abnormalities syndrome (PHACE), and have a higher incidence of subglottic hemangiomas with airway complications.[16,17]

IHs can also be classified as superficial, deep, or compound. Superficial hemangiomas will have the classic bright-red strawberry appearance and appear soft without dependent changes (**Fig. 1**). Deep IH has appearance of a subcutaneous mass and a compound has both. Portions of the IH that are under the skin may appear more dark red or purple. Previous classifications, including strawberry hemangioma, capillary hemangioma or cavernous hemangioma, should not be used.

IHs follow a typical pattern of rapid growth followed by slow involution. They are usually not present at birth, or parents will report a flat, red vascular staining of the skin at the site of a subsequent IH. During the first few months of life, IH will demonstrate rapid expansion in size and, in some cases, may ulcerate, bleed, or cause

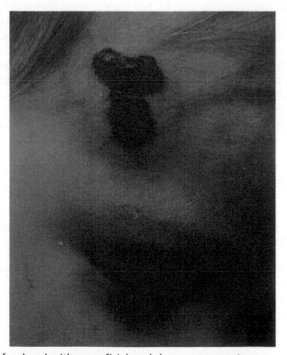

Fig. 1. IH on the forehead with superficial and deep components.

distortion of surrounding tissues and possible lasting cosmetic deformity. By age 5 months, most IHs will grow to 80% of their potential size.

After an initial proliferation stage, there is a period of quiescence followed by slow involution. The bright red of a superficial IH will turn more dusky and gray as it flattens. The involution stage can take years to complete, with approximately 30% of IHs involuting by 3 years, 50% by 5 years, and some lasting until 10 years.[18,19] Although the aberrant vessels naturally involute, there are often residual fibrofatty tissue and telangiectasias that remain, and treatment should be considered.

Management

Propranolol

The dramatic shift in IH treatment after the serendipitous discovery of the effectiveness of propranolol for IH in 2008 by Léauté-Labrèze and colleagues[20] is well described.[21–25] Propranolol is now the first-line treatment of IH, and the threshold for treatment has been decreasing over time. IHs which will cause severe functional or cosmetic deformity should be treated early, including those covering the eye, subglottic, and nasal tip (Cyrano deformity), to prevent complications or vision loss. After the initial case series, there has been an abundance in the literature describing the impressive response to propranolol, with the appropriate shift from initial case reports to randomized controlled trials. A recent trial comparing propranolol to prednisolone showed similar efficacy with significantly fewer adverse events with propranolol, affirming its place as first-line therapy for IH.[23]

The mechanism of action of propranolol in IH is not fully understood but likely is related to VEGF and adrenergic vasoconstriction pathways.[24,25] Propranolol causes involution of the IH, including decrease in size and change from bright red to a more gray, dusky color. These can often be observed within the first few days of treatment. Various protocols have been described, but a consensus statement in 2012 recommends a target dose of 1 to 3 mg/kg/d (usually 2 mg/kg/d) divided 3 times a day, after a screening EKG.[21] Propranolol is most effective during the proliferative phase of IH growth and does not show the same efficacy during the natural involution phase. Patients are typically placed on propranolol for 6 to 12 months, then weaned off. Should rebound growth be observed, propranolol is restarted. For superficial facial lesions without complications, such as on the forehead or conchal bowl, topical timolol cream has shown some effectiveness in preliminary studies.[26,27] It should be noted that there are no Food and Drug Administration–approved treatments for IH, including beta-blockers, which are considered off-label. Approximately 3% of IHs will not respond to propranolol therapy.[28] In a nonresponding lesion biopsy with glucose transporter (GLUT)-1, staining should be strongly considered because lesions that are GLUT-1 negative are not considered IH and will not respond to propranolol.

Subglottic IH typically presents with progressively worsening stridor and airway obstruction in the first few months of life (during the proliferative phase).[29,30] Approximately 50% of patients with subglottic IH will have a cutaneous IH although the converse is not true. Prompt recognition of symptoms and evaluation with laryngoscopy or bronchoscopy is critical. These are typically posterior-lateral, more often on the left, and can be bilateral. In acute distress an endotracheal tube can be carefully advanced past the soft lesion. Previously, tracheostomy, endoscopic laser resection, or open resection was considered, but now intubation with initiation of propranolol is recommended.[31,32] Most lesions will respond, and the patient can be extubated after several days and continued on propranolol as an outpatient.

Surgical management
Even with the paradigm shift of IH treatment with propranolol, it is important to recognize surgery still has a role. Up to 50% of IH will need a procedure at some point, either initial or adjuvant surgical therapy. Often, this is to resect residual fibro-fatty involucrum, or pulsed-dye laser therapy for lasting skin staining. Again, surgical intervention should be considered earlier during the proliferative phase if there is significant deformation of the surrounding tissue, especially cartilage, with functional or cosmetic consequences. It is usually better to resect a problematic hemangioma while it is small than it is to watch it destroy tissue that later needs to be reconstructed.

There are several other types of hemangiomas, which are also benign vascular tumors of capillaries but do not demonstrate the growth/regression pattern of IH. These include noninvoluting congenital hemangioma and rapidly-involuting congenital hemangioma, and they behave as named. Confirmation of diagnosis by a dermatologist is recommended.

VENOUS MALFORMATIONS
Diagnosis

VMs represent the third most common vascular mass in the head and neck after IHs and LMs.[33] By definition, these are present at birth but, depending on the location and growth, may present as late as adulthood. VMs typically present as compressible masses, often with overlying blue or purplish skin staining. On the mucous membranes, these will be soft purple blebs. VMs can present at any site but are more common in the muscle and mucous membranes.[33–37]

Unique characteristics
VMs have several other unique characteristics that aid in diagnosis. These can be elicited to expand with dependent drainage of venous blood into the ectatic veins of the lesion, usually by leaning the patient back and putting the head beneath the heart. The Valsalva maneuver will also cause expansion, and endoscopic evaluation while crying is particularly useful for laryngeal VMs to determine extent of obstruction. In the operating room, the patient can be placed in Trendelenburg position to elicit a similar result.

Additionally, phleboliths may be palpated within the lesion as very firm nodules that may be tender. Acute thrombus formation may cause severe pain with expansion and may be the presenting symptoms of a deep-seated VM.[33] Pain, caused by venous stasis or thrombus, is fairly unique to VMs but may also be seen with AVMs.

Histology
Histologically, VMs are made up of aberrant venous channels in communication with each other. These are tortuous, thin-walled vessels lacking an internal elastic membrane and disorganized smooth muscle cells.[33,38,39] Venous blood from normal vessels enters the lesion and does not easily find an exit, leading to gradual expansion over time. This can invade into adjacent tissue, and the static blood can lead to thrombosis and calcification that is often painful.

Mutations
VMs are typically due to sporadic mutations, but approximately 1% to 5% are familial or genetic. These include cutaneomucosal VM, glomuvenous malformation, and blue rubber bleb nevus syndrome.[40–42] Multifocal VM may have gastrointestinal lesions, with risk for gastrointestinal bleeding, and full evaluation by an experienced dermatologist is recommended.

Ultrasound

Ultrasound of VM is useful for superficial sites and will show a well-demarcated lesion containing compressible hypoechoic tubular channels.[33,43–45] Phleboliths may be present and will appear as echogenic shadowing foci. Doppler ultrasound shows a low-flow lesion as expected. On MRI, VM will appear isointense on T1-weighted sequences and hyperintense on T2-weighted sequences. There is uniform or heterogeneous enhancement, with no large flow voids, which would be present in a high-flow lesion.

Management

Treatment of VM usually involves sclerotherapy or surgery or laser therapy, and often requires a multimodality approach. Most VMs will require treatment at some point. Smaller, well-contained lesions can often be completely cured with a single procedure. For large VMs, complete excision is difficult or has risk of injury to surrounding structures, and recurrence is common. Treatment is guided by the depth of the lesion, proximity to vital structures, and presence of mucosal involvement.

Sclerotherapy

Sclerotherapy typically involves an alcohol-based agent, sodium tetradecyl sulfate foam, or ethanolamine injected directly into the lesion after confirmation of location with fluoroscopy. Lower flow lesions and venous lakes will allow the sclerosing agent to stay in the lesion longer with greater effect without being washed away (as in higher flow lesions). Sclerotherapy has an average of 2 treatments, with most patients requiring 1 to 4 sessions separated by 3 to 12 months.[46,47] Swelling, firmness, and pain are common and last several days. Mucosal or superficial VMs can ulcerate and should be treated with local wound care and an antibiotic with monitoring for subsequent scarring. Other potential complications include peripheral nerve palsy, deep venous thrombosis, and muscle contracture.[48]

Surgery

Surgical treatment of VMs will vary. Some lesions are fairly well defined in the neck and easily separated from surrounding tissue (**Fig. 2**). Others have poorly defined borders and invade normal tissue, leading to a difficult surgery with risk of blood loss. They are generally approached like other head and neck masses, but excision of the involved skin or mucosa needs to be considered when appropriate.

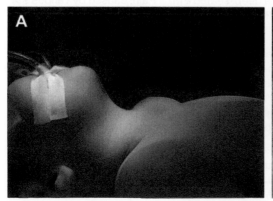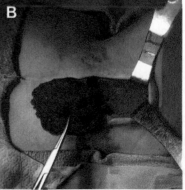

Fig. 2. (*A*) Well-defined VM of the left neck presenting as a neck mass. (*B*) Excision of well-defined left neck VM.

Larger VMs are more challenging, including parotid and masseteric sites. These can be intricately associated with nerves and critical structures. Bipolar nonstick cautery and thrombin-soaked Gelfoam can help to prevent bleeding and protect adjacent nerve structures.[33] Dissection is carried out with caution because the thin-walled ectatic veins will bleed easily. Nonstick bipolar tips (at 25–30 W) can control tedious surface bleeding.

In particular, large VMs involving the parotid should be approached with caution. These will have direct and indirect connections to the draining dural system and internal jugular vein, often intricately wrapping around the facial nerve in the process.[49,50] Although these are venous, they will bleed briskly with risk to the nerve and for major blood loss. Dissection should proceed in the superior to inferior direction to prevent engorgement of the lesion after removing outflowing veins. Bipolar can be used along the surface of the lesion, with multiple ties to contain the VM. Reduction, rather than complete resection, is the goal, and there may come a point (usually many hours into the case), where the patient is better served to contain bleeding and stop the case rather than risk further blood loss or facial palsy.

Laser therapy
Mucosal and aerodigestive VM are amenable to Nd:YAG laser therapy, which has a wavelength of 1064 nm and is suited for the purple color of VM. For airway lesions, the laser fiber is taped to a rigid telescope and the laser applied at 18 to 20 W in a polka-dot pattern, taking care not to connect the dots to prevent mucosal scarring and bleeding (**Fig. 3**).[33] Placing the patient in Trendelenburg position may help make the lesions more obvious. A similar technique can be applied to the oral mucosa, with the fiber threaded through a noncontact laser handpiece (or Fraser suction) at a higher energy of 25 to 30 W. An underwater technique with less thermal damage has been described in which the oral cavity is filled with cold saline during laser application.[51] The Nd:YAG laser can also be used for less accessible VMs, such as in the deep tongue or neck, as an interstitial laser therapy. The fiber is passed through a 14 g needle and into the VM, taking care to stay at least 0.5 cm from any nerve to prevent damage. In this way, selective photothermolysis of the VM can shrink the deep lesion.

LYMPHATIC MALFORMATION
Diagnosis

LMs, which historically have carried many names, including cystic hygroma and lymphangioma, are low-flow malformations of the lymphatic channels and have a highly variable presentation. The abundant lymphatics of the head and neck leads to 75%

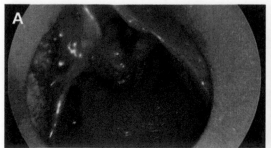
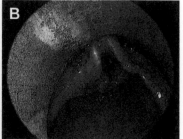

Fig. 3. (A) VM involving left hemilarynx before endoscopic Nd:YAG treatment. (B) VM involving left hemilarynx after 2 sessions of endoscopic Nd:YAG treatment.

of LMs involving this region.[2,52–55] LMs are typically diagnosed before age 2, often prenatally, and large macrocystic lesions can lead to airway obstruction after birth. Diagnosis with prenatal ultrasound and MRI is useful, and an ex utero intrapartum treatment (EXIT) procedure may need to be planned.

LMs are generally classified as macrocystic, microcystic, or mixed, and are often described as a venolymphatic malformation (VLM) if there are both lymphatic and venous components. Macrocystic lesions have cysts greater than 2 cm in diameter and microcysts are less than 2 cm in diameter (**Figs. 4** and **5**).[2,3] It is important to note that there are no histologic difference between macrocystic and microcystic lesions.[54,55] Histologically, all LMs (regardless of cyst size) are made up of ectatic, thin-walled, irregularly shaped vessels of heterogeneous size.[55] There is a complex outer stroma, which includes fibroblasts, leukocytes, and adipocytes. The cause of LMs is unknown, but it is likely related to the failure of developing embryonic lymphatic systems to separate from or connect to the associated venous system.[56] This may also explain the common finding of a mixed VLM of the head and neck.

On examination, LMs have a highly variable appearance. Large macrocysts are often dramatic, and will be less compressible than VMs. LMs can intertwine with normal tissue, including bone and muscles, leading to significant cosmetic and functional morbidity. Mucosal disease will typically have small cystic blebs, often with internal hemorrhage or crusting. LMs can have acute enlargement with infection, even viral upper respiratory infection, or hormone changes at puberty. In rare cases, particularly in the posterior triangle of the neck and adjacent to the skull base, LMs will regress over the first several years of life without treatment.[53]

Staging of lymphatic malformations
LMs are graded I to IV based on the de Serres staging proposal[57]: stage I, unilateral infrahyoid; stage II, unilateral suprahyoid; stage III, unilateral infrahyoid and suprahyoid; and stage IV, bilateral suprahyoid. It is vital for the physician to understand the implications of the different stages of disease. Higher stage disease will tend to have an increased rate of functional impairment, require more complex and frequent treatment, and will be more likely to require long-term tracheostomy dependence. In general, low and lateral is better than high and medial.[56] Suprahyoid (beard) distribution is more likely to be microcystic and interwoven with normal tissue. Mucosal

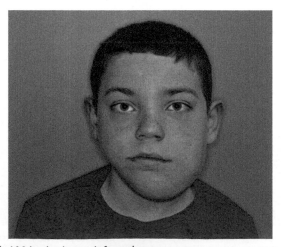

Fig. 4. Macrocystic LM in the lower left neck.

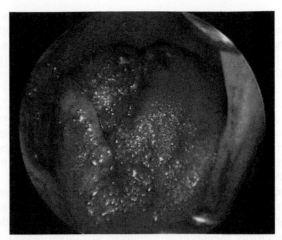

Fig. 5. Microcystic LM of the tongue.

involvement particularly predicts an increased burden of disease and worse response to therapy.[52,56,58]

The Cologne Disease Score as been developed as a useful scoring system to assess LM disease burden.[59,60] This is a simple grading scale to determine the burden of LM disease in relation to respiration, nutrition, speech, and cosmetic appearance. More comprehensive instruments are currently in development, and a national database with standardized patient staging and functional impairment grading is needed.[58,61,62]

Management

The treatment of LMs is complex, highly dependent on the nature of each patient's specific lesion and associated functional impairment. Treatment is aimed at improving function and symptoms, with attempts at objective reduction in size or complete eradication only as secondary goals.[52] The main tenets of treatment are sclerotherapy and surgery, with conservative management measures playing an important role. A recent study comparing primary surgical versus primary sclerotherapy showed no statistically significant difference in effectiveness in the proportion of patients requiring no further treatment. For both modalities, macrocystic lesions tend to be more amenable to treatment.[52]

Conservative Management

It is common for LMs to enlarge significantly with an upper respiratory infection. Higher stage lesions with oral and suprahyoid disease have lesions that are exposed to the oral flora, and oral hygiene is important to prevent recurrent infections and enlargement. There is also evidence of lymphocytopenia in young patients with high-stage malformations.[56,63] Inflammatory episodes will promote new lymphatic vessel growth and expansion of the lesion, with subsequent stasis of flow. The authors treat these episodes promptly with antibiotics (with oral coverage) and glucocorticoids (usually dexamethasone or prednisone), even if the lesion has been previously resected. Early treatment may help prevent permanent enlargement of the lesion.

As with any vascular malformation, LMs will continue to enlarge over time. However, there is a tendency to integrate and expand into normal tissues, including bone, which is seen more often with microcystic disease. Balance must be found on an individual patient basis whether conservative observation outweighs treatment options, and early consideration for sclerotherapy or surgical therapy is warranted. Conservative treatment may include managing complications such as airway obstruction with measures including tracheostomy, tonsillectomy, or conservative tongue reduction.[56]

Sclerotherapy

A variety of sclerotherapy agents have been described in the treatment of LM, with macrocystic lesions showing the most benefit. Under radiographic guidance, the lesion is aspirated, and then a sclerosing agent injected directly into the cyst to induce an inflammatory response. Ideally, this scleroses the internal walls of the cyst together and prevents refilling and expansion with lymphatic fluid.

In the United States, sclerotherapy is usually done with ethanol, sotradecol, or doxycycline. Multiple treatment sessions are often required. Swelling is expected after a session and other complications are not infrequent.[2,56] These include overlying skin breakdown, pain, airway compromise, damage to cranial nerves, and prolonged swelling.[2,62,64] Admission to the ICU may be necessary. All of these potential complications should be discussed with the family before treatment. The agent OK-432 has shown effectiveness in sclerotherapy for LMs but is not approved for use in the United States. Bleomycin is also used with similar efficacy, but concern for pulmonary fibrosis remains.

Interestingly, although sclerotherapy is often used for macrocystic lesions, it may have a role in microcystic lesions as well. This can be done as an interstitial rather than intralesional injection. The sclerotic agent is injected submucosally. This has been described for bleomycin and doxycycline, with bleomycin possibly being more effective. If bleomycin is used, the risk of pulmonary fibrosis needs to be discussed with the family. This presents at doses greater than 400 mg, which is much higher than given during sclerotherapy (usually <10 mg per session). Prevention of hyperoxia during the injection and monitoring pulmonary function will aid with prevention of pulmonary complications. There have been 2 reported deaths after bleomycin injection for venous or LM, both had lesions that had direct connection to systemic vasculature, and large doses were used.

In a small set of patients, the authors have found use for interstitial bleomycin or doxycycline sclerotherapy for aerodigestive microcystic LM. This is particularly helpful in the lip, tongue, floor of mouth, and buccal mucosa, where the microcysts present diffusely on the surface, and surgical resection would result in a functional and cosmetic deficit. Combined with ablation or CO_2 laser therapy, there will be a decrease in the mucosal and deep disease, and may lead to tangible positive results in a historically difficult to treat patient population.

Surgical Management

As with sclerotherapy, surgical excision is more effective when the lesion is focal and macrocystic.[2] In microcystic disease, surgery can be used to debulk the disease and preserve function while creating a more normal appearance. Again, surgical therapy is a balance between removal of disease and preservation of normal tissue. In large lesions, this should be undertaken as a debulking surgery instead of a complete resection if neurovascular structures are at risk. However, when possible, it is important to resect all disease to prevent regrowth.[2] Surgical excision can lead to dense scarring with secondary dysfunction, which is of particular concern in the tongue and airway. Orbital and bony involvement, particularly mandibular, can present with a range of complications and are best managed by a multidisciplinary team of specialists.[56]

Microcystic LMs of the tongue and mucosal surfaces can be difficult to treat and cause severe tongue enlargement with subsequent airway obstruction. Surface and superficial lesions can be managed with local resection, CO_2 laser, or coblation with good results, although multiple sessions are usually required. In some cases, partial tongue resection may be necessary to prevent complications such as airway obstruction or mandibular open bite deformity, and the key-hole or wedge resection can be used. It is important to remain conservative; chasing disease can lead to inadvertent near-glossectomy with disastrous consequences.

Overall, LMs have a highly variable presentation and, therefore, management is individualized. However, future protocols and treatment guidelines depend on the use and reporting of standardized grading scales of disease location, burden, and function. In the management of LMs, many institutions are using a stepped protocol starting with early conservative management, followed by sclerotherapy for persistent symptomatic macrocystic disease without spontaneous resolution, followed by surgery for patients with persistent disease, microcystic disease, or airway compromise.[56,65]

ARTERIOVENOUS MALFORMATIONS
Diagnosis

AVMs are rare but are considered the most dangerous and challenging of vascular malformations.[2,3,66–69] These are high-flow lesions, with aberrant AV connections that bypass the capillary bed. This will recruit more vessels over time, including after resection or embolization, and will invade and destroy adjacent tissue in a relentless fashion.[66–68] These are differentiated from arteriovenous fistulas (AVFs), which are also high-flow lesions with shunting between the venous and arterial system. However, AVFs are typically due to trauma and treated with surgical or embolic therapy with good results.

AVMs have been described as being focal or diffuse. Focal AVMs have a single arterial feeder with a well-defined nidus and usually present as a soft tissue mass with discrete borders in infancy or childhood (**Fig. 6**).[68] These carry a better prognosis due to the ability to completely excise the nidus. Diffuse AVMs will cross and destroy tissue boundaries, are usually discovered in older children or adults, and have a high rate of recurrence after surgical or embolic therapy.[68,70]

Many AVMs are not clinically apparent until adulthood, often after 40 years of age.[2,3,66] Those patients with lesions seen during childhood often report the presence of a vascular blush or staining of the overlying skin. This is often misdiagnosed as a hemangioma. AVMs respond to hormonal changes and can show rapid growth during puberty. Onset at a later age is poorly understood. Trauma and hormonal changes are potential growth triggers, but whether these lesions have been dormant since childhood or represent new malformations is unknown. Extracranial AVMs have a predilection for the midface, oral cavity, and limbs, and AVMs of the external ear are occasionally seen.[67,68,71–73]

Clinically, AVMs are pulsatile, warm, and may have a thrill, which distinguish them from other vascular lesions.[66–69] Intermittent expansion, particularly with hormonal influences, is also characteristic. Skin involvement may present as a vascular stain or blush at birth, with increasing erythema and size with age. This can lead to the misdiagnosis of IH with the false expectation of regression, with possible delay of diagnosis and treatment. Spontaneous, nontraumatic bleeding from a vascular lesion in an older child is suggestive of an AVM.[68] Later stage AVMs present with progressive enlargement, skin mottling, bleeding (potentially life-threatening), soft tissue invasion with disfigurement, ulceration, and pain. AVMs generally follow a course of early

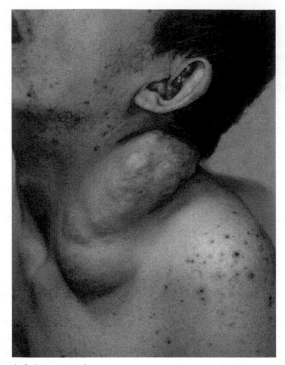

Fig. 6. AVM in the left lower neck.

quiescence, late expansion, and subsequent infiltration and destruction of local soft tissue and bone.[69] There have been no reported cases of spontaneous regression of AVMs.

Staging

A staging system has been developed and modified to help characterize AVMs. In brief

- Stage I: quiescence
- Stage II: active or palpable growth
- Stage III: soft tissue destruction
- Stage IV: heart failure

This has been further modified to include anatomic subsites (number of cervicofacial subunits) and depth of invasion.[7,66,74]

Imaging of AVMs is particularly useful for diagnosis and treatment planning, including magnetic resonance angiography and CT angiography.[69,74,75] Arterial flow voids will be seen on MRI, and angiography may help define the central nidus of the lesion and guide further sclerotherapy.

Management

Embolization and surgical resection are the mainstay of treatment of AVMs, and are usually combined. Smaller, more focal lesions are more amenable to both therapies, which is another argument for treating vascular lesions early while there is still a reasonable expectation for control rather than letting the lesion grow and become more invasive and difficult to excise.[69,76] Embolization agents include absolute ethanol, polyvinyl alcohol, coils, and Onyx.[76,77] This leads to selective destruction of the feeding vessels with decreased flow and temporary control of the lesion. However, recurrence rates are high, and embolization is usually followed by surgical extirpation 24 to 48 hours later.[69,76,78]

Surgical therapy is effective for smaller, focal lesions; however, diffuse AVMs have a high rate of recurrence even after aggressive surgical steps.[69,78,79] Partial treatment tends to only worsen the disease acutely.[68] Superselective preoperative embolization with Onyx, which will spark with cauterization, can help decrease blood flow and define the borders of the lesion. Large lesions may require staged excisions with serial local tissue flaps or complex free flap reconstruction.

The goal of surgical excision is complete resection of the AVM. Any AVM left behind will eventually expand and become a problem. However, the surgeon should expect significant bleeding, and the treatment should be no worse than the disease with consideration of life-threatening factors.[68,79] Nonstick bipolar cautery and Gelfoam with thrombin can aid with intraoperative bleeding. Surgical excision is the best chance for cure in small and medium malformations, and has the best chance of controlling diffuse lesions.[68] The high rate of recurrence (up to 93% in diffuse lesions) has encouraged surgeons to approach the excision with the mindset of a neoplasm rather than a benign vascular lesion. Using the same mentality as neoplastic or other vascular lesions, several pharmacotherapy interventions have been tried, including propranolol, vincristine, and Marmistat (a matrix metalloproteinase inhibitor); however, at this point none are considered reliable treatment options for AVM.[68,80]

SUMMARY

Vascular malformations represent a complex and highly variable group of head and neck masses for which correct diagnosis is of the utmost importance. A thorough history and examination can usually lead to diagnosis, which is confirmed with imaging. The decision-making process of whether and when to treat these lesions requires expertise across multiple disciplines, and will be dually rewarding and frustrating. Using the guidelines described above, the clinician can set a realistic expectation and plan for each individual patient.

REFERENCES

1. Mulliken J, Glowacki J. Hemangiomas and vascular malformations in infants and children: a classification based on endothelial characteristics. Plast Reconstr Surg 1982;69(3):412–20.
2. Buckmiller L, Richter G, Suen J. Diagnosis and management of hemangiomas and vascular malformations of the head and neck. Oral Dis 2010;16(5):405–18.
3. Eivazi B, Werner J. Management of vascular malformations and hemangiomas of the head and neck-an update. Curr Opin Otolaryngol Head Neck Surg 2013; 21(2):157–63.
4. Drolet B, Esterly N, Frieden I, et al. Hemangiomas in children. N Engl J Med 1999; 341:173–81.
5. Haggstrom A, Drolet B, Baselga E, et al. Prospective study of infantile hemangiomas: demographic, prenatal, and perinatal characteristics. J Pediatr 2007;150:291–4.
6. Greene AK, Kim S, Rogers G, et al. Risk of vascular anomalies with Down syndrome. Pediatrics 2008;121:e135–40.
7. Kohout MP, Hansen M, Pribaz J, et al. Arteriovenous malformations of the head and neck: natural history and management. Plast Reconstr Surg 1998;102: 643–54.

8. Lei Z, Huang X, Sun Z, et al. Surgery of lymphatic malformations in oral and cervicofacial regions in children. Oral Surg Oral Med Oral Pathol Oral Radiol Endod 2007;104:338–44.

9. Bai Y, Jia J, Huang X, et al. Sclerotherapy of microcystic lymphatic malformations in oral and facial regions. J Oral Maxillofac Surg 2009;67:251–6.

10. Kilcline C, Frieden I. Infantile hemangiomas: how common are they? A systematic review of the medical literature. Pediatr Dermatol 2008;25(2):168–73.

11. Hartzell L, Buckmiller L. Current management of infantile hemangiomas and their common associated conditions. Otolaryngol Clin North Am 2012;45:545–56.

12. Huoh K, Rosbe K. Infantile hemangiomas of the head and neck. Pediatr Clin North Am 2013;60(4):937–49.

13. North P, Waner M, Mizeracki A, et al. A unique microvascular phenotype shared by juvenile hemangiomas and human placenta. Arch Dermatol 2001;137(5): 559–70.

14. Badi A, Kerschner J, North P, et al. Histopathologic and immunophenotypic profile of subglottic hemangioma: multicenter study. Int J Pediatr Otorhinolaryngol 2009;73(9):1187–91.

15. Horii K, Drolet B, Frieden I, et al. Prospective study of the frequency of hepatic hemangiomas in infants with multiple cutaneous infantile hemangiomas. Pediatr Dermatol 2011;28(3):245–53.

16. Rosbe K, Suh K, Meyer A, et al. Propranolol in the management of airway infantile hemangiomas. Arch Otolaryngol Head Neck Surg 2010;136(7):658–65.

17. Orlow S, Isakoff M, Blei F. Increased risk of symptomatic hemangiomas of the airway in association with cutaneous hemangiomas in a "beard" distribution. J Pediatr 1997;131(4):643–6.

18. Margileth A, Museles M. Cutaneous hemangiomas in children: diagnosis and conservative management. JAMA 1965;194(5):523–63.

19. Ronchese F. The spontaneous involution of cutaneous vascular tumors. Am J Surg 1953;86(4):376–86.

20. Léauté-Labrèze C, Dumas de la Roque E, Hubiche T, et al. Propranolol for severe hemangiomas of infancy. N Engl J Med 2008;358:2649–51.

21. Drolet B, Frommelt P, Chamlin S, et al. Initiation and use of propranolol for infantile hemangioma: report of a consensus conference. Pediatrics 2013;131(1): 128–40.

22. Parikh S, Darrow D, Grimmer J, et al. Propranolol use for infantile hemangiomas American Society of Pediatric Otolaryngology Vascular Anomalies Task Force Practice Patterns. JAMA Otolaryngol Head Neck Surg 2013;139(2):153–6.

23. Bauman N, McCarter R, Guzzetta P, et al. Propranolol vs prednisolone for symptomatic proliferating infantile hemangiomas: a randomized clinical trial. JAMA Otolaryngol Head Neck Surg 2014;140(4):323.

24. Ji Y, Chen S, Li K, et al. Upregulated autocrine vascular endothelial growth factor (VEGF)/VEGF receptor-2 loop prevents apoptosis in haemangioma-derived endothelial cells. Br J Dermatol 2014;170(1):78–86.

25. England R, Banerjee D, Shawber C, et al. Propranolol action is mediated via the beta-2 adrenergic receptor in hemangioma stem cells. Plast Reconstr Surg 2013; 131(5):62.

26. Moehrle M, Léauté-Labrèze C, Schmidt V, et al. Topical timolol for small hemangiomas of infancy. Pediatr Dermatol 2012;30(2):245–9.

27. Semkova K, Kazandjieva J. Topical timolol maleate for treatment of infantile haemangiomas: preliminary results of a prospective study. Clin Exp Dermatol 2012; 38(2):143–6.

28. Buckmiller L, Munson P, Dyamenahalli U, et al. Propranolol for infantile hemangiomas: early experience at a tertiary vascular anomalies center. Laryngoscope 2010;120(4):676–81.
29. Truong M, Perkins J, Messner A, et al. Propranolol for the treatment of airway hemangiomas: a case series and treatment algorithm. Int J Pediatr Otorhinolaryngol 2010;74(9):1043–8.
30. Bajaj Y, Kapoor K, Ifeacho S, et al. Great Ormond Street Hospital treatment guidelines for use of propranolol in infantile isolated subglottic haemangioma. J Laryngol Otol 2013;127(3):295–8.
31. O-Lee TJ, Messner A. Subglottic hemangioma. Otolaryngol Clin North Am 2008; 41(5):903–11.
32. Benoit M, North P, McKenna M, et al. Facial nerve hemangiomas: vascular tumors or malformations? Otolaryngol Head Neck Surg 2010;142(1):108–14.
33. Richter G, Braswell L. Management of venous malformations. Facial Plast Surg 2012;28(6):603–10.
34. Rosbe K, Hess C, Dowd C, et al. Masseteric venous malformations: diagnosis, treatment, and outcomes. Otolaryngol Head Neck Surg 2010;143:779–83.
35. Eivazi B, Wiegand S, Teymoortash A, et al. Laser treatment of mucosal venous malformations of the upper aerodigestive tract in 50 patients. Lasers Med Sci 2010;25:571–6.
36. Glade R, Richter G, James C, et al. Diagnosis and management of pediatric cervicofacial venous malformations: retrospective review from a vascular anomalies center. Laryngoscope 2010;120(2):229–35.
37. Konez O, Burrows P, Mulliken J. Cervicofacial venous malformations. MRI features and interventional strategies. Interv Neuroradiol 2002;8:227–34.
38. Dompmartin A, Vikkula M, Boon L. Venous malformation: update on aetiopathogenesis, diagnosis and management. Phlebology 2010;25(5):224–35.
39. North P, Mihm M. Histopathological diagnosis of infantile hemangiomas and vascular malformations. Facial Plast Surg Clin North Am 2001;9(4):505–24.
40. Steiner F, FitzJohn T, Tan S. Surgical treatment for venous malformation. J Plast Reconstr Aesthet Surg 2013;66(12):1741–9.
41. Boon L, Mulliken J, Enjolras O, et al. Glomuvenous malformation (glomangioma) and venous malformation: distinct clinicopathologic and genetic entities. Arch Dermatol 2004;140(8):971–6.
42. Vikkula M, Boon L, Mulliken J, et al. Molecular basis of vascular anomalies. Trends Cardiovasc Med 1998;8(7):281–92.
43. Trop I, Dubois J, Guibaud L, et al. Soft-tissue venous malformations in pediatric and young adult patients: diagnosis with doppler US 1. Radiology 1999;212:841–5.
44. Flors L, Leiva-Salinas C, Maged I, et al. MR imaging of soft-tissue vascular malformations: diagnosis, classification, and therapy follow-up. Radiographics 2011; 31(5):1321–40.
45. McCafferty I, Jones R. Imaging and management of vascular malformations. Clin Radiol 2011;66(12):1208–18.
46. Gurgacz S, Zamora L, Scott A. Percutaneous sclerotherapy for vascular malformations: a systematic review. Ann Vasc Surg 2014;28(5):1335–49. pii: S0890-5096(14) 00062–4.
47. Leung M, Leung L, Fung D, et al. Management of the low-flow head and neck vascular malformations in children: the sclerotherapy protocol. Eur J Pediatr Surg 2013;24(1):97–101.
48. Burrows P, Mason K. Percutaneous treatment of low flow vascular malformations. J Vasc Interv Radiol 2004;15(5):431–45.

49. Achache M, Fakhry N, Varoquaux A, et al. Management of vascular malformations of the parotid area. Eur Ann Otorhinolaryngol Head Neck Dis 2013;130(2):55–60.
50. Colletti G, Colombo V, Mattassi R, et al. The strangling technique to treat large cervicofacial venous malformations: a preliminary report. Head Neck 2013; 36(10):E94–8.
51. Crockett D, Meier J, Wilson K, et al. Treatment of oral cavity venous malformations with the Nd:YAG laser using the underwater technique. Otolaryngol Head Neck Surg 2013;149(6):954–6.
52. Balakrishnan K, Menezes M, Chen B, et al. Primary surgery vs primary sclerotherapy for head and neck lymphatic malformations. JAMA Otolaryngol Head Neck Surg 2014;140(1):41–5.
53. Perkins J, Maniglia C, Magit A, et al. Clinical and radiographic findings in children with spontaneous lymphatic malformation regression. Otolaryngol Head Neck Surg 2008;138(6):772–7.
54. Chen E, Hostikka S, Oliaei S, et al. Similar histologic features and immunohistochemical staining in microcystic and macrocystic lymphatic malformations. Lymphat Res Biol 2009;7(2):75–80.
55. Perkins J, Manning S, Tempero R, et al. Lymphatic malformations: current cellular and clinical investigations. Otolaryngol Head Neck Surg 2010;142(6):789–94.
56. Manning S, Perkins J. Lymphatic malformations. Curr Opin Otolaryngol Head Neck Surg 2013;21(6):571–5.
57. De Serres L, Sie K, Richardson M. Lymphatic malformations of the head and neck. Arch Otolaryngol Head Neck Surg 1995;121(5):577–82.
58. Balakrishnan K, Edwards T, Perkins J. Functional and symptom impacts of pediatric head and neck lymphatic malformations developing a patient-derived instrument. Otolaryngol Head Neck Surg 2012;147(5):925–31.
59. Wittekindt C, Michel O, Streppel M, et al. Lymphatic malformations of the head and neck: introduction of a disease score for children, Cologne Disease Score (CDS). Int J Pediatr Otorhinolaryngol 2006;70(7):1205–12.
60. Wiegand S, Eivazi B, Zimmermann A. Evaluation of children with lymphatic malformations of the head and neck using the cologne disease score. Int J Pediatr Otorhinolaryngol 2009;73(7):955–8.
61. Perkins J, Coltrera M. Relational databases for rare disease study: application to vascular anomalies. Arch Otolaryngol Head Neck Surg 2008;134(1):62–6.
62. Adams M, Saltzman B, Perkins J. Head and neck lymphatic malformation treatment. Otolaryngol Head Neck Surg 2012;147(4):627–39.
63. Tempero R, Hannibal M, Finn L, et al. Lymphocytopenia in children with lymphatic malformation. Arch Otolaryngol Head Neck Surg 2006;132:93–7.
64. Churchill P, Otal D, Pemberton J, et al. Sclerotherapy for lymphatic malformations in children: a scoping review. J Pediatr Surg 2011;46:912–22.
65. Gilony D, Schwartz M, Shpitzer T, et al. Treatment of lymphatic malformations: a more conservative approach. J Pediatr Surg 2012;47:1837–42.
66. Richter G, Suen J. Clinical course of arteriovenous malformations of the head and neck: a case series. Otolaryngol Head Neck Surg 2010;142(2):184–90.
67. Erdmann M, Jackson J, Davies D, et al. Multidisciplinary approach to the management of head and neck arteriovenous malformations. Ann R Coll Surg Engl 1995;77:53.
68. Richter G, Suen J. Pediatric extracranial arteriovenous malformations. Curr Opin Otolaryngol Head Neck Surg 2001;19(6):455–61.
69. Richter G, Friedman A. Hemangiomas and vascular malformations: current theory and management. Int J Pediatr 2012;2012:645678 Article ID 645678.

70. Liu A, Mulliken J, Zurakowski D, et al. Extracranial arteriovenous malformations: natural progression and recurrence after treatment. Plast Reconstr Surg 2010; 125:1185–94.
71. Wu J, Bisdorff A, Gelbert F, et al. Auricular arteriovenous malformation: evaluation, management, and outcome. Plast Reconstr Surg 2005;115(4):985–95.
72. Wiegand S, Tiburtius J, Zimmermann A, et al. Localization and treatment of lingual venous and arteriovenous malformations. Vasc Med 2014;19(1):49–53.
73. Richter G, Suen J, North P. Arteriovenous malformations of the tongue: a spectrum of disease. Laryngoscope 2007;117(2):328–35.
74. Ziyeh S, Strecker R, Berlis A, et al. Dynamic 3D MR angiography of intra- and extracranial vascular malformations at 3T: a technical note. AJNR Am J Neuroradiol 2005;26(3):630–4.
75. Tao Q, Lv B, Bhatia K, et al. Three-dimensional CT angiography for the diagnosis and assessment of arteriovenous malformations in the oral and maxillofacial region. J Craniomaxillofac Surg 2010;28(1):32–7.
76. Dmytriw A, Ter Brugge K, Krings T, et al. Endovascular treatment of head and neck arteriovenous malformations. Neuroradiology 2014;56(3):227–36.
77. Thiex R, Wu I, Mulliken J, et al. Safety and clinical efficacy of onyx for embolization of extracranial head and neck vascular anomalies. AJNR Am J Neuroradiol 2011;32(6):1082–6.
78. Fearon J. Discussion: extracranial arteriovenous malformations: natural progression and recurrence after treatment. Plast Reconstr Surg 2010;125(4):1195–6, 2010.
79. Visser A, FitzJohn T, Tan S. Surgical management of arteriovenous malformation. J Plast Reconstr Aesthet Surg 2011;64(3):283–91.
80. Burrows P, Mulliken J, Fishman S, et al. Pharmacological treatment of a diffuse arteriovenous malformation of the upper extremity in a child. J Craniofac Surg 2009;20(Suppl 1):597–602.

Pediatric Thyroid Nodules and Malignancy

Kris R. Jatana, MD[a], Donald Zimmerman, MD[b],*

KEYWORDS

- Pediatric thyroid • Thyroid nodule • Thyroid cancer • Neck mass
- Pediatric thyroidectomy

KEY POINTS

- Pediatric thyroid cancer occurs more frequently than in the past, so an understanding of risk factors and available diagnostic testing is critical.
- Pediatric thyroid nodules behave differently than adult nodules, as the rate of malignancy in pediatric nodules may be as high as 25% compared with the rate of 5% in adult nodules.
- Fine-needle aspiration cytology can be helpful when definitive, but the diagnostic category "indeterminate" presents a clinical challenge.
- Experienced pediatric endocrinologists and thyroid surgeons should mange thyroid nodules in children.

INTRODUCTION

It has been reported that between 1973 and 2004, the incidence of thyroid cancer in patients younger than 20 years increased by 1.1% per year based on the Surveillance, Epidemiology, and End Results registry at the National Cancer Institute.[1]

Pediatric thyroid nodules exhibit several differences compared with nodules in adults. The prevalence of nodules in adults ranges from about 5% by physical examination to up to 35% by ultrasound scan and up to 65% in autopsy studies. However, there is limited knowledge of the prevalence of thyroid nodules in the pediatric population.[2] Although several studies have looked at this issue, many have used different diagnostic approaches, so it is difficult to know the true prevalence of malignant thyroid nodules. A study in the United States found that the prevalence of palpable thyroid nodules in children was 1.5%.[3] A recent ultrasound study in Japan found

No conflicts of interest or financial disclosures.
[a] Department of Otolaryngology-Head and Neck Surgery, Nationwide Children's Hospital, The Ohio State University, 555 South 18th Street, Suite 2A, Columbus, OH 43205, USA; [b] Department of Pediatrics, Lurie Children's Hospital, Northwestern University Feinberg School of Medicine, 225 East Chicago Avenue, Chicago, IL 60611, USA
* Corresponding author.
E-mail address: DZimmerman@luriechildrens.org

Otolaryngol Clin N Am 48 (2015) 47–58
http://dx.doi.org/10.1016/j.otc.2014.09.005
0030-6665/15/$ – see front matter © 2015 Elsevier Inc. All rights reserved.

Abbreviations	
ETT	Endotracheal tube
FNA	Fine-needle aspiration
MEN	Multiple endocrine neoplasia
TSH	Thyroid-stimulating hormone

that thyroid cysts were present in 56.88% and thyroid nodules in 1.65%. Cysts and nodules with diameters greater than 5 mm occurred in 4.58% and 1.01%, respectively.[4] One factor affecting detection on physical examination is nodule location; a posteriorly located nodule may be missed in some patients and only found on ultrasound examination. Pediatric thyroid carcinoma incidence was higher in women, highest in the 15- to 19-year age group, and more common in whites compared with African Americans in the Surveillance, Epidemiology, and End Results database between 1973 and 2007. It has been reported that there is a distinct difference between the rate of malignancy of thyroid nodules in adults and children. Although approximately 5% of adult nodules are malignant, 26.4% (range, 9.2%–50%) of pediatric nodules are malignant.[5]

Pediatric thyroid malignancies are nearly all well-differentiated subtypes of papillary, follicular, and medullary. Anaplastic carcinoma is typically seen in older adults.

As in adults, papillary carcinoma is the most common subtype of thyroid carcinoma in the pediatric population. Follicular cancer is second in prevalence, and medullary is least prevalent. Pediatric patients with papillary thyroid cancer typically present at a more advanced stage than do adults. However, pediatric patients do have better outcomes.[6]

Pediatric thyroid surgery is extremely safe, especially when performed at a high-volume endocrine surgery center. Pediatric centers often select surgical treatment for benign nodular thyroid disease because of the less-intensive follow-up required with this approach. In addition, pediatric thyroid surgeons choose total thyroidectomy over limited resection. This may reflect increasing confidence in the safety and efficacy of surgery.[7]

The differential diagnosis for cystic thyroid lesions includes benign cystic degeneration, thyroglossal duct cyst, parathyroid cyst, branchial cleft cyst, follicular adenoma, chronic lymphocytic thyroiditis, multinodular goiter, and thyroid carcinoma.[8]

PATHOPHYSIOLOGY AND ETIOLOGY
Radiation

Radiation—especially for the treatment of primary pediatric malignancies—has been associated with a higher rate of thyroid cancer.[9] A fairly recent example of radiation effects on the thyroid come from Chernobyl when the incidence of thyroid cancer in younger children correlated to radiation exposure in the form of various radioactive isotopes of iodine. Typically, a papillary cancer was present in these patients. Radiation treatment to the head, neck, and upper chest for treatment of other childhood malignancies has been associated with the development of a secondary thyroid malignancy. The risk of thyroid cancer increases in proportion to increasing radiation doses up to 20 to 29 Gy but then decreases with higher doses. It is likely that higher radiation doses result in cell death rather than resulting in carcinogenic mutations. There is also some evidence that chemotherapy may be a contributing factor, but this has not been well elucidated in children.[10]

Genetics

In addition, some patients are genetically prone to thyroid malignancy development. This is most evident in multiple endocrine neoplasia (MEN) type 2 in which medullary thyroid carcinoma is nearly ubiquitous. More recently, nonmedullary thyroid cancer has been described in several familial settings.[11]

CLINICAL PRESENTATION/EXAMINATION

A detailed history and physical examination is needed. Both benign and malignant nodules can present with variable states of thyroid function: euthyroid, hypothyroid, or hyperthyroid. Symptoms associated with hypothyroidism include:

- Fatigue
- Weight gain
- Cold intolerance
- Constipation
- Dry skin

Symptoms associated with hyperthyroidism include:

- Sweating
- Heat intolerance
- Anxiety
- Rapid heart rate/palpitations
- Frequent stools
- Insomnia
- Tremors

A family history of thyroid neoplasms or a family history of inherited condition or syndromes that are associated with thyroid cancer and exposure to ionizing radiation are important risk factors for the development of pediatric thyroid cancer. Familial conditions that may be associated with thyroid nodules and malignancy are listed in **Table 1**. In addition to these conditions, nonmedullary thyroid carcinoma may occur without other tumors or abnormalities.

Table 1
Thyroid nodule and cancer-related inherited conditions

	Gene Involved	Features
Cowden	PTEN tumor suppressor	Thyroid, GI, breast, uterine tumors
Familial adenomatous polyposis	APC gene (AD)	Increased risk of thyroid cancer, GI polyps with increased risk of malignant transformation
Gardner	APC gene (AD)	Increased risk thyroid cancer, jaw osteomas, GI polyps with increased risk of malignant transformation
Peutz-Jeghers	STK11 gene (AD)	Increased risk thyroid cancer, GI hamartomas, pigmented oral lesions
MEN 2A	RET proto-oncogene (AD)	Medullary thyroid carcinoma, pheochromocytoma, parathyroid
MEN 2B	RET proto-oncogene (AD)	Medullary thyroid carcinoma, pheochromocytoma, mucosal neuromas, Marfanoid

Abbreviations: AD, autosomal dominant; GI, gastrointestinal.

On physical examination, vital signs can suggest altered thyroid function. Brady-cardia and narrow pulse pressure are often seen in hypothyroidism, whereas tachy-cardia and widened pulse pressure are characteristic of hyperthyroidism. Height percentile is particularly useful when compared with weight percentile (hyperthyroid-ism is often characterized by height percentile greater than weight percentile and hy-pothyroidism by weight percentile greater than height percentile). Growth velocity is also informative (accelerated in hyperthyroidism and slowed in hypothyroidism.) Phys-iognomy can reveal associated syndromes. The most characteristic is the Marfanoid habitus (long arms and legs) and lumpy-bumpy lips and tongue characteristic of MEN type 2B.

Both thorough palpation of the thyroid gland and of all levels of the neck for lymph-adenopathy are critical.

DIAGNOSTIC PROCEDURES
Laboratory Studies

The levels of thyroid-stimulating hormone (TSH) in 125 pediatric patients with benign and malignant nodules were retrospectively evaluated by Mussa and colleagues. The TSH level in those with malignant nodules was significantly higher (3.23 ± 1.59 vs 1.64 ± 0.99; $P<.001$) and although not diagnostic, could help make the decision to proceed with cytology evaluation sooner. Pediatric thyroid cancer is nearly all well differenti-ated and, therefore, more likely to be TSH dependent (except for medullary thyroid cancer).

Thyroid Ultrasound Scan

Thyroid ultrasound scan is inexpensive, radiation free, quick, and requires no sedation in children. Thyroid ultrasound scan should be performed in all patients with thyroid nodules.

Concerning features observed on ultrasound scan include microcalcifications, indistinct margins, variable echogenicity, transverse blood flow pattern, and lymph node alterations.[12–14]

Fine-Needle Aspiration

All pediatric solid thyroid nodules greater than 1 cm in diameter should be biopsied by FNA. Those nodules that are between 0.5 cm and 1 cm should be biopsied by FNA if any other historical, physical examination, or ultrasonographic risk factors are present (**Box 1**). An experienced cytopathologist is critical to making clear management deci-sions on FNAs of thyroid nodules.

In a review of 218 FNAs in patients aged 10 to 21 years, 54% were found to be benign, 8% were malignant, and the remaining 37% were suspicious or unsatis-factory specimens. This modality had a sensitivity of 100% and a specificity of 65%.

If surveillance is elected, and there is evidence of nodule growth on ultrasound ex-amination, then FNA biopsy is indicated. Up to 40% of FNA biopsies will be in the inde-terminate category. This finding presents a clinical management dilemma, as some of these lesions will harbor malignancy. Using molecular testing of FNA samples in this category may prove to be most useful.[15] Several genetic tests have been used, including the Veracyte Afirma gene analysis and Asuragen miRInform molecular panel. A peripheral blood assay looking for TSH receptor mRNA is also available. Such tests may help risk stratification of patients who may benefit from total thyroidectomy rather than just doing thyroid lobectomy.

Box 1
Risk factors for thyroid malignancy

Clinical history

• Prior ionizing radiation exposure

• Family history of thyroid cancer

• Family history of thyroid cancer–associated conditions

Physical examination findings

• Palpable firm lymphadenopathy

• Hard or fixed nodules

• Features of ganglioneuromatosis (MEN 2B)

Ultrasonography findings

• Indistinct margins of nodules

• Microcalcifications

• Nodule growth while on levothyroxine

• Transverse blood flow pattern

• Lymph node alterations

The presence of thyroid tissue on an FNA of a cervical lymph node should raise concern of metastatic thyroid cancer in the setting of normally positioned thyroid gland. In this situation, ultrasound scan is needed to further assess the thyroid gland for any nodules.

Thyroid Scintigraphy

Technetium Tc 99 m, iodohippurate sodium I 131, or sodium iodide I 123 scintigraphy (nuclear medicine scan) can detect ectopic thyroid tissue and also help confirm the presence or absence of thyroid tissue in the normal location. This is useful in setting of an ectopic thyroid, such as a lingual thyroid. Papillary carcinoma may be found in about 5% of hyperthyroid nodules.[5]

SURVEILLANCE OF THYROID NODULES

Of greatest importance is regular clinical and ultrasound monitoring of putatively benign thyroid nodules to observe growth, abnormal neighboring lymph nodes, or calcification (**Fig. 1**).

MULTIPLE ENDOCRINE NEOPLASIA 2A AND 2B

The RET proto-oncogene is a transmembrane tyrosine kinase receptor located on chromosome 10q11.2. It has autosomal dominant transmission, so when one parent is affected, then a 50% risk exists in a child. Patients with MEN 2B have malignant transformation of C cells very early in life compared with those with MEN 2A. The current National Comprehensive Cancer Network panel guidelines state to perform prophylactic thyroidectomy by age 5 years for MEN 2A and at diagnosis or during the first year of life for MEN 2B. The American Thyroid Association guidelines suggest all patients with MEN 2B during childbearing years, should consider prenatal genetic counseling; they also suggest doing prophylactic thyroidectomy for highest-risk mutations (M918T and A883F) as early as possible within first year of life. Shankar and

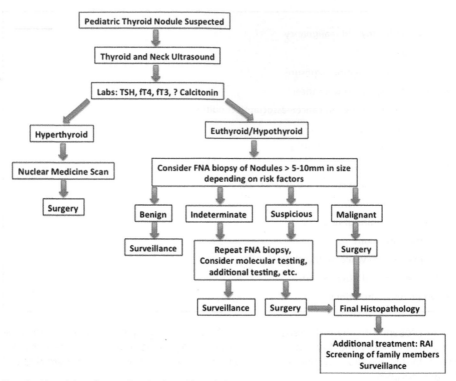

Fig. 1. Algorithm for pediatric thyroid nodules.

colleagues[16] suggest that with parental history of known MEN 2B, RET proto-oncogene testing should be done soon after birth, and if positive prophylactic thyroidectomy should be done in first 30 days of life. They found a 2.5-mm focus of medullary thyroid carcinoma after doing thyroidectomy at age 9 weeks. The earliest reported metastatic medullary thyroid cancer in MEN 2B was at age 3 months. Obtaining calcitonin levels in these patients is recommended; however, there are limited data describing the normal range at age younger than 6 months. Patients with MEN 2A can be divided into medium and lower risk individuals based on specific mutations in the RET proto-oncogene. Those with intermediate-risk mutations are advised to undergo prophylactic thyroidectomy by age 5 years. The specific mutations are described in the thyroid cancer guidelines of the American Thyroid Association.[17] By doing early thyroidectomy in MEN 2, it may be possible to potentially avoid the central neck lymph node dissection, which is associated with higher postoperative rates of hypoparathyroidism and recurrent laryngeal nerve injury. An experienced thyroid surgeon at a tertiary care pediatric medical center should perform surgery in these younger patients.

Medullary thyroid carcinoma tends to metastasize early, and given that it is resistant to chemotherapy and radiation, surgical intervention is the primary treatment modality.

MISCELLANEOUS CONDITIONS
Branchial Cleft Anomalies

Both third and fourth branchial cleft anomalies can directly involve the thyroid gland. It is possible that these could present as isolated nodules in the thyroid if the rest of the anomaly is decompressed. Often these children will present with recurrent neck/thyroid abscesses or thyroiditis. Esophogram can be helpful in looking for a pyriform sinus fistula in these patients (95% left sided, 4% right, <1% bilateral), but direct laryngoscopy to visualize the tract is often needed. The treatment options include endoscopic cautery of the pyriform sinus to reduce contamination of the tract or open excision of the fistula including thyroid lobectomy. The older age of the patient, size of the fistula, and presence of underlying food debris in the thyroid gland are likely contributing factors for needing open surgical intervention.

Thyroglossal Duct Cyst Carcinoma

A thyroglossal duct cyst that arises from remnants of the embryologic thyroglossal duct, is the most common congenital midline mass seen in the pediatric population. The standard treatment, a Sistrunk operation, involves removing the cyst, tract, midportion of the hyoid bone, and a portion of tongue base musculature. The recurrence rate has decreased to 2% to 4% when this operation is performed. An ultrasound scan is typically performed preoperatively to assess the presence of normal thyroid gland specifically and rest of the midline neck. The diagnosis of carcinoma within the cyst or tract is very rare (less than 1% of cases), and it usually shows up as an incidental finding on final pathologic analysis of the specimen. Approximately 26 cases of this entity have been reported in children, and 215 in literature overall, as it is most common in the fourth decade of life. Nearly all these pediatric cases are papillary carcinoma, but some have been mixed papillary/follicular subtypes.[18] Less commonly, squamous cell, Hurthle cell, follicular, and anaplastic have been reported in adults. Medullary carcinoma is not found in these remnants, as it comes from parafollicular C cells, neural crest origin. Synchronous carcinoma of the thyroglossal duct cyst and thyroid gland are extremely rare.[19] The treatment options have been debated, including Sistrunk alone and Sistrunk with concomitant total thyroidectomy. Central neck lymph node dissections are considered in these cases. Routine surveillance with ultrasound examinations of patients with an initially normal thyroid gland has been performed[18]; however, recent evidence suggests that prognosis may be better when total thyroidectomy is performed.[20]

Ectopic Thyroid

Based on embryologic variations, ectopic thyroid tissue can be found in sites along the descent of the thyroglossal duct, with the most common site (90%) being the lingual region. In general, this ectopic thyroid gland is not capable of functioning normally and results in a 33% to 62% rate of hypothyroidism. A lingual thyroid can cause globus sensation, dysphagia, hemoptysis, or airway obstruction in some patients. An ectopic thyroid gland is typically managed conservatively, and there is less than 1% risk of malignancy.

Medical management with levothyroxine supplementation can be effective in reducing the size of the ectopic tissue and any compressive symptoms.[21] [131]I ablation would require high doses and is not an ideal option for pediatric patients given unknown long-term risks. Surgical resection of the lingual thyroid gland can be accomplished with transoral microscopic surgery, transoral robotic surgery, or open surgical resection.[22,23] The age of the patient and anatomic ability for microscopic dissection or the robotic arms to properly fit help guide decision making for a transoral endoscopic approach. Regarding pediatric patients, a recent report described a transoral microscopic approach in an 11-year-old patient and transoral robotic approach in a 14-year-old patient.[22]

SURGICAL INTERVENTION
Preoperative Assessment

It is important for the thyroid surgeon to do a complete head and neck physical examination, including assessment of the vocal cord function either by direct flexible or indirect mirror laryngoscopy. A collaborative approach for treatment planning with both the pediatric endocrinologist and the pediatrician is important. Surgeon-directed ultrasound scan can be helpful in surgical planning and mapping of any cervical lymphadenopathy.

Nerve Monitoring

Intraoperative recurrent laryngeal nerve monitoring during thyroidectomy is done at most institutions. Currently, the smallest commercially available monitoring endotracheal tube (ETT) is 5.0, which is still too large for younger pediatric patients. The Nerveana system (Ventura, CA) uses a laryngeal surface electrode sticker that can be placed on smaller-sized ETTs. The Medtronic Xomed (Jacksonville, FL) has hookwire electrodes that are partially covered with Teflon. These electrodes can be placed by the pediatric thyroid surgeon with direct laryngoscopy into the vocalis muscles for intraoperative electromyography monitoring. It is important to check the monitoring system and electrode placement to make sure it is functioning appropriately before the start of thyroidectomy. A nerve stimulator can be used to stimulate the RLN as needed for identification and preservation during thyroidectomy. In addition to the ETT size limitations, the disadvantage of the monitoring ETT is that twisting of the tube/ventilator circuit during the surgery can cause the contact electrodes to be displaced after initial placement. The hookwire electrodes placed into directly into the vocalis muscle may be more reliable. This hookwire monitoring technique has been reported in 17 pediatric patients who underwent thyroid surgery, with 1 vocal cord paresis out of 32 nerves at risk, which ultimately returned to normal function.[24] Regardless, nerve monitoring is not a replacement for a pediatric thyroid surgeon's technical skills and understanding of surgical anatomy.

Surgical Intervention

An experienced surgeon comfortable with the meticulous dissection and preservation of the recurrent laryngeal nerve, identification of the parathyroid glands, and central and modified radical neck dissections should perform pediatric thyroidectomy. Central neck dissection should be considered in all malignancies, and a modified radical neck dissection should be considered when additional lymphadenopathy outside the central neck is present. The decision to perform thyroid lobectomy versus total thyroidectomy is a collaborative decision with the pediatric endocrinologist and surgeon. In experienced surgical hands, the risk of complications from total thyroidectomy is low. When preoperative or intraoperative pathologic analysis is not conclusive and malignancy is found on final pathology for lobectomy, then a patient should return to the operating room for completion thyroidectomy.

Preservation of the neurovascular structures within the neck is the goal. If total thyroidectomy or a completion is performed, then calcium levels should be monitored every 4 to 8 hours until confirmation of stability. Ionized calcium is typically a better assessment of the calcium unless albumin levels have already been checked to confirm that the total calcium level will be accurate for monitoring. Communication postoperatively with the pediatric endocrinologist is important for the management of hypocalcemia from transient or permanent hypoparathyroidism and thyroid hormone replacement (**Fig. 2**).

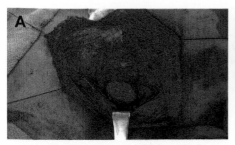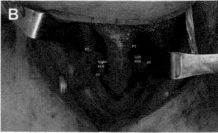

Fig. 2. A 10-year-old boy presented with cervical lymphadenopathy enlarging over 1 year. FNA shows metastatic papillary thyroid carcinoma. Ultimately, he underwent total thyroidectomy, central neck dissection, bilateral modified radical neck dissections, and superior mediastinal dissections. All parathyroid glands and recurrent laryngeal nerves were preserved. Postoperatively he had transient hypocalcemia and went on to get radioactive iodine and is still disease free at 3 years.

Postoperative Management

Immediately after total thyroidectomy surgery, monitoring of calcium levels is usually performed every 4 to 8 hours until stability is reached. A lower parathyroid hormone level postoperatively may be predictive of prolonged calcium or vitamin D supplementation.[25] Thyroid hormone supplementation after total thyroidectomy is necessary, and if the patient requires radioactive iodine therapy, the wean of the medication should be coordinated with the endocrinologist.

After thyroidectomy, studies are performed to determine if all thyroid tumor has been removed. Measurement of thyroglobulin, the protein produced by thyroid follicular cells that serve as the source of tyrosine for production of thyroid hormones, helps determine the amount of residual thyroid tissue (including the benign thyroid remnant and any thyroid cancer.) Often, postoperative whole-body radioiodine scanning is performed with ^{123}I once circulating levels of TSH have increased to 30 mIU/L after thyroidectomy or after recombinant TSH injection (if thyroid hormone replacement has been initiated.) In addition, ultrasonography of the neck is used to ascertain adequate removal of thyroid tissue and suspicious lymph nodes. Routine administration of therapeutic ^{131}I for thyroid remnant ablation is rarely indicated in thyroid tumors regarded as low risk for producing mortality. These studies are repeated at regular intervals, although radioiodine scans may be omitted if other study findings are reassuring (**Box 2**).

Box 2
Surgical complications

- Bleeding/neck hematoma, including potential vascular injury to carotid artery or internal jugular vein
- Nerve injuries, both sensory and motor
- Wound infection
- Hypertrophic scar
- Hypothyroidism in setting of lobectomy, risk very low
- Hypocalcemia (secondary to hypoparathyroidism), can be transient or permanent
- Vocal cord paresis/paralysis (temporary or permanent) from recurrent laryngeal nerve injury, unilateral or bilateral; if bilateral may require a tracheostomy tube because of airway obstruction

CLINICAL OUTCOMES IN THE LITERATURE
Children's Hospital of Boston

Scholz and colleagues[26] published a review of pediatric thyroid surgery over 35 years (n = 175) from Children's Hospital of Boston, and the indications for surgery included:

- Nodules, 83%
- Hyperthyroidism, 7%
- Goiter, 7%
- MEN 2, 2%

Most common in females between the ages of 10 and 17 years.

Of the patients who had thyroid nodules, 35.6% had malignancy. Complications from their review included hypocalcemia (6.9%) and vocal cord paralysis (1.7%).[26]

Mayo Clinic Study

Another large pediatric review was recently published from the Mayo Clinic experience (n = 177) over a 20-year period. Their most common surgical indications were:

- Hyperthyroidism, 40%
- Nodules, 39%
- MEN 2, 12%
- Goiter, 6%

Overall, 26.5% had thyroid malignancy. Reported complications included transient hypocalcemia (32.7%), permanent hypocalcemia (2.3%), and transient vocal cord paralysis (2.3%). There were no cases of permanent vocal cord paralysis.[27]

A central neck dissection is found to be associated with higher rates of hypocalcemia and vocal cord paralysis.[28] Some evidence indicates that children younger than 6 years undergoing thyroidectomy have higher complication rates,[29] and an experienced multidisciplinary team approach is best.

REFERENCES

1. Hogan AR, Zhuge Y, Perez EA, et al. Pediatric thyroid carcinoma: incidence and outcomes in 1753 patients. J Surg Res 2009;156:167–72.
2. Dean DS, Gharib H. Epidemiology of thyroid nodules. Best Pract Res Clin Endocrinol Metab 2008;22:901–11.
3. Rallison ML, Dobyns BM, Meikle AW, et al. Natural history of thyroid abnormalities: prevalence, incidence, and regression of thyroid diseases in adolescents and young adults. Am J Med 1991;91:363–70.
4. Hayashida N, Imaizumi M, Shimura H, et al. Thyroid ultrasound findings in children from three Japanese prefectures: aomori, yamanashi and nagasaki. PLoS One 2013;8:e83220.
5. Niedziela M. Pathogenesis, diagnosis and management of thyroid nodules in children. Endocr Relat Cancer 2006;13:427–53.
6. Kiratli PO, Volkan-Salanci B, Gunay EC, et al. Thyroid cancer in pediatric age group: an institutional experience and review of the literature. J Pediatr Hematol Oncol 2013;35:93–7.
7. Burke JF, Sippel RS, Chen H. Evolution of pediatric thyroid surgery at a tertiary medical center. J Surg Res 2012;177:268–74.
8. Yoskovitch A, Laberge JM, Rodd C, et al. Cystic thyroid lesions in children. J Pediatr Surg 1998;33:866–70.

9. Rose J, Wertheim BC, Guerrero MA. Radiation treatment of patients with primary pediatric malignancies: risk of developing thyroid cancer as a secondary malignancy. Am J Surg 2012;204:881–6 [discussion: 886–7].

10. Cohen A, Rovelli A, Merlo DF, et al. Risk for secondary thyroid carcinoma after hematopoietic stem-cell transplantation: an EBMT Late Effects Working Party Study. J Clin Oncol 2007;25:2449–54.

11. Richards ML. Thyroid cancer genetics: multiple endocrine neoplasia type 2, non-medullary familial thyroid cancer, and familial syndromes associated with thyroid cancer. Surg Oncol Clin N Am 2009;18:39–52, viii.

12. Dinauer CA, Breuer C, Rivkees SA. Differentiated thyroid cancer in children: diagnosis and management. Curr Opin Oncol 2008;20:59–65.

13. Papini E, Guglielmi R, Bianchini A, et al. Risk of malignancy in nonpalpable thyroid nodules: predictive value of ultrasound and color-Doppler features. J Clin Endocrinol Metab 2002;87:1941–6.

14. Drozd VM, Lushchik ML, Polyanskaya ON, et al. The usual ultrasonographic features of thyroid cancer are less frequent in small tumors that develop after a long latent period after the Chernobyl radiation release accident. Thyroid 2009;19:725–34.

15. Zimmerman D. Thyroid carcinoma in children and adolescents: diagnostic implications of analysis of the tumor genome. Curr Opin Pediatr 2013;25:528–31.

16. Shankar RK, Rutter MJ, Chernausek SD, et al. Medullary thyroid cancer in a 9-week-old infant with familial MEN 2B: implications for timing of prophylactic thyroidectomy. Int J Pediatr Endocrinol 2012;2012:25.

17. Cooper DS, Doherty GM, Haugen BR, et al. Revised American Thyroid Association management guidelines for patients with thyroid nodules and differentiated thyroid cancer. Thyroid 2009;19:1167–214.

18. Pfeiffer MS, Kim GH, Krishnan M. Thyroglossal duct papillary carcinoma in a 15-year old female and review of pediatric cases of thyroglossal duct carcinoma. Int J Pediatr Otorhinolaryngol 2014;78:135–8.

19. Cherian MP, Nair B, Thomas S, et al. Synchronous papillary carcinoma in thyroglossal duct cyst and thyroid gland: case report and review of literature. Head Neck 2009;31:1387–91.

20. Pellegriti G, Lumera G, Malandrino P, et al. Thyroid cancer in thyroglossal duct cysts requires a specific approach due to its unpredictable extension. J Clin Endocrinol Metab 2013;98:458–65.

21. Dutta D, Kumar M, Thukral A, et al. Medical management of thyroid ectopia: report of three cases. J Clin Res Pediatr Endocrinol 2013;5:212–5.

22. Howard BE, Moore EJ, Hinni ML. Lingual thyroidectomy: the mayo clinic experience with transoral laser microsurgery and transoral robotic surgery. Ann Otol Rhinol Laryngol 2014;123:183–7.

23. Pellini R, Mercante G, Ruscito P, et al. Ectopic lingual goiter treated by transoral robotic surgery. Acta otorhinolaryngol Ital 2013;33:343–6.

24. Cheng J, Kazahaya K. Endolaryngeal hookwire electrodes for intraoperative recurrent laryngeal nerve monitoring during pediatric thyroid surgery. Otolaryngol Head Neck Surg 2013;148:572–5.

25. Grodski S, Serpell J. Evidence for the role of perioperative PTH measurement after total thyroidectomy as a predictor of hypocalcemia. World J Surg 2008;32:1367–73.

26. Scholz S, Smith JR, Chaignaud B, et al. Thyroid surgery at Children's Hospital Boston: a 35-year single-institution experience. J Pediatr Surg 2011;46:437–42.

27. Kundel A, Thompson GB, Richards ML, et al. Pediatric endocrine surgery: a 20-year experience at the Mayo Clinic. J Clin Endocrinol Metab 2014;99:399–406.
28. Kloos RT, Eng C, Evans DB, et al. Medullary thyroid cancer: management guidelines of the American Thyroid Association. Thyroid 2009;19:565–612.
29. Sosa JA, Tuggle CT, Wang TS, et al. Clinical and economic outcomes of thyroid and parathyroid surgery in children. J Clin Endocrinol Metab 2008;93:3058–65.

Malignant Cervical Masses in Children

Matthew T. Brigger, MD, MPH, CDR, MC, USN[a,b,*], Michael J. Cunningham, MD[c,d]

KEYWORDS

- Malignancy • Neck • Pediatric • Cervical mass

KEY POINTS

- The timely diagnosis of malignant cervical masses in children necessitates a high level of suspicion.
- The care of children with malignant cervical masses requires a multidisciplinary approach.
- Staging systems provide a basis for counseling, risk stratification, and treatment planning for children with cervical malignancies.
- Recent advances in molecular genetics, tumor biology, and treatment strategies are changing the management of head and neck malignancies in children.

INTRODUCTION

Cervical masses commonly occur in the pediatric population. Although most are benign processes of inflammatory or congenital origin, a high level of suspicion is necessary given that more than 10% of all biopsied masses prove to be malignant.[1] A working knowledge of the diagnostic possibilities is requisite, as is recognition of the potential short-term and long-term implications for children and their families.

EPIDEMIOLOGY

Similar to the overall rate of pediatric cancer, the incidence of pediatric head and neck malignancies seems to be increasing based on the National Cancer Institute (NCI)

The views expressed in this article are those of the authors and do not necessarily reflect the official policy or position of the Department of the Navy, the Department of Defense, or the US Government.

[a] Department of Otolaryngology – Head and Neck Surgery, Naval Medical Center San Diego, 34520 Bob Wilson Drive, Suite 200, San Diego, CA 92134, USA; [b] Uniformed Services University of the Health Sciences, Bethesda, MD, USA; [c] Department of Otolaryngology and Communication Enhancement, Boston Children's Hospital, Boston, MA, USA; [d] Department of Otology and Laryngology, Harvard Medical School, Boston, MA, USA
* Corresponding author. Department of Otolaryngology – Head and Neck Surgery, Naval Medical Center San Diego, 34520 Bob Wilson Drive, Suite 200, San Diego, CA 92134.
E-mail address: matt.brigger@alumni.vanderbilt.edu

Otolaryngol Clin N Am 48 (2015) 59–77
http://dx.doi.org/10.1016/j.otc.2014.09.006
0030-6665/15/$ – see front matter Published by Elsevier Inc.

Abbreviations: pediatric malignant cervical masses	
BL	Burkitt lymphoma
CNS	Central nervous system
CT	Computed tomography
EBV	Epstein-Barr virus
EES	Extraskeletal Ewing sarcoma
FNA	Fine-needle aspiration
HL	Hodgkin lymphoma
INSS	International Neuroblastoma Staging System
IRS	Intergroup Rhabdomyosarcoma Studies
MRI	Magnetic resonance imaging
NCI	National Cancer Institute
NHL	Non-Hodgkin lymphoma
PET	Positron emission tomography
REAL	Revised European-American Lymphoma
RMS	Rhabdomyosarcoma
RS	Reed-Sternberg
SEER	Surveillance, Epidemiology and End Results
TNM	Tumor-node-metastasis
WHO	World Health Organization

Surveillance, Epidemiology, and End Results (SEER) tumor registry.[2] Estimates of the number of pediatric primary malignancies arising in the head and neck vary from 5% to 12% depending on whether or not retinoblastoma is included.[2–4]

Reviews of childhood cervical malignancies have shown several histopathologic trends.[2,5] Lymphomas are the predominant neoplasms of the head and neck region. Soft tissue sarcomas, specifically rhabdomyosarcoma (RMS), are the next most common, whereas skeletal sarcomas are comparatively rare. Thyroid carcinomas and salivary gland malignancies are less frequently reported. A summary of SEER pathologic diagnoses of pediatric cervicofacial neoplasms between 1973 and 2010 is provided in **Table 1**. Pediatric head and neck cancer incidence rates vary significantly according to age, gender, race, ethnicity, and geography.[2] In particular, age at presentation shows a variety of tendencies, as listed in **Table 2**.

EVALUATION

The evaluation of a child with a suspected cervical malignancy requires a thorough diagnostic approach, often requiring multiple modalities. A comprehensive history establishes the presentation, progression, and associated symptoms of the lesion as well as systemic manifestations. The most common presentation of a cervical malignancy is simply an asymptomatic mass. Attention to the child's past history of risk factors such as prior radiation therapy, exposure to carcinogenic or immunosuppressive drugs, a previous primary malignancy, and a family history of childhood cancer or systemic cancer predisposition is useful.[6–8] All children with a suspected malignancy require a complete otolaryngologic and systemic examination, frequently including an endoscopic assessment of the upper aerodigestive tract.

Imaging

Imaging is an important adjunct in the evaluation of suspected malignancies to precisely define the principal lesion and detect additional primary or metastatic sites of disease for accurate clinical staging. Ultrasonography provides an initial modality

Table 1
Pediatric head and neck malignancies (NCI SEER tumor database, 1973–2010)

Pathologic Diagnosis	Number of Malignancies		
	Total	Male	Female
Acinar cell carcinoma	133	45	88
Adenocarcinoma	39	21	18
Adenoid cystic	37	12	25
Germ cell	58	25	33
Lymphoma	2239	1395	844
Hodgkin lymphoma	1399	800	599
Non-Hodgkin lymphoma	840	595	245
Melanoma	581	316	265
Mucoepidermoid	276	120	156
Neural malignancies	3277	1739	1538
Neuroblastoma	1447	810	637
Retinoblastoma	1533	794	739
Other neural malignancies	297	135	162
Skeletal sarcoma	256	150	106
Osteosarcoma	98	58	40
Chondrosarcoma	50	32	18
Ewing sarcoma	77	41	36
Other skeletal sarcomas	31	19	12
Soft tissue sarcoma	1030	536	494
RMS	755	395	360
Non-RMS soft tissue sarcomas	275	141	134
Squamous cell carcinoma	149	95	54
Thyroid carcinoma	2763	541	2222
Follicular	250	43	207
Medullary	132	55	77
Papillary	2381	443	1938
Total	10,838	4995	5843

Table 2
Age distribution at presentation of children with head and neck malignancies

	Average Age (y)	Age Range (y)
Malignant teratoma	—	NB
Neuroblastoma	1.9	NB–5
RMS	6.4	NB–17
Non-Hodgkin lymphoma	8.0	2–18
Other sarcomas	8.1	NB–18
Hodgkin lymphoma	11.8	4–19
Thyroid carcinoma	12.4	6–18
Nasopharyngeal carcinoma	14.4	9–18
Salivary gland malignancies	15.2	7–8

Abbreviation: NB, newborn.

From Cunningham MJ, Myers EM, Bluestone CD. Malignant tumors of the head and neck in children: a twenty-year review. Int J Pediatr Otorhinolaryngol 1987;13:282; with permission.

that is readily available and not associated with the risks of radiation, contrast administration, or sedation. Ultrasonography allows determination of mass location and consistency as well as vascular flow characteristics. However, the improved anatomic detail provided by computed tomography (CT) or MRI is often required for both diagnostic and therapeutic decision making. CT has traditionally been the imaging modality of choice for many otolaryngologists given the ease of acquisition combined with an excellent ability to assess the degree of tumor extension within and across anatomic planes, provide differentiation between solid and cystic masses, and evaluate osseous erosion. Concerns about diagnostic radiation exposure in children have significantly increased the use of MRI. MRI offers additional advantages, including better contrast of tissues of similar densities, better delineation of neoplasms from surrounding soft tissue structures, and the avoidance of intravenous iodinated contrast material. The need for sedation and the lack of osseous detail present significant drawbacks in some patients. Functional imaging with PET with 18-F-fluoro-2-deoxy-D-glucose can additionally be used to evaluate both primary and metastatic tumor response to treatment, as well as to screen for neoplastic disease recurrence.[9,10]

Fine-needle Aspiration

Fine-needle aspiration (FNA) biopsy is common in the evaluation of adult head and neck malignancies, particularly thyroid and salivary gland lesions.[11–13] The reliability of an FNA biopsy diagnosis is highly dependent on the expertise of the cytopathologist and often proves challenging to obtain, particularly in young children, without the need for sedation. When necessary, the open biopsy of a cervical mass is performed in either excisional or incisional fashion depending on the size, location, and differential diagnosis of the lesion. The planning of an excisional or incisional biopsy must take into account potential implications with respect to future definitive resection from both a therapeutic and cosmetic standpoint.

Multidisciplinary Approach

Childhood head and neck malignancies require a multidisciplinary team approach to provide treatment. In addition to otolaryngologists, the team often includes pediatricians, medical oncologists, radiation oncologists, diagnostic and interventional radiologists, pediatric surgeons, and additional pediatric surgical specialists. Supportive services include speech language pathologists, nutritionists, child psychologists, social workers, and child life specialists. Most institutions treating children with head and neck cancer do so in the setting of a multidisciplinary tumor board to coordinate comprehensive therapy.

LYMPHATIC MALIGNANCY

Cervical lymphadenopathy in children is typically of benign infectious or inflammatory cause. However, neoplasms of the lymphatic system must be kept in mind as part of the differential diagnosis.

Hodgkin Lymphoma

Hodgkin lymphoma (HL) is a malignant neoplasm of the lymphatic system with a bimodal age distribution, one peak occurring during adolescence and young adulthood, and another peak after the age of 50 years. HL is uncommon in preadolescent children and rarely occurs in children younger than 5 years old.[14]

Epidemiology

Although no definitive causal factors are known, there is an association between Epstein-Barr virus (EBV) infection and HL. Increased titers of EBV-induced antibodies have been documented in patients with HL, and there is an increased risk of developing HL following a confirmed bout of infectious mononucleosis.[15,16] HL is distinguished histopathologically by the presence of Reed-Sternberg (RS) cells, which are multinucleated cells with large nucleoli and a halo or clear zone around the nucleolus. The RS cell seems to be most commonly of germinal center B-cell origin, but cases of T-cell origin have been described.[17,18]

Classification of Hodgkin lymphoma

The Rye classification was historically the most common method to designate the various types of HL based on the cellular background: lymphocyte predominant, lymphocyte depletion, nodular sclerosis, and mixed cellularity. Recognition that nodular lymphocyte-predominant HL differs both morphologically and immunophenotypically from the other classic subtypes of HL led to an alternative pathologic classification, called the Revised European-American Lymphoma (REAL) classification system. This schema divides HL into 2 broad categories: classic HL and nodular lymphocyte-predominant HL.[19,20] The REAL classification was eventually adopted into the World Health Organization (WHO) classification, the latter currently serving as the most widely accepted means to describe hematopoietic and lymphoid neoplasms.[21]

Clinical features of Hodgkin lymphoma

Although extranodal primary sites of origin such as the lymphoid tissue of the Waldeyer ring have been described, HL arises within lymph nodes in more than 90% of childhood, adolescent, and young adult cases.[22,23] The typical patient with HL has asymmetric lymphadenopathy that is firm, rubbery, and nontender. The cervical, supraclavicular, and mediastinal lymph nodes are the most frequent sites of presentation. Extranodal involvement occurs with disease progression, the spleen, liver, lung, bone, and bone marrow being the common organ systems affected. At presentation, 25% to 30% of children with HL have nonspecific systemic symptoms, termed B-symptoms, including unexplained fever, night sweats, weight loss, weakness, anorexia, and pruritus.[16]

Staging of Hodgkin lymphoma

The Ann Arbor staging system (Table 3) is used to stratify risk for patients with HL. This staging system is based on the premise that HL progresses from a unifocal lymph node site, spreads via lymphatics to contiguous lymph node groups, and then involves extralymphatic sites principally by hematogenous dissemination.[24] Pretreatment staging of HL consists of a combination of history, physical examination findings, and both anatomic and functional imaging. Bone marrow aspirate with biopsy is necessary for patients with clinical stage III or IV disease and for patients of any stage with B-symptoms.[16]

Management of Hodgkin lymphoma

The treatment of HL varies according to stage. Surgery often plays little role beyond initial diagnostic biopsy; multimodal chemotherapy and radiation constitute the primary therapies. Patients with HL who relapse may be candidates for autologous stem cell transplantation.[25] With current therapeutic regimens, more than 90% of all patients with HL, regardless of stage, initially achieve a complete remission. Prolonged remission and cure is achieved in approximately 90% of patients with early stage I and II disease and in 35% to 60% of patients with advanced stage III and IV

Table 3
Ann Arbor staging classification of HL

Stage[a]	Definition
I	Involvement of a single lymph node region (I) or of a single extralymphatic organ or site (I_E)
II	Involvement of 2 or more lymph node regions on the same side of the diaphragm (II) or localized involvement of extralymphatic organ or site and of 1 or more lymph node regions on the same side of the diaphragm (II_E). An optional recommendation is that the numbers of node regions involved be indicated by a subscript (eg, II_3)
III	Involvement of lymph node regions on both sides of the diaphragm (III), which may also be accompanied by localized involvement of extralymphatic organ or site (III_E) or by involvement of the spleen (III_S), or both (III_{SE})
IV	Diffuse or disseminated involvement of 1 or more extralymphatic organs or tissues with or without associated lymph node enlargement. The reason for classifying the patient as stage IV should be identified further by defining site by symbols

[a] Each stage is subdivided into A and B categories indicating the absence or presence, respectively, of documented unexplained fever, night sweats, or weight loss (>10% of body weight in the prior 6 months).

disease.[16,26] Histopathologic findings also have prognostic implications. Patients with lymphocyte-predominant lesions have the most favorable survival, followed In prognostic order by the nodular sclerosis, mixed cellularity, and lymphocyte depletion subtypes.[26]

Non-Hodgkin Lymphoma

Non-Hodgkin lymphoma (NHL) designates a heterogeneous group of solid primary neoplasms of the lymphatic system. In children, NHL most commonly occurs between the ages of 2 to 12 years and shows a male predilection.[27,28] Both congenital and acquired immunodeficiency disorders predispose to the development of NHL.

Classification of non-Hodgkin lymphoma

The classification of NHL continues to evolve. In the 1950s, Hicks and colleagues[29] unified older classification systems by recognizing the resemblance of malignant lymphoma cells to their benign lymphocytic or histiocytic counterparts that became known as the Rappaport classification.[30] Subsequent advances in immunophenotyping allowed separation of NHL into categories of B-cell, T-cell, and true histiocytic origins.[31] In 2001 and 2008 the WHO developed and subsequently updated an evidence-based classification system using a combination of tumor morphology; immunophenotyping; and genetic, molecular, and clinical features for all neoplasms of lymphatic origin.[21] This system is currently the most robust and widely used classification scheme for all lymphomas.

Clinical features of non-Hodgkin lymphoma

The clinical features of NHL reflect the site of origin of the primary tumor and the extent of local and systemic disease. Asymptomatic lymphadenopathy is the most common initial presentation, with approximately 45% of patients having head and neck involvement at diagnosis.[32,33] Nodal growth may be rapid, but insidious presentations more often occur.

Childhood NHL additionally differs from adult NHL in that it has a greater likelihood of being composed of unfavorable cell types, a tendency toward both leukemic transformation and hematogenous dissemination, and a higher risk of central nervous system (CNS) involvement.[28,34] Constitutional signs and symptoms that correlate with advanced disease include fever, weight loss, malaise, pancytopenia resulting from bone marrow infiltration, and neurologic manifestations.

Staging for non-Hodgkin lymphoma
The Ann Arbor staging classification for HL (see **Table 3**) is often still applied to patients with NHL. Alternatively the St Jude classification system (**Table 4**), first described in 1980, is commonly used.[35] The St Jude classification system attempts to account for the characteristic extranodal presentations and tendency toward hematogenous dissemination, bone metastases, and CNS involvement in childhood NHL.[34–36] The staging of NHL of the head and neck requires a comprehensive history and physical examination, serologic testing including complete blood count and lactate dehydrogenase level, chest radiograph, bone marrow biopsy, and cerebrospinal fluid analysis in addition to appropriate head and neck imaging typically by means of CT and often MRI.[37] More recently, PET has shown utility for disease staging and for following disease progression during treatment.[38]

Stage I NHL is infrequently diagnosed in the pediatric age group. Approximately 80% of children with NHL have advanced stage II, III, or IV disease.[35,36] As in HL, surgery plays little role in NHL management beyond diagnostic biopsy and occasional surgical debulking in the setting of aerodigestive tract compression.[39] The principal treatment of nearly all stages of cervical NHL is systemic chemotherapy; the rapid doubling time of high-grade NHL makes it highly chemosensitive.[32,33] Radiation therapy has a limited role in the treatment of NHL. Treatment of relapse consists of high-dose chemotherapy; bone marrow transplantation may be considered.[28]

Prognosis
Prognosis is principally associated with disease stage and response to initial therapy. The overall 5-year disease-free survival rate for NHL of the head and neck approximates 70% to 76%.[32,33] The event-free survival rate for NHL, irrespective of site of origin, is 85% to 95% for stage I and II disease and 50% to 85% for stage III and IV

Table 4
St Jude NHL classification system

Stage	Criteria for Extent of Disease
I	A single tumor (extranodal) or single anatomic area (nodal), with the exclusion of mediastinum or abdomen
II	A single tumor (extranodal) with regional node involvement Two or more nodal areas on the same side of the diaphragm Two single (extranodal) tumors with or without regional node involvement on the same side of the diaphragm A primary gastrointestinal tract tumor, usually in the ileocecal area, with or without involvement of associated mesenteric nodes only
III	Two single tumors (extranodal) on opposite sides of the diaphragm Two or more nodal areas above and below the diaphragm All the primary intrathoracic tumors (mediastinal, pleural, thymic) All extensive primary intra-abdominal disease All paraspinal or epidural tumors, regardless of other tumor sites
IV	Any of the earlier criteria with initial CNS and/or bone marrow involvement

Adapted from Murphy SB, Fairclough DL, Hutchison RE, et al. Non-Hodgkin's lymphomas of childhood: an analysis of the histology, staging, and response to treatment of 338 cases at a single institution. J Clin Oncol 1989;7(2):186–93.

disease, depending on the histologic type.[28] Given the observation that most childhood NHL is characterized by T-cell or B-cell differentiation, immunotherapy may have a future therapeutic role.

Burkitt Lymphoma

Burkitt lymphoma (BL) is an NHL deserving special attention because of its predilection for children and distinct epidemiologic and clinical features.[40,41] Epidemiologic differences separate BL into endemic and a sporadic types. Endemic BL is generally limited to equatorial Africa and is characterized by serologic evidence supporting a causal role for EBV. Almost all patients with endemic BL show high antibody titers to EBV determinant antigens, and 80% to 90% of their tumor cells contain copies of the EBV DNA genome; in contrast, only 15% to 20% of patients with the sporadic form of BL show this EBV association.[42]

Clinical features

BL almost exclusively affects children, with a predilection for boys.[40,41] However, the clinical characteristics of endemic BL differ greatly from those of the sporadic form. Endemic BL is diagnosed at an average age of 9 years and characteristically occurs as a facial mass originating from the jaw.[43,44] In contrast, sporadic BL is associated with slightly older children (average age 12 years) and usually presents in the abdomen.[45] Approximately one-quarter of sporadic BL cases involve the head and neck. Asymptomatic cervical lymph node enlargement is the most common presentation; jaw involvement as seen in endemic BL is comparatively rare.

Staging for Burkitt lymphoma

Staging work-up for BL is similar to that used in other NHLs. The primary treatment modality for both endemic and sporadic BL is chemotherapy. Surgery is typically limited to diagnostic biopsy purposes. The exception to this rule is surgical reduction of tumor bulk, which has been shown to improve survival in abdominal BL; a similar role for tumor debulking or resection of head and neck BL has not been defined.[44,46] Event-free survival rates at 3 and 5 years for both endemic and sporadic BL are 85% to 95% for limited disease and 75% to 85% for advanced disease; relapse rates are lower and survival rates significantly higher in patients with a smaller tumor burden at presentation.[47] For localized disease limited to the head and neck, a 90% long-term survival is reported.[48] Children younger than 12 years of age do significantly better than older patients, and high anti-EBV antigen titers in patients with sporadic BL seem to be associated with more favorable prognoses.[45,47]

SOFT TISSUE AND SKELETAL MALIGNANCY

Soft tissue malignancies of mesenchymal derivation present significant diagnostic and therapeutic dilemmas. These tumors are classified by the tissue of origin and have various degrees of clinical aggressiveness.

Rhabdomyosarcoma

RMS is the most common soft tissue malignancy in the pediatric age group, accounting for 50% to 70% of all childhood sarcomas.[49–51] The incidence of RMS diagnosis is 4.5 cases per million children per year.[52] According to the Intergroup Rhabdomyosarcoma Studies (IRS), 35% of pediatric RMS presents in the head and neck. Approximately 70% of these children manifest their disease before 12 years of age, and 43% present at an age younger than 5 years. There is no apparent sex predilection. RMS is 4 times more common in white children than in any other racial group.[53]

Epidemiology

Although most cases of RMS are sporadic, there seem to be both environmental and genetic risk factors. Implicated environmental exposures of variable relevance include parental smoking, in utero radiation exposure, advanced maternal age, a maternal history of prior spontaneous abortions, and recreational drug use by the mother.[54–57] Several familial syndromes including Li-Fraumeni syndrome, Beckwith-Wiedemann syndrome, and Costello syndrome have been associated with increased risk for pediatric RMS.[58–60]

Histology

RMS has a spectrum of histopathologic subtypes. These subtypes include embryonal (54%), alveolar (18.5%), undifferentiated (6.5%), and botryoid (4.5%).[61] In the head and neck, RMS is anatomically categorized as orbital, parameningeal, and nonparameningeal.[62,63] Parameningeal sites include the nasopharynx, paranasal sinuses, middle ear, and infratemporal fossa. All other cervicofacial sites are considered nonparameningeal.[64]

Metastases

Metastatic spread of RMS occurs by lymphatic and hematogenous routes.[51,65] The incidence of cervical lymph node metastases varies depending on the primary head and neck site, and approximately 13% of patients with RMS of the head and neck present with distant metastases to lung, bone, and bone marrow.[66]

Staging in rhabdomyosarcoma

Staging of RMS is based on a combination of factors. These factors include histologic subtype, tumor-node-metastasis (TNM) grade based on location and size, and clinicopathologic grouping determined by resectability of local and regional disease.[67–69] Staging allows stratification into low-risk, moderate-risk, and high-risk groups. A TNM-based staging system modified by the IRS accounts for size, location, regional disease, and metastatic disease (**Table 5**).

Treatment guidelines for rhabdomyosarcoma

Treatment guidelines established by the IRS emphasize the superiority of multimodality therapy. Using multimodality treatment principles, the 3-year relapse-free survival rates have increased to 91% for orbital primary disease, 46% for parameningeal

Table 5
TNM classification of RMS modified by the IRS group

Stage	Site	T	Size	N	M
I	Orbit, head, and neck, excluding parameningeal sites; genitourinary but not bladder or prostate	T1 or T2	A or B	Any N	M0
II	Bladder, prostate, T1 or T2 extremity, cranial parameningeal sites, other	T1 or T2	A	N0 or Nx	M0
III	Bladder, prostate, T1 or T2 extremity, cranial parameningeal sites, other	T1 or T2	A B	N1 Any N	M0
IV	All	T1 or T2	A or B	N0 or N1	M1

TNM and the size of the tumor are defined as follows: A, a tumor less than or equal to 5 cm; B, a tumor greater than 5 cm; M0, no distant metastasis; M1, metastasis present; N0, clinically involved lymph nodes; N1, regionally involved lymph nodes; Nx, clinical status of lymph nodes unknown; T1, confined to the site of origin; T2, extension or fixation to surrounding structures.

Adapted from Pappo AS, Shapiro DN, Crist WM. Biology and therapy of pediatric rhabdomyosarcoma. J Clin Oncol 1995;13:2123; with permission.

primary disease, and 75% for other head and neck sites.[66] Surgical extirpation of the primary tumor is indicated when such removal imposes no major functional disability and when excision of the primary tumor permits either the elimination of postoperative radiation therapy or a reduction in radiation dose. This indication applies to many non-orbital and nonparameningeal head and neck sites.[70]

Because the anatomic location in the head and neck often precludes complete resection, radiation therapy is commonly recommended. Recent advances in proton beam therapy techniques have allowed more precise dosing delivery and sparing of uninvolved critical structures.

Almost all patients with head and neck RMS, regardless of resectability, receive systemic chemotherapy. Chemotherapy is typically administered postoperatively to patients with small resectable lesions. Preoperative chemotherapy may be administered to children with larger lesions to decrease tumor volume before excision. Completely excised lesions with a clinically negative neck generally require no treatment beyond chemotherapy and observation. Children with a clinically positive neck benefit from neck dissection with additional radiotherapy.[67] Radiation therapy is also indicated for any incompletely excised tumors.

The histopathologic subtype is an important variable, with embryonal histology having a more favorable prognosis than other histologic subtypes.[71] Advances in molecular pathology focusing on chromosomal translocations have yielded valuable implications for diagnosis and prognosis.[72,73] The specific chromosomal abnormalities may prove to be useful targets for molecular therapy in the future.[73]

Overall, children with localized disease receiving combination therapy have a 5-year survival rate of 70%. However, such rates are highly specific to individuals based on the multiple prognostic factors outlined earlier.

Nonrhabdomyosarcoma Sarcomas

Soft tissue sarcomas other than RMS account for 3% to 5% of all malignant neoplasms in children.[51,74] A bimodal age distribution curve with incidence peaks in children younger than 5 years of age and in adolescence is characteristic of almost all of these lesions.[75] The soft tissue sarcomas of infants and young children primarily occur in the head and neck region, whereas lesions in adolescents predominantly arise in the trunk and extremities. In general, with the exception of fibrosarcoma, soft tissue sarcomas show a tendency toward both local recurrence and metastatic hematogenous spread. This behavior dictates a multimodality therapeutic approach similar to that used in patients with RMS.[76–79] Complete surgical excision with negative margins is the treatment of choice. Radiation and chemotherapy are typically reserved for cases of incomplete resection or unresectable disease.[80,81]

Fibrosarcoma

Fibrosarcoma is the most common sarcoma histology after RMS, accounting for 11% of all soft tissue sarcomas of childhood.[51] Although fibrosarcoma is primarily an adolescent malignancy of the extremities, approximately 15% to 20% of fibrosarcomas occur in the head and neck, predominantly in infants and young children.[75] Fibrosarcoma may also arise in older children as a secondary neoplasm following radiation therapy.[82]

On histopathology, fibrosarcoma consists of malignant fibroblasts associated with variable collagen or reticulin production. Fibrosarcoma is unique among the soft tissue sarcomas because metastatic disease in infants and young children is uncommon. Lymph node metastases and hematogenous metastases to lung and bone are reported in less than 10% for children younger than age 10 years, whereas rates approach 50% in patients older than 15 years.[83,84]

Therapy is primarily directed at local disease control. Complete surgical excision, when possible, is advocated. Maintenance of function at the expense of inadequate margins or incompletely resected disease is often necessary in childhood head and neck cases. In such situations, gross tumor resection is followed by local radiation therapy or chemotherapy.[85] Preoperative chemotherapy may also be used to decrease the size of the tumor in an attempt to enhance the likelihood of complete resection.[86] The incidence of local recurrence varies greatly, with reported rates between 17% and 43%.[86] The 5-year survival rate of infants and young children with fibrosarcoma is between 80% and 90%.

Extraskeletal Ewing Sarcoma

Extraskeletal Ewing sarcoma (EES), also called primitive neuroectodermal tumor, is a malignant soft tissue tumor identical in histologic appearance to Ewing sarcoma of bone. The specific cell of origin of EES is suspected to be a primitive mesenchymal stem cell.[87] Most individuals with EES are younger than 30 years at the time of diagnosis with an average age at presentation of 15 years.[88] In the head and neck, EES typically arises within soft tissues adjacent to the cervical spine and presents with pain, tenderness, and neurologic disturbances related to spinal cord compression.[89]

Treatment of EES generally consists of surgical excision alone or in combination with radiotherapy or chemotherapy. Mortality is high because of local recurrence as well as pulmonary and osseous metastases. The multimodality IRS protocols used in the treatment of RMS have been applied to both adults and children with EES.[88] In 2 retrospective evaluations of patients with EES, positive prognostic factors for disease-free survival include age less than 16 years, complete wide resection, higher hemoglobin and lower lactate dehydrogenase levels, and aggressive use of multiagent chemotherapy followed by either surgical resection or radiation therapy.[88,90]

Additional Soft Tissue Sarcomas

Additional soft tissue sarcomatous neoplasms of the head and neck region in children include malignant hemangioendothelioma, hemangiopericytoma, Kaposi sarcoma, malignant peripheral nerve sheath tumors, synovial sarcoma, leiomyosarcoma, liposarcoma, alveolar soft sarcoma, and malignant fibrous histiocytoma.[51,91] The use of surgery and radiation therapy to control local disease, with the adjuvant administration of systemic chemotherapy to prevent metastases, seems applicable to these rare lesions as well.

Desmoid-type Aggressive Fibromatosis

Although histologically benign, desmoid-type aggressive fibromatosis deserves special mention. This locally infiltrative clonal fibroblastic proliferation typically arises in the deep soft tissues. The lesions are rare, with an annual incidence of 2 to 4 per 1 million for all sites, but 10% to 15% occur in the head and neck.[92–94] Most head and neck desmoid-type aggressive fibromatosis involve the mandible; in descending order of frequency the submandibular area, neck, tongue, sinuses, upper lip, and hard palate can also be involved.[95] A variety of causes, including genetic predisposition, surgical trauma, Gardner syndrome, and endocrine factors, have been implicated but not conclusively verified.[94,96–102] These lesions are prone to local recurrence but do not metastasize. The primary treatment approach has been complete surgical resection with a low incidence of recurrence if negative margins are obtained. However, their infiltrative nature makes comprehensive resection potentially disfiguring, with surgical recurrence rates approximating 50% in the head and neck region.[95] Adjuvant therapies, including chemotherapy, radiotherapy, hormonal therapy, and even nonsteroidal antiinflammatories, have been given in recurrent and unresectable disease with variable, but generally low, levels of success.[95,103–106]

Neuroendocrine Malignancy

Neurogenic tumors of the head and neck include benign and malignant lesions, both of which generally present as lateral neck masses. Excluding CNS neoplasms, tumors originating from neural crest cells represent the most important neural cause of head and neck malignancies. Neurogenic tumors of neural crest origin are typically associated with the sympathetic chain and may present with associated sympathetic nervous system manifestations.

Neuroblastoma/Ganglioneuroma/Ganglioneuroblastoma

Neuroblastoma is the third most common pediatric malignancy and is the most common extracranial solid tumor malignancy in children less than 5 years of age; 40% of neuroblastoma cases are diagnosed in children less than 1 year of age.[107] Neuroblastoma is the most common histologic subtype of neuroblastic tumors, a category that also includes ganglioneuroblastomas and ganglioneuromas. These three histologic subtypes represent different developmental stages of the same disease process, ranging from the least differentiated (neuroblastoma) to most differentiated (ganglioneuroma).[108] The tumors show a decreasing metastatic potential based on increasing degree of differentiation. Most cervical neuroblastoma lesions are metastases from sites below the diaphragm.[109]

Although a solid neck mass is the most common presentation, respiratory distress and feeding difficulties may occur because of direct tracheal and esophageal compression or involvement of cranial nerves IX, X, XI, or XII.

Reflecting their neural crest derivation and typical sympathetic chain origin, neuroblastomas produce a measurable increase in catecholamine levels in 70% to 90% of patients. High catecholamine levels have been correlated with immature histology, large primary tumors, and advanced disease; increased lactate dehydrogenase levels are an additional unfavorable laboratory finding.[110] Molecular genetic markers, including proto-oncogene N-myc amplification, DNA ploidy, deletion of chromosome 1p, and expression of the TRK gene, have prognostic significance, allowing stratification of patients into low-risk, intermediate-risk, or high-risk groups.[111–113]

The International Neuroblastoma Staging System (**Table 6**) is based on extent of disease at presentation and degree of resection. The choice of single-modality or multimodality therapy depends on the risk stratification of the patient. Surgical biopsy is initially necessary to establish the diagnosis and to help stage the disease from a molecular genetics screening standpoint. In patients without N-myc amplification, complete tumor excision obviates adjuvant chemotherapy with evidence that near-complete resection with residual microscopic or even macroscopic disease may not adversely affect survival.[114] Multiagent chemotherapy is generally indicated in patients after incomplete resection of primary cervical neuroblastoma, in patients with metastatic disease to the head and neck from other primary sites, and in patients with resectable disease but positive N-myc amplification.

Prognosis is influenced principally by age, stage, and tumor N-myc amplification status.[110,113] Overall 3-year event-free survival rates for International Neuroblastoma Staging System (INSS) stage I, II, and IV-S disease range from 75% to 90% in infants, and rates for stage III and IV disease are 80% to 90% and 60% to

Table 6 INSS classification	
Stage 1	Localized tumor with complete gross excision, with or without microscopic residual disease; representative ipsilateral lymph nodes negative for tumor microscopically (nodes attached to and removed with the primary tumor may be positive)
Stage 2A	Localized tumor with incomplete gross excision; representative ipsilateral nonadherent lymph nodes negative for tumor microscopically
Stage 2B	Localized tumor with or without complete gross excision, with ipsilateral nonadherent lymph nodes positive for tumor. Enlarged contralateral lymph nodes must be negative microscopically
Stage 3	Unresectable unilateral tumor infiltrating across the midline, with or without regional lymph node involvement; or localized unilateral tumor with contralateral regional lymph node involvement; or midline tumor with bilateral extension by infiltration (unresectable) or by lymph node involvement
Stage 4	Any primary tumor with dissemination to distant lymph nodes, bone, bone marrow, liver, skin, and/or other organs (except as defined for stage 4S)
Stage 4S	Localized primary tumor (as defined for stages 1, 2A, or 2B), with dissemination limited to skin, liver, and/or bone marrow (limited to infants <1 y of age)

Adapted from Brodeur GM, Pritchard J, Berthold F, et al. Revisions of the international criteria for neuroblastoma diagnosis, staging, and response to treatment. J Clin Oncol 1993;11(8):1470.

75%, respectively; for children older than 1 year, the rates are 50% and 15% for stage III and IV disease, respectively.[110,111]

OUTCOMES OF TREATMENT WITH LONG-TERM SURVIVORS

The marked success of pediatric head and neck oncologic intervention, with resultant long-term survival of successfully treated children, has revealed the potential deleterious aspects of such therapies. The survivors of childhood head and neck cancer have a demonstrable increase in growth arrest, hypothyroidism, sterility, and pulmonary fibrosis.[16,115] Those treated in multimodality fashion are at particular risk for the development of second malignancies involving the lung, gastrointestinal tract, breast, and thyroid, as well as both acute lymphoblastic leukemia and NHL.[15,16,116]

FUTURE DEVELOPMENTS

Advances in both diagnostic and therapeutic regimens over the past 30 years have resulted in good progress toward treating childhood neoplastic disease. The continual evolution of classification systems accounting for not only histology but also molecular genetics has redefined treatment algorithms. Current efforts to better understand the biological basis of malignancy have facilitated much of this progress. Of prime importance is the increased understanding of the role of the immune system in the genesis of neoplastic disease. Oncologists have exploited the protective nature of the immune system by targeting antigens expressed by tumor cells with monoclonal antibodies to allow the specific delivery of therapy to neoplastic cells while protecting normal cell types. With the unlocking of the human genome and the ability to rapidly analyze chromosomal abnormalities, treatment stratification based on genetic prognostic profiling is already a reality for some malignancies. The future of cancer therapy is likely to see significant improvement beyond surgical extirpation and ablative chemotherapy and radiation toward a more nuanced approach.

REFERENCES

1. Torsiglieri AJ Jr, Tom LW, Ross AJ 3rd, et al. Pediatric neck masses: guidelines for evaluation. Int J Pediatr Otorhinolaryngol 1988;16(3):199–210.
2. Albright JT, Topham AK, Reilly JS. Pediatric head and neck malignancies: US incidence and trends over 2 decades. Arch Otolaryngol Head Neck Surg 2002;128(6):655–9.
3. Healy GB. Malignant tumors of the head and neck in children: diagnosis and treatment. Otolaryngol Clin North Am 1980;13(3):483–8.
4. Xue H, Horwitz JR, Smith MB, et al. Malignant solid tumors in neonates: a 40-year review. J Pediatr Surg 1995;30(4):543–5.
5. Cunningham MJ, Myers EN, Bluestone CD. Malignant tumors of the head and neck in children: a twenty-year review. Int J Pediatr Otorhinolaryngol 1987; 13(3):279–92.
6. Meadows AT, Silber J. Delayed consequences of therapy for childhood cancer. CA Cancer J Clin 1985;35(5):271–86.
7. Zahm SH, Devesa SS. Childhood cancer: overview of incidence trends and environmental carcinogens. Environ Health Perspect 1995;103(Suppl 6): 177–84.
8. Smulevich VB, Solionova LG, Belyakova SV. Parental occupation and other factors and cancer risk in children: I. Study methodology and non-occupational factors. Int J Cancer 1999;83(6):712–7.
9. Greven KM, Keyes JW Jr, Williams DW 3rd, et al. Occult primary tumors of the head and neck: lack of benefit from positron emission tomography imaging with 2-[F-18]fluoro-2-deoxy-D-glucose. Cancer 1999;86(1):114–8.
10. Sandlund JT. Burkitt lymphoma: staging and response evaluation. Br J Haematol 2012;156(6):761–5.
11. De Keyser LF, Van Herle AJ. Differentiated thyroid cancer in children. Head Neck Surg 1985;8(2):100–14.
12. Derias NW, Chong WH, O'Connor AF. Fine needle aspiration cytology of a head and neck swelling in a child: a non-invasive approach to diagnosis. J Laryngol Otol 1992;106(8):755–7.
13. Mobley DL, Wakely PE Jr, Frable MA. Fine-needle aspiration biopsy: application to pediatric head and neck masses. Laryngoscope 1991;101(5):469–72.
14. Ultmann JE, Moran EM. Clinical course and complications in Hodgkin's disease. Arch Intern Med 1973;131(3):332–53.
15. Alexander FE, Jarrett RF, Lawrence D, et al. Risk factors for Hodgkin's disease by Epstein-Barr virus (EBV) status: prior infection by EBV and other agents. Br J Cancer 2000;82(5):1117–21.
16. Hudson MM, Donaldson SS. Hodgkin's disease. Pediatr Clin North Am 1997; 44(4):891–906.
17. Seitz V, Hummel M, Marafioti T, et al. Detection of clonal T-cell receptor gamma-chain gene rearrangements in Reed-Sternberg cells of classic Hodgkin disease. Blood 2000;95(10):3020–4.
18. Marafioti T, Hummel M, Foss HD, et al. Hodgkin and Reed-Sternberg cells represent an expansion of a single clone originating from a germinal center B-cell with functional immunoglobulin gene rearrangements but defective immunoglobulin transcription. Blood 2000;95(4):1443–50.

19. Harris NL. Hodgkin's lymphomas: classification, diagnosis, and grading. Semin Hematol 1999;36(3):220–32.
20. Harris NL, Jaffe ES, Stein H, et al. A revised European-American classification of lymphoid neoplasms: a proposal from the International Lymphoma Study Group. Blood 1994;84(5):1361–92.
21. Campo E, Swerdlow SH, Harris NL, et al. The 2008 WHO classification of lymphoid neoplasms and beyond: evolving concepts and practical applications. Blood 2011;117(19):5019–32.
22. Dailey SH, Sataloff RT. Lymphoma: an update on evolving trends in staging and management. Ear Nose Throat J 2001;80(3):164–70.
23. Urquhart A, Berg R. Hodgkin's and non-Hodgkin's lymphoma of the head and neck. Laryngoscope 2001;111(9):1565–9.
24. Carbone PP, Kaplan HS, Musshoff K, et al. Report of the Committee on Hodgkin's Disease Staging Classification. Cancer Res 1971;31(11):1860–1.
25. Verdeguer A, Pardo N, Madero L, et al. Autologous stem cell transplantation for advanced Hodgkin's disease in children. Spanish group for BMT in children (GETMON), Spain. Bone Marrow Transplant 2000;25(1):31–4.
26. Colby TV, Hoppe RT, Warnke RA. Hodgkin's disease: a clinicopathologic study of 659 cases. Cancer 1982;49(9):1848–58.
27. Armitage JO. Treatment of non-Hodgkin's lymphoma. N Engl J Med 1993; 328(14):1023–30.
28. Sandlund JT, Downing JR, Crist WM. Non-Hodgkin's lymphoma in childhood. N Engl J Med 1996;334(19):1238–48.
29. Hicks EB, Rappaport H, Winter WJ. Follicular lymphoma; a re-evaluation of its position in the scheme of malignant lymphoma, based on a survey of 253 cases. Cancer 1956;9(4):792–821.
30. Jones SE, Fuks Z, Bull M, et al. Non-Hodgkin's lymphomas. IV. Clinicopathologic correlation in 405 cases. Cancer 1973;31(4):806–23.
31. Lukes RJ, Collins RD. Immunologic characterization of human malignant lymphomas. Cancer 1974;34(Suppl 4):1488–503.
32. La Quaglia MP. Non-Hodgkin's lymphoma of the head and neck in childhood. Semin Pediatr Surg 1994;3(3):207–15.
33. Roh JL, Huh J, Moon HN. Lymphomas of the head and neck in the pediatric population. Int J Pediatr Otorhinolaryngol 2007;71(9):1471–7.
34. Murphy SB, Fairclough DL, Hutchison RE, et al. Non-Hodgkin's lymphomas of childhood: an analysis of the histology, staging, and response to treatment of 338 cases at a single institution. J Clin Oncol 1989;7(2):186–93.
35. Murphy SB. Classification, staging and end results of treatment of childhood non-Hodgkin's lymphomas: dissimilarities from lymphomas in adults. Semin Oncol 1980;7(3):332–9.
36. Murphy SB. Childhood non-Hodgkin's lymphoma. N Engl J Med 1978;299(26): 1446–8.
37. Chabner BA, Fisher RI, Young RC, et al. Staging of non-Hodgkin's lymphoma. Semin Oncol 1980;7(3):285–91.
38. A predictive model for aggressive non-Hodgkin's lymphoma. The International Non-Hodgkin's Lymphoma Prognostic Factors Project. N Engl J Med 1993; 329(14):987–94.
39. Whalen TV, La Quaglia MP. The lymphomas: an update for surgeons. Semin Pediatr Surg 1997;6(1):50–5.
40. Kearns DB, Smith RJ, Pitcock JK. Burkitt's lymphoma. Int J Pediatr Otorhinolaryngol 1986;12(1):73–84.

41. Ziegler JL. Burkitt's lymphoma. N Engl J Med 1981;305(13):735–45.
42. Takada K. Role of Epstein-Barr virus in Burkitt's lymphoma. Curr Top Microbiol Immunol 2001;258:141–51.
43. Magrath IT. African Burkitt's lymphoma. History, biology, clinical features, and treatment. Am J Pediatr Hematol Oncol 1991;13(2):222–46.
44. Miron I, Frappaz D, Brunat-Mentigny M, et al. Initial management of advanced Burkitt lymphoma in children: is there still a place for surgery? Pediatr Hematol Oncol 1997;14(6):555–61.
45. Levine PH, Kamaraju LS, Connelly RR, et al. The American Burkitt's Lymphoma Registry: eight years' experience. Cancer 1982;49(5):1016–22.
46. Kemeny MM, Magrath IT, Brennan MF. The role of surgery in the management of American Burkitt's lymphoma and its treatment. Ann Surg 1982;196(1):82–6.
47. Magrath I, Lee YJ, Anderson T, et al. Prognostic factors in Burkitt's lymphoma: importance of total tumor burden. Cancer 1980;45(6):1507–15.
48. Link MP, Donaldson SS, Berard CW, et al. Results of treatment of childhood localized non-Hodgkin's lymphoma with combination chemotherapy with or without radiotherapy. N Engl J Med 1990;322(17):1169–74.
49. Donaldson SS. Rhabdomyosarcoma: contemporary status and future directions. The Lucy Wortham James Clinical Research Award. Arch Surg 1989;124(9):1015–20.
50. MacArthur CJ, McGill TJ, Healy GB. Pediatric head and neck rhabdomyosarcoma. Clin Pediatr (Phila) 1992;31(2):66–70.
51. Miser JS, Pizzo PA. Soft tissue sarcomas in childhood. Pediatr Clin North Am 1985;32(3):779–800.
52. Ries LA, Smith MA, Gurney JG, et al. Cancer incidence and survival among children and adolescents: United States SEER Program. 1975-1995. Bethesda (MD): National Cancer Institute; 1999.
53. McGill T. Rhabdomyosarcoma of the head and neck: an update. Otolaryngol Clin North Am 1989;22(3):631–6.
54. Grufferman S, Schwartz AG, Ruymann FB, et al. Parents' use of cocaine and marijuana and increased risk of rhabdomyosarcoma in their children. Cancer Causes Control 1993;4(3):217–24.
55. Grufferman S, Wang HH, DeLong ER, et al. Environmental factors in the etiology of rhabdomyosarcoma in childhood. J Natl Cancer Inst 1982;68(1):107–13.
56. Hartley AL, Birch JM, McKinney PA, et al. The Inter-Regional Epidemiological Study of Childhood Cancer (IRESCC): case control study of children with bone and soft tissue sarcomas. Br J Cancer 1988;58(6):838–42.
57. Ghali MH, Yoo KY, Flannery JT, et al. Association between childhood rhabdomyosarcoma and maternal history of stillbirths. Int J Cancer 1992;50(3):365–8.
58. Dagher R, Helman L. Rhabdomyosarcoma: an overview. Oncologist 1999;4(1):34–44.
59. Smith AC, Squire JA, Thorner P, et al. Association of alveolar rhabdomyosarcoma with the Beckwith-Wiedemann syndrome. Pediatr Dev Pathol 2001;4(6):550–8.
60. Hennekam RC. Costello syndrome: an overview. Am J Med Genet C Semin Med Genet 2003;117C(1):42–8.
61. Barr FG. Soft tissue tumors: Alveolar rhabdomyosarcoma. Atlas Genet Cytogenet Oncol Haematol 2009;13(12):981–5.
62. Crist W, Gehan EA, Ragab AH, et al. The Third Intergroup Rhabdomyosarcoma Study. J Clin Oncol 1995;13(3):610–30.
63. Daya H, Chan HS, Sirkin W, et al. Pediatric rhabdomyosarcoma of the head and neck: is there a place for surgical management? Arch Otolaryngol Head Neck Surg 2000;126(4):468–72.

64. Wiener ES. Head and neck rhabdomyosarcoma. Semin Pediatr Surg 1994;3(3): 203–6.
65. Raney RB Jr, Zimmerman RA, Bilaniuk LT, et al. Management of craniofacial sarcoma in childhood assisted by computed tomography. Int J Radiat Oncol Biol Phys 1979;5(4):529–34.
66. Lawrence W Jr, Hays DM, Heyn R, et al. Lymphatic metastases with childhood rhabdomyosarcoma. A report from the Intergroup Rhabdomyosarcoma Study. Cancer 1987;60(4):910–5.
67. Raney RB Jr, Tefft M, Newton WA, et al. Improved prognosis with intensive treatment of children with cranial soft tissue sarcomas arising in nonorbital parameningeal sites. A report from the Intergroup Rhabdomyosarcoma Study. Cancer 1987;59(1):147–55.
68. Maurer HM, Moon T, Donaldson M, et al. The Intergroup Rhabdomyosarcoma Study: a preliminary report. Cancer 1977;40(5):2015–26.
69. Donaldson SS, Belli JA. A rational clinical staging system for childhood rhabdomyosarcoma. J Clin Oncol 1984;2(2):135–9.
70. Kraus DH, Saenz NC, Gollamudi S, et al. Pediatric rhabdomyosarcoma of the head and neck. Am J Surg 1997;174(5):556–60.
71. Meza JL, Anderson J, Pappo AS, et al. Analysis of prognostic factors in patients with nonmetastatic rhabdomyosarcoma treated on intergroup rhabdomyosarcoma studies III and IV: the Children's Oncology Group. J Clin Oncol 2006; 24(24):3844–51.
72. Pappo AS, Shapiro DN, Crist WM. Rhabdomyosarcoma. Biology and treatment. Pediatr Clin North Am 1997;44(4):953–72.
73. Oda Y, Tsuneyoshi M. Recent advances in the molecular pathology of soft tissue sarcoma: implications for diagnosis, patient prognosis, and molecular target therapy in the future. Cancer Sci 2009;100(2):200–8.
74. Grovas A, Fremgen A, Rauck A, et al. The National Cancer Data Base report on patterns of childhood cancers in the United States. Cancer 1997;80(12):2321–32.
75. Chabalko JJ, Creagan ET, Fraumeni JF Jr. Epidemiology of selected sarcomas in children. J Natl Cancer Inst 1974;53(3):675–9.
76. Wanebo HJ, Koness RJ, MacFarlane JK, et al. Head and neck sarcoma: report of the Head and Neck Sarcoma Registry. Society of Head and Neck Surgeons Committee on Research. Head Neck 1992;14(1):1–7.
77. Eavey RD, Janfaza P, Chapman PH, et al. Skull base dumbbell tumor: surgical experience with two adolescents. Ann Otol Rhinol Laryngol 1992;101(11):939–45.
78. Jenkin D, Sonley M. Soft-tissue sarcomas in the young: medical treatment advances in perspective. Cancer 1980;46(3):621–9.
79. Fernandez Sanroman J, Alonso del Hoyo JR, Diaz FJ, et al. Sarcomas of the head and neck. Br J Oral Maxillofac Surg 1992;30(2):115–8.
80. Nasri S, Mark RJ, Sercarz JA, et al. Pediatric sarcomas of the head and neck other than rhabdomyosarcoma. Am J Otolaryngol 1995;16(3):165–71.
81. Blakely ML, Spurbeck WW, Pappo AS, et al. The impact of margin of resection on outcome in pediatric nonrhabdomyosarcoma soft tissue sarcoma. J Pediatr Surg 1999;34(5):672–5.
82. Wexler LH, Helman LJ. Pediatric soft tissue sarcomas. CA Cancer J Clin 1994; 44(4):211–47.
83. Chung EB, Enzinger FM. Infantile fibrosarcoma. Cancer 1976;38(2):729–39.
84. Stout AP. Fibrosarcoma in infants and children. Cancer 1962;15:1028–40.
85. Requena C, Miranda L, Canete A, et al. Congenital fibrosarcoma simulating congenital hemangioma. Pediatr Dermatol 2008;25(1):141–4.

86. Palumbo JS, Zwerdling T. Soft tissue sarcomas of infancy. Semin Perinatol 1999; 23(4):299–309.
87. Variend S. Small cell tumours in childhood: a review. J Pathol 1985;145(1):1–25.
88. Ahmad R, Mayol BR, Davis M, et al. Extraskeletal Ewing's sarcoma. Cancer 1999;85(3):725–31.
89. Gustafson RO, Maragos NE, Reiman HM. Extraskeletal Ewing's sarcoma occurring as a mass in the neck. Otolaryngol Head Neck Surg 1982;90(4):491–3.
90. Venkitaraman R, George MK, Ramanan SG, et al. A single institution experience of combined modality management of extra skeletal Ewings sarcoma. World J Surg Oncol 2007;5:3.
91. Restrepo JP, Handler SD, Saull SC, et al. Malignant fibrous histiocytoma. Otolaryngol Head Neck Surg 1987;96(4):362–5.
92. Wilkins SA Jr, Waldron CA, Mathews WH, et al. Aggressive fibromatosis of the head and neck. Am J Surg 1975;130(4):412–5.
93. Masson JK, Soule EH. Desmoid tumors of the head and neck. Am J Surg 1966; 112(4):615–22.
94. Reitamo JJ, Scheinin TM, Hayry P. The desmoid syndrome. New aspects in the cause, pathogenesis and treatment of the desmoid tumor. Am J Surg 1986; 151(2):230–7.
95. Pena S, Brickman T, Sthilaire H, et al. Aggressive fibromatosis of the head and neck in the pediatric population. Int J Pediatr Otorhinolaryngol 2014;78(1):1–4.
96. Rao BN, Horowitz ME, Parham DM, et al. Challenges in the treatment of childhood fibromatosis. Arch Surg 1987;122(11):1296–8.
97. Ayala AG, Ro JY, Goepfert H, et al. Desmoid fibromatosis: a clinicopathologic study of 25 children. Semin Diagn Pathol 1986;3(2):138–50.
98. Skubitz KM, Skubitz AP. Gene expression in aggressive fibromatosis. J Lab Clin Med 2004;143(2):89–98.
99. McKinnon JG, Neifeld JP, Kay S, et al. Management of desmoid tumors. Surg Gynecol Obstet 1989;169(2):104–6.
100. Faulkner LB, Hajdu SI, Kher U, et al. Pediatric desmoid tumor: retrospective analysis of 63 cases. J Clin Oncol 1995;13(11):2813–8.
101. Janinis J, Patriki M, Vini L, et al. The pharmacological treatment of aggressive fibromatosis: a systematic review. Ann Oncol 2003;14(2):181–90.
102. Tejpar S, Nollet F, Li C, et al. Predominance of beta-catenin mutations and beta-catenin dysregulation in sporadic aggressive fibromatosis (desmoid tumor). Oncogene 1999;18(47):6615–20.
103. Teshima M, Iwae S, Hirayama Y, et al. Nonsteroidal anti-inflammatory drug treatment for desmoid tumor recurrence after surgery. Otolaryngol Head Neck Surg 2012;147(5):978–9.
104. Sharma A, Ngan BY, Sandor GK, et al. Pediatric aggressive fibromatosis of the head and neck: a 20-year retrospective review. J Pediatr Surg 2008;43(9):1596–604.
105. Morris LG, Sikora AG, Kuriakose MA, et al. Tamoxifen therapy for aggressive fibromatosis of the posterior triangle of the neck. Otolaryngol Head Neck Surg 2007;136(4):674–6.
106. Longhi A, Errani C, Battaglia M, et al. Aggressive fibromatosis of the neck treated with a combination of chemotherapy and indomethacin. Ear Nose Throat J 2011;90(6):E11–5.
107. Woods WG, Gao RN, Shuster JJ, et al. Screening of infants and mortality due to neuroblastoma. N Engl J Med 2002;346(14):1041–6.
108. Moukheiber AK, Nicollas R, Roman S, et al. Primary pediatric neuroblastic tumors of the neck. Int J Pediatr Otorhinolaryngol 2001;60(2):155–61.

109. Brown RJ, Szymula NJ, Lore JM Jr. Neuroblastoma of the head and neck. Arch Otolaryngol 1978;104(7):395–8.
110. Castleberry RP. Predicting outcome in neuroblastoma. N Engl J Med 1999; 340(25):1992–3.
111. Castleberry RP. Biology and treatment of neuroblastoma. Pediatr Clin North Am 1997;44(4):919–37.
112. Alvarado CS, London WB, Look AT, et al. Natural history and biology of stage A neuroblastoma: a Pediatric Oncology Group Study. J Pediatr Hematol Oncol 2000;22(3):197–205.
113. Bagatell R, Rumcheva P, London WB, et al. Outcomes of children with intermediate-risk neuroblastoma after treatment stratified by MYCN status and tumor cell ploidy. J Clin Oncol 2005;23(34):8819–27.
114. Cecchetto G, Mosseri V, De Bernardi B, et al. Surgical risk factors in primary surgery for localized neuroblastoma: the LNESG1 study of the European International Society of Pediatric Oncology Neuroblastoma Group. J Clin Oncol 2005; 23(33):8483–9.
115. Hudson MM, Donaldson SS. Treatment of pediatric Hodgkin's lymphoma. Semin Hematol 1999;36(3):313–23.
116. Carbone A, Weiss LM, Gloghini A, et al. Hodgkin's disease: old and recent clinical concepts. Ann Otol Rhinol Laryngol 1996;105(9):751–8.

Endoscopic Endonasal Surgery for Sinonasal and Skull Base Lesions in the Pediatric Population

Jeffrey C. Rastatter, MD[a,b,*], Carl H. Snyderman, MD, MBA[c,d,*],
Paul A. Gardner, MD[d], Tord D. Alden, MD[e,f],
Elizabeth Tyler-Kabara, MD, PhD[d,g]

KEYWORDS

• Pediatric • Endoscopic • Endonasal • Skull base surgery • Cranial • Reconstruction

KEY POINTS

• Endoscopic endonasal approaches to the skull base can be used safely to manage sinonasal and skull base lesions in pediatric patients.

• Understanding the age-dependent pneumatization patterns of the paranasal sinuses, particularly the sphenoid sinus, is critical for planning a safe endonasal approach in pediatric patients.

• Techniques to minimize and control intraoperative blood loss are critical in pediatric patients owing to their overall lower blood volume compared with adult patients.

Continued

Disclosures: Dr C.H. Snyderman is a consultant for SPIWay, LLC and Dr P.A. Gardner is a consultant for Integra LifeSciences.
[a] Division of Pediatric Otolaryngology, Ann & Robert H. Lurie Children's Hospital of Chicago, 225 East Chicago Avenue, Box 25, Chicago, IL 60611, USA; [b] Department of Otolaryngology–Head and Neck Surgery, Northwestern University Feinberg School of Medicine, NMH/Galter Room 15-200, 675 N Saint Clair, Chicago, IL 60611, USA; [c] Department of Otolaryngology, Eye & Ear Institute, University of Pittsburgh School of Medicine, 200 Lothrop Street, Suite 500, Pittsburgh, PA 15213, USA; [d] Department of Neurological Surgery, University of Pittsburgh School of Medicine, 200 Lothrop Street, PUH B-400, Pittsburgh, PA, 15213, USA; [e] Division of Pediatric Neurosurgery, Ann & Robert H. Lurie Children's Hospital of Chicago, 225 East Chicago Avenue, Box 28, Chicago, IL 60611, USA; [f] Department of Neurological Surgery, Northwestern University Feinberg School of Medicine, NMH/Arkes Family Pavilion Suite 2210, 676 N Saint Clair, Chicago, IL 60611, USA; [g] Division of Pediatric Neurosurgery, Children's Hospital of Pittsburgh of the University of Pittsburgh Medical Center, 4401 Penn Avenue, Pittsburgh, PA, 15224, USA
* Corresponding authors. Division of Pediatric Otolaryngology, Ann & Robert H. Lurie Children's Hospital of Chicago, 225 East Chicago Avenue, Box 25, Chicago, IL 60611. Department of Otolaryngology, Eye & Ear Institute, University of Pittsburgh School of Medicine, 200 Lothrop Street, Suite 500, Pittsburgh, PA 15213.
E-mail addresses: jrastatter@luriechildrens.org; snydermanch@upmc.edu

Continued

- The potential size of a nasoseptal flap is smaller in pediatric patients, and careful preoperative and intraoperative planning helps to ensure the appropriateness of its use for skull base reconstruction.
- Teamwork, surgeon experience, and surgical navigation are all important for safe and effective pediatric endoscopic skull base surgery.

 A video of an endoscopy demonstrating a congenital skull base lesion accompanies this article http://www.oto.theclinics.com/

INTRODUCTION

Pediatric sinonasal and skull base lesions encompass a diverse range of pathologies and conditions that have a myriad of presentations, depending on the child's age, location of the lesion, and disease-specific characteristics. The diagnosis and management of these lesions can be complex and demands an understanding of sinonasal and skull base embryology, developmental anatomy, location-specific symptoms, and disease-specific characteristics and behavior. Comprehensive and safe management of these lesions requires a team approach of medical and surgical services with extensive training and experience. Surgical management in particular demands extensive clinical training supplemented by cadaveric dissection to gain the requisite knowledge of the 3-dimensional anatomy, specialized instrumentation, and teamwork necessary for optimal outcomes and safety.

Historically, skull base surgery was only performed by open, external approaches and craniotomies to reach various areas of the cranial base. These procedures are well-described, have a role in contemporary surgery, and have been safely performed in adult and pediatric patients.[1,2] Transnasal approaches to the skull base developed later, using a microscope for visualization and driven largely by advances with pituitary surgery.[3] More recently, endoscopic endonasal approaches (EEAs) to the skull base have developed, driven partially by advances in instrumentation and experience related to endoscopic sinus surgery and pituitary surgery.[4]

EEAs to the skull base, initially employed for adult pituitary surgery, are now also used to safely approach varied pathologies in more distant skull base locations in the coronal and sagittal planes.[5–7] As technology, instrumentation, and surgeon experience have progressed, endoscopic endonasal techniques are being used more often in pediatric skull base surgery, as demonstrated by the increasing number of publications on this topic related to pediatric patients as case reports[8–12] and even some case series.[13–15] This review aims to illustrate the current state of diagnosis and management of pediatric sinonasal and skull base lesions, particularly related to EEAs, resection, and reconstruction.

EMBRYOLOGY AND DEVELOPMENT

A working knowledge of sinonasal and skull base embryology is important for understanding how this complex anatomy forms leading up to birth, and serves as a basis for understanding how this anatomy grows and develops from birth to adulthood. Errors in normal embryologic development lead to some of the pathologies encountered by the skull base surgeon. Descriptions of the embryologic basis of specific lesions are discussed later in the section detailing individual lesions and pathologies. Although some important aspects are described herein, more detailed descriptions of sinonasal and skull base embryology are well-documented elsewhere.[16,17]

Sinonasal Embryology and Development

The pneumatized paranasal sinuses can provide access to the skull base when performing an EEA. An understanding of the age-dependent growth and pneumatization patterns are critical to safe surgical planning.

In the fourth week of gestation, ectoderm from the frontonasal process contributes to the nasal capsule. The lateral walls of the nasal capsule enlarge, grooves begin to form, and by 9 to 10 weeks gestation, 6 ridges or ethmoturbinals are evident. The first through fourth ethmoturbinals form the uncinate process, portions of the ethmoid bulla, attachment of the middle turbinate to the lateral nasal wall, and attachment of the superior turbinate to the lateral nasal wall, respectively. The fifth and sixth ethmoturbinals obliterate or contribute to a supreme turbinate. The furrow between the first and second ethmoturbinal contributes to the ethmoid infundibulum.

The maxillary sinus begins development around 9 to 10 weeks gestation as a lateral outgrowth from the ethmoid infundibulum, is present at birth, and shows a biphasic growth pattern with increased growth between 0 to 3 years and 6 to 12 years of life. It reaches full adult size around age 18 years. The ethmoid sinuses begin development shortly after the maxillary sinuses, first with the anterior cells as evaginations from the nasal wall in the middle meatus and later the posterior cells as evaginations from the nasal wall in the superior meatus. The ethmoid sinus is present at birth, and growth and pneumatization continue until around the age of 12 years. The frontal sinus begins development around the fourth month of gestation as an upward extension from the frontal recess. Not notable at birth, the frontal sinus can been seen on x-ray at age 2 years, invades the frontal bone around 5 years, and reaches an adult size in late adolescence.[18]

The sphenoid sinus plays a central role both physically and conceptually when planning and executing EEAs to the skull base. Most such approaches begin with a bilateral wide sphenoidotomy and identification of key landmarks within the sphenoid sinus. Around the fourth week of gestation, the sphenoid sinus begins development as paired evaginations from the sphenoethmoidal recess. Pneumatization begins at the anterior inferior sphenoid face and proceeds posteriorly well into adolescence. A recent study showed that by age 6 to 7 years, the sphenoid face is fully pneumatized and the planum sphenoidale is nearly 90% pneumatized. Pneumatization into the clival recess was seen at age 10 years, but the majority of specimens (84%) showed no dorsum sellae pneumatization. A "sellar" type pneumatization pattern was characteristic of 6- to 13-year-olds.[19]

Skull Base Embryology and Development

The human skull develops from 3 components: The membranous neurocranium that forms the flat bones of the skull, the cartilaginous neurocranium or chondrocranium that forms the majority of the skull base, and the viscerocranium that forms the facial skeleton. Around the fourth month of gestation, the skull base begins development from the chondrocranium. The anterior and posterior skull base develops from embryologically distinct tissues. Separated by the sella turcica, the anterior skull base arises from neural crest cells, and the posterior skull base develops from the paraxial mesoderm.[16] The anterior skull base serves as a scaffold for the facial skeleton and grows at a faster rate than the posterior skull base. Surgery of the skull base has the potential to impact craniofacial growth and development.

SURGICAL ANATOMY

A thorough understanding of the 3-dimensional sinonasal and skull base anatomy is critical for performing safe surgery. This knowledge is gained from extensive study of pictures, models, and cadaveric dissection, as well as surgical experience. The skull base is divided into 3 parts by bony landmarks on the cranial side (**Fig. 1**)—anterior, middle, and posterior—and each part is related to cranial and extracranial components (**Table 1**).[20] The nasal side of the skull base is better subdivided based on sinonasal landmarks and surgical modules in the sagittal and coronal planes.[5–7]

It is important to understand the anatomy from both the cranial and endonasal viewpoints, and to be able to conceptualize the anatomic structure of both sides (cranial and endonasal) when viewing from one side of the skull base. For example, when viewing the cribriform plate endonasally, one must recognize that the frontal lobe and olfactory tract lie on the cranial side.

ANTERIOR CRANIAL BASE
Cranial Aspect

The anterior cranial base is composed of the frontal, ethmoid, and sphenoid bones. From anterior to posterior, it extends from the inner surface of the frontal bones to the sphenoid ridges, which are joined medially by the chiasmatic groove.[20] The optic

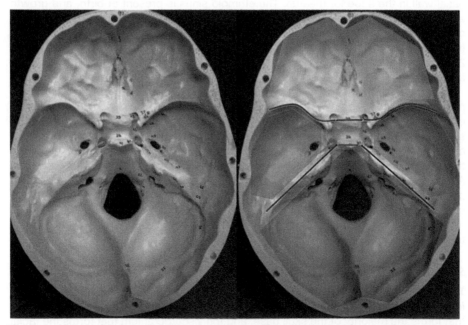

Fig. 1. A skull model demonstrating the cranial surface of the skull base with the anterior cranial fossa (*light green shading*) separated from the middle cranial fossa (*yellow and blue shading*) by a line along the sphenoid ridges (*curved blue lines*) and chiasmatic groove (*red line*). The medial portion of the middle cranial fossa (*blue shading*) includes the sella turcica and grooves for the internal carotid arteries within the cavernous sinuses on either side. The lateral portion of the middle cranial fossa is also represented (*yellow shading*). The posterior cranial fossa (*pink shading*) is separated from the middle cranial fossa by a line along the petrous ridges (*purple line*) and the dorsum sellae (*green line*).

Table 1
Cranial and extracranial components of the skull base

Component	Anterior Skull Base	Middle Skull Base	Posterior Skull Base
Intracranial	Anterior cranial fossa, frontal lobes	Middle cranial fossa, temporal lobes, pituitary fossa, cavernous sinuses	Posterior cranial fossa, brainstem, cerebellum
Osteology	Frontal bone, ethmoid bone, sphenoid bone (planum sphenoidale)	Sphenoid bone, temporal bones	Sphenoid bone, temporal bones, occipital bone
Foramina	Optic canal, foramen cecum, olfactory foramina, ethmoid foramina	Vidian canal, foramen rotundum, foramen ovale, foramen spinosum, internal auditory canal	Hypoglossal canal, foramen magnum, jugular foramen
Extracranial	Frontal and ethmoid sinuses, nasal cavity, orbit, lacrimal apparatus	Sphenoid and maxillary sinuses, nasopharynx, fossa of Rosenmueller, pterygopalatine fossa, infratemporal fossa, parapharyngeal space, infrapetrosal space	Nasopharynx
Major vessels	Anterior and posterior ethmoid arteries, ophthalmic artery, fronto-orbital artery, anterior cerebral artery, anterior communicating artery, artery of Heubner	Middle cerebral artery, internal carotid artery, hypophyseal arteries, Vidian artery, internal maxillary artery, sphenopalatine artery, middle meningeal artery, accessory meningeal artery	Vertebral artery, basilar artery, superior cerebellar artery, posterior cerebral artery
Major nerves	Olfactory bulb, olfactory tract (Cranial nerve I)	Cranial nerves II, III, IV, V, and VI; cavernous sinus nerves; Vidian nerve	Cranial nerves IX, X, XI, and XII

canal is formed by the orbital process of the frontal bone and lesser wing of the sphenoid bone and transmits the optic nerve and ophthalmic artery.

In the midline from anterior to posterior, the frontal bone, ethmoid bone, and sphenoid bones are joined at suture lines. The ethmoid bone from medial to lateral includes the crista galli, cribriform plate, and fovea ethmoidalis (ethmoid roof). More laterally, the frontal bone forms the majority of the anterior cranial base. The frontal lobes of the brain fill the anterior cranial fossa with the rectus gyri medially and the orbital gyri laterally. The frontoorbital artery lies on the inferior medial surface of the frontal lobe, and the olfactory bulb and tract lie on the cribriform plate opposing the frontal lobe's inferior surface. The falx cerebri separates the cerebral hemispheres and attaches to the crista galli. The superior sagittal sinus runs along the superior edge of the falx cerebri and connects to an emissary vein at the foramen cecum just anterior to the crista galli.

Endonasal Aspect

From an endonasal perspective, the anterior two thirds of the midline anterior cranial base relates to the ethmoid bone and sinus (cribriform plate, fovea ethmoidalis) and the posterior one third relates to the sphenoid sinus and planum sphenoidale. The anterior ethmoid foramen transmits the anterior ethmoid artery in a lateral course just caudal to where the anterior cranial base curves superiorly into the frontal sinus. At times, this artery can be found away from the skull base on a bony mesentery, placing it at risk of injury during surgery. The posterior ethmoid foramen, often located at the junction of the fovea ethmoidalis and planum sphenoidale, transmits the posterior ethmoid artery. Both anterior and posterior ethmoid arteries are branches of the ophthalmic artery, and both foramina are within the frontoethmoid suture.[5]

MIDDLE CRANIAL BASE
Cranial Aspect

The middle cranial base is composed of the sphenoid and temporal bones. From anterior to posterior, it extends from the sphenoid ridges and chiasmatic groove to the petrous ridges and dorsum sellae.[20] The medial region is largely composed of the body of the sphenoid bone and includes the sella turcica. The sella turcica includes, from anterior to posterior, the tuberculum sellae, anterior clinoid processes, hypophyseal fossa (housing the pituitary gland), and dorsum sellae with posterior clinoid processes. The cavernous sinus, a venous channel, lies immediately lateral to each side of the sella turcica and transmits the cavernous segment of the carotid artery and cranial nerves III, IV, V1, and VI. The temporal lobes of the brain fill the middle cranial fossae.[20]

More laterally, the middle fossa transmits the other branches of the trigeminal nerves through foramen rotundum and foramen ovale. The middle meningeal artery enters via foramen spinosum. The floor of the middle fossa overlies the horizontal petrous internal carotid artery and contains the geniculate ganglion with its exposed greater superficial petrosal nerve branch which extends over the horizontal internal carotid artery to the vidian nerve.

Endonasal Aspect

The undersurface of the middle cranial base relates to the following 4 defined spaces: Pterygopalatine fossa, infratemporal fossa, parapharyngeal space, and infrapetrosal space. These spaces are dense with important structures and many neurovascular elements that traverse the skull base via foramina. The detailed boundaries and contents of these spaces are described elsewhere and are beyond the scope of this article. From an endoscopic endonasal perspective, the pterygopalatine fossa and infratemporal fossa are more approachable, often after removal of the medial and posterior maxillary sinus walls. From the nasal cavity a natural pathway can be followed laterally through the sphenopalatine foramen to the pterygopalatine fossa, and then further lateral through the pterygomaxillary fissure to the infratemporal fossa. Within the sphenoid sinus, the anterior face of the hypophyseal fossa can be easily seen with sufficient sinus pneumatization.

POSTERIOR CRANIAL BASE
Cranial Aspect

The posterior cranial base is composed of the sphenoid, temporal, and occipital bones. From anterior to posterior, it extends from the petrous ridges and dorsum sellae to the inner surface of the occipital bone. The posterior cranial fossa is the most inferiorly located fossa, lies between the tentorium cerebelli and foramen magnum, and houses the brainstem and cerebellum. The internal acoustic meatus transmits cranial nerves

VII and VIII, the jugular foramen transmits the internal jugular vein and cranial nerves IX, X, and XI, and the hypoglossal canal transmits cranial nerve XII.[20]

Endonasal Aspect

From an endonasal perspective the posterior cranial base relates to the clivus and can be divided into 3 segments[6]:

1. Superior segment from the dorsum sellae and posterior clinoids to the sellar floor;
2. Middle segment from the sellar floor to the sphenoid sinus floor (clival recess); and
3. Inferior segment from the sphenoid sinus floor to the foramen magnum.

The superior segment relates intracranially with cranial nerve III, the posterior cerebral artery, and the superior cerebellar artery; the middle segment relates to cranial nerve VI, the anterior inferior cerebellar artery, and the basilar artery; and the inferior segment relates to cranial nerves IX, X, and XII and the vertebrobasilar junction.[7]

SPHENOID SINUS ANATOMY

The endonasal anatomy of the sphenoid sinus deserves emphasis owing to the central role it plays in planning and executing endonasal skull base surgery. The majority of EEAs begin with a wide bilateral sphenoidotomy (removal of the sphenoid face from planum to floor and laterally to each lateral recess, the sphenoid rostrum, and the intersinus septations) and identification of anatomic landmarks. A completely pneumatized sphenoid sinus (late adolescent or adult) often will have the following endoscopic landmarks:

1 Midline from superior to inferior: Planum sphenoidale, tuberculum sellae, sellar floor, clival recess; and
2 Laterally from superior to inferior: Optic canal, lateral opticocarotid recess, parasellar carotid artery, paraclival carotid artery (**Fig. 2**).

The lateral opticocarotid recess is a pneumatization of the optic strut, a strip of bone on the cranial side that separates the optic nerve and superior orbital fissure, extending to the sphenoid sinus from the anterior clinoid process.

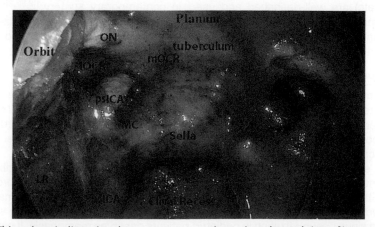

Fig. 2. This cadaveric dissection demonstrates an endoscopic endonasal view of important skull base landmarks and anatomy seen after wide bilateral sphenoidectomy. lOCR, lateral opticocarotid recess; LR, lateral recess; MC, middle clinoid; mOCR, medial opticocarotid recess; ON, optic nerve; pclCA, paraclival internal carotid artery; psICA, parasellar internal carotid artery.

Understanding the age-dependent progression of sphenoid sinus pneumatization is critical when performing surgery in pediatric patients. Many of the endoscopic landmarks notable with complete pneumatization can be difficult or impossible to visualize upon initially entering the sinus in young patients with incomplete pneumatization. Surgeon experience, surgical navigation, and careful bone removal are essential when identifying sphenoid anatomy in an incompletely pneumatized sinus.[19] An appropriate understanding of the related anatomy, combined with accurate image guidance and careful exposure allows for efficient identification of critical structures, regardless of degree of pneumatization.

SPECIAL ANATOMIC CONSIDERATIONS FOR PEDIATRIC SKULL BASE SURGERY

Along with variable sphenoid sinus pneumatization, the smaller size of the pediatric sinonasal anatomy can pose limitations on the ability to approach the skull base endonasally. Until the age of 6 to 7, the nasal aperture is significantly narrower compared with that in adults and may pose limitations for an EEA in very young patients. Further, intercarotid artery distances within the clivus at the level of the cavernous sinus are statistically narrower in children relative to adults. More inferiorly, intercarotid artery distances at the level of the superior clivus are stable throughout life.[19] Knowledge of the anatomic location of sinonasal and skull base growth centers is important, because disturbance of these centers can impact craniofacial growth. For example, the spheno-occipital synchondrosis is among the primary skull base growth centers and closes at the completion of skull base ossification around age 12 to 16 years.[16]

SURGICAL TECHNIQUE: APPROACH AND RESECTION

Pediatric skull base surgery has a rich history. Over the last several decades, various approaches and techniques have been described and mastered by surgeons to address pathology in essentially any skull base location.[21] Initially described in adults, application of skull base approaches to pediatric patients are first found in the literature from the 1980s and 1990s.[22–24] Open surgical approaches, both transfacial (craniofacial) and transcranial (bifrontal, frontotemporal, orbitozygomatic, lateral temporal, preauricular infratemporal, retrosigmoid, suboccipital, transmastoid, translabyrinthine, etc) are well-described and used in contemporary surgery.[1,2,25,26] In the 1990s, microscopic transnasal transsphenoidal approaches were popularized and are still in use currently.[3,27] The focus of this article is on the more recent developments with EEAs to the skull base in the pediatric population.

Endoscopic Skull Base Surgery: The Sagittal and Coronal Planes

Approaches to the skull base from the endoscopic endonasal perspective can be categorized by individual surgical modules as first described by the University of Pittsburgh Center for Cranial Base Surgery (**Table 2**).[28] The modules are described by the named portion of the skull base that serves as the site of operation or point of entry into the intracranial cavity.

In the sagittal plane, from rostral to caudal the modules include transcribriform, transplanum, transsellar, transclival, and transodontoid. Most of these approaches begin with a wide bilateral sphenoidotomy and identification of key landmarks as described in the sphenoid sinus anatomy section. The need to account for variable sphenoid sinus pneumatization in pediatric patients deserves reemphasis. If nasoseptal flap (NSF) reconstruction is planned, the flap is raised before wide sphenoidotomy, thereby preserving the flap pedicle and blood supply. This is discussed further elsewhere in this article.

Table 2	
Classification of endoscopic approaches	
Sagittal Plane	**Coronal Plane**
Transfrontal	Transorbital
Transcribriform	Petrous apex (medial transpetrous)
Transplanum (suprasellar/subchiasmatic)	Lateral transcavernous
Transsphenoidal (sellar/medial transcavernous)	Transpterygoid
Transclival (Posterior clinoid, mid clivus, foramen magnum)	Transpetrous (superior, inferior)
Transodontoid	Transcondylar
	Parapharyngeal space

The sphenoid sinus can be approached and opened directly after lateralization of the nasal turbinates. If more exposure is needed for visualization or instrumentation, bilateral posterior ethmoidectomies and removal of 1 or both middle turbinates is performed. We often remove the right middle turbinate and use this side as the primary entry point for the endoscope. Wide sphenoidotomy and posterior septectomy with or without bilateral posterior ethmoidectomies are often sufficient exposure for a transsellar or transplanum approach. Rostrally, anterior ethmoid cells need to be removed for a transcribriform surgery, and caudally the sphenoid sinus floor and soft tissue over the clivus requires removal for a transclival or transodontoid approach.

In the coronal plane, the described modules allow extension of the surgical approach laterally. The first step is often a transpterygoid module, which involves wide removal of the medial maxillary wall; removal of the posterior maxillary sinus wall, thereby exposing the pterygopalatine fossa; and extension of sphenoid sinus floor removal laterally into the pterygoid base. The vidian canal is a key landmark in the pterygoid base, serving as an approximate location of the foramen lacerum and carotid artery deeper in the bone, and a starting point for locating the foramen rotundum with further dissection lateral and superior to the vidian canal.[29] Dissection can proceed from "known to unknown" more deeply and laterally, allowing access to the petrous apex and middle cranial fossa. These approaches require a comfort level with identifying and working around critical neurovascular anatomy including the carotid artery. Further details regarding these approaches can be found elsewhere.[5–7,13,14,29–33]

Endoscopic Skull Base Surgery: Hemostatic Control and Surgical Goals

Endoscopic endonasal pediatric skull base surgery requires expert control of bleeding and a clear vision of the surgical goals. Even in the absence of high-flow bleeding, the robust vascularity of the nose and sinuses can lead to oozing and substantial blood loss over time. Oozing and low-flow venous bleeding can often be controlled with combinations of pressure, hemostatic agents, cautery, or warm saline irrigation.[34] High-flow bleeding, whether venous (cavernous sinus) or arterial (sphenopalatine artery, vidian artery, carotid artery, etc), requires immediate attention. Arterial or high-flow bleeding can sometimes be controlled by similar methods. Larger arteries demand experience and teamwork to allow proper visualization and control. Carotid artery injury and bleeding can be catastrophic, and injury can be avoided by thorough anatomic knowledge and good surgical technique. Carotid artery injuries can sometimes be repaired, but often require nasal packing and endovascular sacrifice.[35–37] Preoperative selective embolization or arterial ligation of external carotid branches early in a surgery can also limit intraoperative blood loss.

Endoscopic Skull Base Surgery: Imaging and Surgical Navigation

Preoperative study of imaging, typically both computed tomography (CT) and MRI, is critical for surgical planning. With pediatric patients, CT demonstrates the size and state of pneumatization of the sinuses. Intraoperative image-guided navigation is also strongly recommended and arguably essential. For surgical navigation, we typically use a fine-cut CT angiography (good bone and vascular detail) as the reference study and merge an MRI (good soft tissue and tumor detail). During surgery, the CT angiography and MRI can be viewed individually or fused. MRI is often the study of choice for following patients postoperatively, because it does not involve radiation and fast sequences can often be done without sedation, even in young patients.

Endoscopic Skull Base Surgery: Team Surgery and the Learning Curve

A team approach including medical and surgical specialists is important for the overall management of these complicated pediatric skull base lesions. A 2-surgeon team, often consisting of an otolaryngologist and a neurosurgeon working together, provides advantages over either operating alone. The initial approach to the sphenoid sinus, raising of the NSF when indiated, and completion of the wide sphenoidotomy are performed by 1 surgeon, typically the otolaryngologist. The wide sphenoidotomy and posterior septectomy allow the transition to 2 surgeons (4 hands) working simultaneously, as instruments introduced through either nostril (binarial method) provide access to both sides of the posterior nasal space and skull base. A 2-surgeon uninarial method is described, but the binarial method is appropriate for the majority of endoscopic endonasal skull base procedures. Further details of the equipment and positioning (surgeon and patient) for these surgeries can be found elsewhere.[5] Learning to function well as a surgical team and learning the complex anatomy and instrumentation required to safely execute these surgeries demands extensive practice and experience. A stepwise progression of a surgical team, starting with mastering the more straightforward procedures before attempting more complicated approaches, has been recommended.[28]

SKULL BASE RECONSTRUCTION AFTER ENDOSCOPIC SURGERY

Advances in skull base reconstruction after endoscopic surgery have allowed surgeons to perform more extensive initial resections while maintaining acceptable rates of postreconstruction cerebrospinal fluid (CSF) leak or other potential complications. For relatively small postoperative defects (<1 cm) with minimal or no CSF leak, free grafts of fascia (underlay and/or overlay of the exposed dura mater), fat, muscle, mucosa, cartilage, bone, or a combination of these materials may be successful. For larger skull base defects or moderate- to high-flow CSF leaks, vascularized (pedicled) tissue to augment the reconstruction is preferable. Options for vascularized tissue include sinonasal flaps and scalp flaps (**Table 3**). Sinonasal flaps include nasoseptal,[38–40] inferior turbinate,[41] and middle turbinate flaps.[42] Scalp flaps include pericranial,[43] galeopericranial, temporoparietal fascial,[44] and temporalis muscle flaps. Further reading on advanced uses of these vascularized flaps can be found elsewhere.[44–46] Reconstructions are held in place during the healing phase by thin coverings of tissue glues such as Tisseel (Baxter, Deerfield, IL, USA) or DuraSeal (Covidien, Dublin, Ireland), and nasal packing with absorbable or nonabsorbable materials for variable lengths of time (surgeon and defect size and flow dependent). Lumbar drains are sometimes used postoperatively with repair of high-flow CSF defects.

Flap	Blood Supply
Table 3	
Vascularized sinonasal and scalp flaps	
Sinonasal	
Nasoseptal flap	Posterior septal arteries
Inferior turbinate flap	Branches of the sphenopalatine artery
Middle turbinate flap	Branches of the sphenopalatine artery
Scalp	
Pericranial flap/galeopericranial flap	Supraorbital and supratrochlear arteries
Temporoparietal fascial flap	Superficial temporal artery
Temporalis muscle flap	Deep temporal arteries

Nasoseptal Flap

First described in 2006,[38] the NSF has become the "work horse" for adult and, more recently, pediatric skull base reconstruction after endoscopic endonasal surgery. Pedicled on the posterior septal branches of the sphenopalatine artery, this mucoperiosteal and mucoperichondrial flap is robust and reaches most skull base locations (**Fig. 3**). The pedicle courses across the inferior sphenoid sinus face, and flap harvest

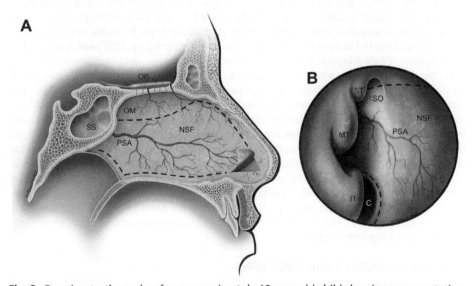

Fig. 3. Drawing to the scale of an approximately 10-year-old child showing representative anatomy for designing a nasoseptal flap for reconstruction of the skull base. The sagittal (A) and endoscopic (B) views demonstrate the posteriorly based pedicle supplied by the posterior septal branch (sometimes branches) of the sphenopalatine artery. The *dotted lines* represent the location of the mucosal incisions. In the sagittal view (A), note the designed preservation of the olfactory mucosa located posterior superior on the nasal septum. The endoscopic view (B) shows the superior incision originating from the level of the natural sphenoid os, and the inferior incision following the edge and curvature of the choanal arch to the nasal floor. C, choanae; IT, inferior turbinate; MT, middle turbinate; NSF, nasoseptal flap; OB, olfactory bulb; OM, olfactory mucosa; PSA, posterior septal artery; SO, sphenoid os; SS, sphenoid sinus; ST, superior turbinate.

should occur before wide sphenoidotomy as removal of the sphenoid face before harvest could interrupt the pedicle.

CSF leak rates after endoscopic reconstruction with an NSF have become comparable with open surgical techniques in the adult literature.[39] Pediatric series of NSF reconstructions are less robust owing to lesser pediatric patient volumes (lower incidence of conditions requiring skull base resection compared with adult patients) and many surgeons first choosing to master the technique in adults before applying it to children. Recent series suggest a success rate similar to adult NSF reconstructions or open reconstructions in pediatric patients.[13,40]

The maximal size of an NSF that can be harvested depends on nasal growth, an important consideration with pediatric patients. A recent study of craniofacial CT scans suggest that although the width of the NSF is likely sufficient at any age, the length may be insufficient for a transsellar/transplanum defect until age 6 to 7 years, a transcribriform defect until age 9 to 10 years, and insufficient for a clival defect at all pediatric ages.[47] However, we have used NSF reconstructions successfully in patients as young as 4 years old with a transsellar/transplanum defect. In very young patients, or with patients in whom the NSF is not available, other reconstruction flaps or free grafts should be considered.

COMPLICATIONS IN SKULL BASE SURGERY

Potential complications after skull base surgery, particularly endoscopic endonasal surgery, are variable and in part related to the age of the patient, nature of the disease treated (size, type, location of the lesion), extent of the surgical intervention, and choice of reconstructive method (free graft vs pedicle flap). Possible complications include those related to sinonasal function, neurovascular injury, CSF leak, central nervous system (CNS) infection (meningitis, cerebritis, abscess), and damage to CNS tissue (endocrinopathy, motor, or sensory dysfunction). Short-term sinonasal dysfunction requiring scheduled debridement and saline irrigation is expected, but long-term issues are possible and include synechiae, nasal obstruction, chronic sinusitis, septal perforation, and altered olfaction. Neurovascular complications include intraoperative hemorrhage, stroke, and cranial nerve dysfunction (vision loss, diplopia, hoarseness, dysphagia, and dysarthria). Postoperative CSF leak is best managed by revision surgery and repair to avoid meningitis. An important consideration in pediatric patients is the potential impact of skull base surgery on craniofacial growth. Based on our experience with open skull base surgery and sinus surgery for inflammatory disease, it seems endoscopic skull base surgery can be done safely with little impact on craniofacial growth, but further longitudinal studies are required to definitively understand the long-term impact.

SELECTED PATHOLOGIES AND CONDITIONS

Conditions and pathologies that impact the pediatric skull base are numerous and diverse. This section is not an exhaustive list of all conditions, but rather serves to highlight some of the more frequently encountered lesions (**Table 4**).

Anterior Cranial Base

Congenital midline nasal mass
Midline nasal masses are rare lesions that occur anywhere from the tip of the nose to the glabellar region. Approximately 60% of these are dermoid cysts, with gliomas or encephaloceles the next most likely in the differential diagnosis. The etiology is thought to be a developmental failure of separation of the dural (neuroectoderm) diverticulum

Table 4
Selected pediatric sinonasal and skull base lesions

Anterior Cranial Base/Nasal Cavity/Maxillary Sinus/Orbit	Middle Cranial Base/Sphenoid/ Sella/Infratemporal Fossa	Posterior Cranial Base
Meningoencephalocele	Meningoencephalocele	Chordoma
Nasal dermoid	Pituitary adenoma	Vestibular schwannoma
Glioma	Craniopharyngioma	Epidermoid cyst
Mucocele	Cholesterol granuloma	Glomus jugulare
Juvenile nasopharyngeal angiofibroma	Trigeminal schwannoma	Osteomyelitis
Fibrous dysplasia	Juvenile nasopharyngeal angiofibroma	Chondrosarcoma
Fibro-osseous tumors	Sarcomas	
Esthesioneuroblastoma		

through the foramen cecum from the overlying skin.[48] There may be a pit in the nasal skin, often at the osseocartilaginous junction (rhinion). An intracranial component is found in 5% to 45% of nasal dermoids.[49,50] They present as an isolated pit, lump, or swelling, possibly with signs of infection. An intracranial component is at risk of intracranial infection (meningitis, abscess). Untreated, further growth can lead to infection, cosmetic nasal deformity, or intracranial mass effect. CT and MRI are complementary and both may be helpful in making the diagnosis. A bifid crista galli on CT is suggestive of a skull base defect and intracranial involvement, and MRI can demonstrate the extent of intracranial involvement.[51] Surgical excision is the treatment of choice. The approach depends on the location, skin involvement, and extent of the lesion, and options include external incisions (ellipse around the pit, external rhinoplasty, bicoronal), craniotomy, and more recently endoscopic endonasal or endoscopic-assisted surgery.[49,52]

Encephalocele

Congenital or acquired defects in the skull base can lead to encephaloceles, herniation of intracranial contents into the sinonasal spaces. These lesions are described by the herniated contents, such as meningocele (meninges, CSF) or meningoencephalocele (meninges, CSF, brain tissue) most commonly.[53] Congenital lesions may be incidentally noted on imaging for other reasons, or present with nasal obstruction, infection (meningitis, CNS infection) or CSF rhinorrhea (**Fig. 4**, Video 1). Acquired lesions are usually owing to trauma. Workup includes nasal endoscopy, full neurologic evaluation, endocrine evaluation depending on the location and symptoms, and imaging with both CT and MRI. Although some acquired traumatic skull base defects resolve with conservative measures, most congenital encephaloceles require surgical intervention.[54] The goals of surgery are to resolve nasal obstruction, provide a watertight division between the sinonasal and intracranial cavities, and minimize injury to any CNS contents in or near the encephalocele. The surgical approach depends on the size of the patient and size/location of the lesion. Open approaches (craniotomy, transpalatal) may be required, but endoscopic endonasal repairs are often possible, even in children under age 2 years.[55]

Middle Cranial Base: Sellar and Suprasellar

Pituitary adenoma

Pituitary tumors are relatively rare in children.[56] They may present as an incidental finding on imaging for other reasons, or may be symptomatic from endocrinopathy

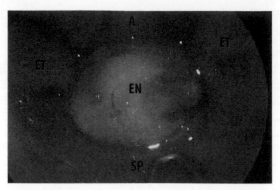

Fig. 4. Endoscopic view of the nasopharynx in an 11-month-old child who presented with nasal obstruction. The nasal airway is obstructed by an encephalocele (EN) situated between the Eustachian tubes (ET) laterally, the soft palate (SP) anteriorly, and the adenoid (A) posteriorly. View is from a 120° telescope introduced orally. See also Video 1.

related to a functional adenoma or hypofunctional gland, or symptoms related to mass effect of the lesion (visual changes, headache, nausea; **Fig. 5**). Contrary to adults, most pituitary adenomas in children are functional. The most common is prolactinoma followed by corticotropinoma and somatotropinoma. Nonfunctioning adenomas, thyroid-stimulating hormone–secreting and gonadotropin-secreting adenomas constitute 3% to 6% of childhood pituitary adenomas. Surgery is indicated for the majority of tumors, with the goals of surgery being total resection with preservation or restoration of endocrine and CNS function. MRI is indicated preoperatively and for postoperative surveillance. CT may be useful preoperatively in selected cases when bone detail of the sphenoid sinus/sellar region is desired. An EEA is appropriate in most patients with decreased morbidity relative to transseptal microscopic approaches.[57,58]

Craniopharyngioma
Thought to arise from epithelial remnants of Rathke's pouch, craniopharyngioma is the most common pediatric benign tumor in the sellar/parasellar region, representing 50%

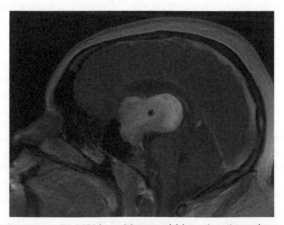

Fig. 5. Sagittal post contrast T1 MRI in a 14-year-old boy showing a large sellar/suprasellar pituitary macroadenoma (*asterisk*) with posterior extension to the interpeduncular cistern.

of pediatric sellar tumors. Although benign, these tumors can cause significant morbidity and pose management challenges owing to size, location, and a tendency to recur even years after treatment.[59] Composed of both solid and cystic components, these tumors can present with endocrinopathy and CNS changes related to mass effect. MRI can help to define the extent of the tumor. When possible, optimal management includes total resection with preservation and restoration of endocrine and CNS function. An alternative strategy for some larger lesions with hypothalamic involvement is debulking or subtotal resection with postoperative radiation therapy. Even with optimal management, permanent endocrinopathy or CNS dysfunction may result, and recurrence can occur months or years after treatment. Long-term surveillance is essential. The surgical approach depends on the size and extent of the tumor and the experience and preference of the surgical team. Open (pterional, subfrontal) and transnasal (microscopic, endoscopic) strategies have been described.[60–62]

Rathke's cleft cyst

Rathke's cleft cyst is a benign cystic lesion that must be differentiated from a craniopharyngioma or cystic pituitary adenoma. A small, nonenhancing, intracystic nodule is considered pathognomonic.[63] These lesions can often be followed conservatively, but when symptomatic (headache, vision loss, endocrine dysfunction) are managed surgically by cyst drainage. An EEA is usually feasible with decreased morbidity compared with an open approach.

Pterygopalatine Fossa/Infratemporal Fossa

Juvenile nasopharyngeal angiofibroma

Juvenile nasopharyngeal angiofibroma is a benign, highly vascular tumor that arises from cells in the area of the sphenopalatine foramen. The specific cell of origin and etiology are not certain. Growth of these lesions is well-described and traverses natural sinonasal pathways and bony foramina, potentially involving the nasal cavity, nasopharynx, pterygoplalatine fossa, infratemporal fossa, clivus, planum, orbit, or middle cranial fossa.[64] Presentation, almost always in a teenage male, may include epistaxis or nasal obstruction, and possibly visual or CNS symptoms for extensive lesions. Physical examination and imaging (CT and MRI) can be highly suggestive of the diagnosis and sufficient to plan a management strategy (**Fig. 6**). Biopsy should be avoided because significant bleeding can result. Various staging systems have been described based on the extent of disease (imaging and clinical examination), the details of which are beyond the scope of this review article.[65,66] The treatment of choice when possible is surgical resection, usually with preoperative embolization to limit intraoperative blood loss. Radiation has been described for treatment of primary or residual disease, but long-term effects of such treatment must be considered. It is the authors' preference to avoid radiation treatment in the vast majority of cases. The surgical approach may be open or endoscopic.[67] Endoscopic resections have been described for even extensive lesions, and this is the authors' preferred approach for the majority of these tumors.

Posterior Cranial Base: Clival

Chordoma

Chordoma is a locally aggressive, osseous tumor of the embryologic notochord that can present with destructive involvement of the skull base, most commonly the clivus, and often shows overtly malignant behavior, with metastatic disease in 10% to 20% of cases. CT and MRI can define the extent of the lesion, and diagnosis is confirmed by identifying 1 of 3 histologic subtypes on biopsy (classical, chondroid, dedifferentiated;

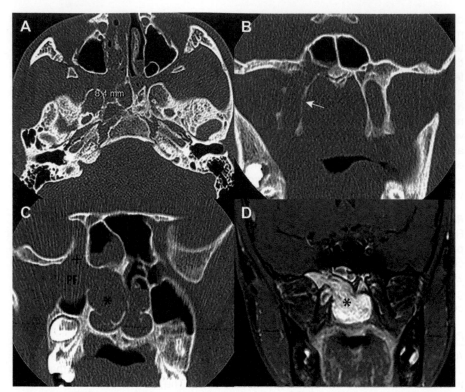

Fig. 6. Computed tomography (CT) and MRI views of a 14-year-old boy with a large juvenile nasopharyngeal angiofibroma (*asterisk*). (*A*) Axial CT view demonstrating widening of the right pterygopalatine fossa (*green line*). (*B* and *C*) Coronal CT views demonstrating bone erosion of the right skull base and pterygoid plates (*white arrow*), and involvement of the right pterygopalatine fossa (PF) and nasal cavity. Note the communication with the inferior orbital fissure (+).(*D*) Coronal MRI view showing extension of the lesion to the middle cranial fossa abutting the right temporal lobe.

Fig. 7). Total resection is the treatment of choice, but this is often challenging owing to involvement or close association with critical structures (internal carotid artery encasement, brainstem proximity). Radiation therapy and possibly chemotherapy have a role in management of residual or recurrent disease. Open or endoscopic approaches are well-described, and often multiple procedures are required to gain local control. The average survival is 54% at age 5 years, and worse prognosis is seen in patients younger than 5 years old.[24,68]

Variable Location

Fibrous dysplasia

Fibrous dysplasia is a bone growth abnormality where normal bone is replaced by fibroosseous, often expansile tissue.[69] Skull base involvement with fibrous dysplasia can impinge on neurovascular structures, leading to neuropathy and functional loss, notably optic nerve compression and visual loss (**Fig. 8**).[70] Observation is recommended in the absence of neural compromise. Optic nerve decompression is advisable in cases of acute or progressive visual deterioration.[71] External craniotomy approaches

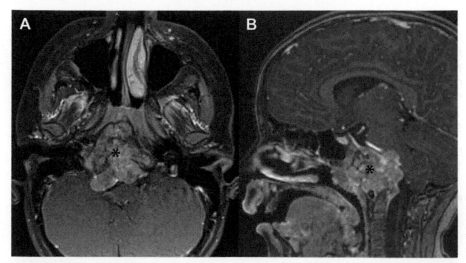

Fig. 7. Axial (*A*) and sagittal (*B*) post contrast T1 MRI views. A 10-year-old girl demonstrating a clival chordoma (*asterisk*) extending posteriorly to the prepontine and premedullary cisterns.

for optic nerve decompression are well-described and still relevant. EEAs and management of skull base fibrous dysplasia are also documented.[72]

Considerations with malignant lesions

Malignant tumors of the pediatric skull base are rare but may include rhabdomyosarcoma or nonrhabdosarcomas. The role of the skull base surgeon in these cases is variable, ranging from biopsy to guide chemotherapy and radiation (rhabdomyosarcoma); resection or debulking to downstage the lesion in preparation for chemotherapy or radiation therapy or both; surgery to relieve symptoms; and rarely, total resection for some nonrhabdosarcomas of appropriate size and location. It is critical to define the goals of treatment before surgery in these cases.

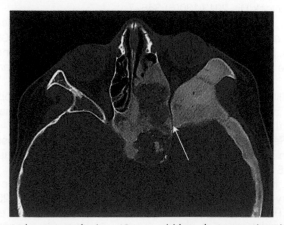

Fig. 8. Axial computed tomography in a 12-year-old boy demonstrating sinonasal and skull base fibrous dysplasia causing severe left optic canal stenosis (*white arrow*).

SUMMARY

Endoscopic endonasal surgery of the skull base continues to grow and develop as new technologies and techniques are introduced. More frequently, these techniques are being applied to pediatric patients for a variety of skull base conditions and pathologies. With appropriate surgeon experience and current technology, EEAs have been shown to be safe and feasible in all but the youngest of patients.

SUPPLEMENTARY DATA

Supplementary data related to this article can be found online at http://dx.doi.org/10.1016/j.otc.2014.09.007.

REFERENCES

1. Kennedy JD, Haines SJ. Review of skull base surgery approaches: with special reference to pediatric patients. J Neurooncol 1994;20:291–312.
2. Gil Z, Constantini S, Spektor S, et al. Skull base approaches in the pediatric population. Head Neck 2005;27:682–9.
3. Kern EB, Laws ER Jr. The transseptal approach to the pituitary gland. Rhinology 1978;16:59–78.
4. Jankowski R, Auque J, Simon C, et al. Endoscopic pituitary tumor surgery. Laryngoscope 1992;102:198–202.
5. Kassam A, Snyderman CH, Mintz A, et al. Expanded endonasal approach: the rostrocaudal axis. Part I. Crista galli to the sella turcica. Neurosurg Focus 2005; 19:E3.
6. Kassam A, Snyderman CH, Mintz A, et al. Expanded endonasal approach: the rostrocaudal axis. Part II. Posterior clinoids to the foramen magnum. Neurosurg Focus 2005;19:E4.
7. Kassam AB, Gardner P, Snyderman C, et al. Expanded endonasal approach: fully endoscopic, completely transnasal approach to the middle third of the clivus, petrous bone, middle cranial fossa, and infratemporal fossa. Neurosurg Focus 2005;19:E6.
8. Gassab E, Krifa N, Kedous S, et al. Endoscopic endonasal management of congenital intranasal meningocele in a 2-month-old infant. Eur Ann Otorhinolaryngol Head Neck Dis 2013;130(6):345–7.
9. Kanaan HA, Gardner PA, Yeaney G, et al. Expanded endoscopic endonasal resection of an olfactory schwannoma. J Neurosurg Pediatr 2008;2:261–5.
10. Kanowitz SJ, Bernstein JM. Pediatric meningoencephaloceles and nasal obstruction: a case for endoscopic repair. Int J Pediatr Otorhinolaryngol 2006;70: 2087–92.
11. Salmasi V, Blitz AM, Ishii M, et al. Expanded endonasal endoscopic approach for resection of a large skull base aneurysmal bone cyst in a pediatric patient with extensive cranial fibrous dysplasia. Childs Nerv Syst 2011;27:649–56.
12. Salmasi V, Reh DD, Blitz AM, et al. Expanded endonasal endoscopic approach for resection of a skull base low-grade smooth muscle neoplasm. Childs Nerv Syst 2012;28:151–8.
13. Chivukula S, Koutourousiou M, Snyderman CH, et al. Endoscopic endonasal skull base surgery in the pediatric population. J Neurosurg Pediatr 2013;11:227–41.
14. Kassam A, Thomas AJ, Snyderman C, et al. Fully endoscopic expanded endonasal approach treating skull base lesions in pediatric patients. J Neurosurg 2007;106:75–86.

15. Locatelli D, Rampa F, Acchiardi I, et al. Endoscopic endonasal approaches to anterior skull base defects in pediatric patients. Childs Nerv Syst 2006;22: 1411–8.
16. Gruber DP, Brockmeyer D. Pediatric skull base surgery. 1. Embryology and developmental anatomy. Pediatr Neurosurg 2003;38:2–8.
17. Sadler TW. Langman's medical embryology. Philadelphia: Lippincott Williams & Wilkins; 2009.
18. Bailey B, editor. Head and neck surgery – otolaryngology. Philadelphia: Lippincott Williams & Wilkins; 2001.
19. Tatreau JR, Patel MR, Shah RN, et al. Anatomical considerations for endoscopic endonasal skull base surgery in pediatric patients. Laryngoscope 2010;120: 1730–7.
20. Rhoton AL Jr. The anterior and middle cranial base. Neurosurgery 2002;51: S273–302.
21. Teo C, Dornhoffer J, Hanna E, et al. Application of skull base techniques to pediatric neurosurgery. Childs Nerv Syst 1999;15:103–9.
22. Borba LA, Al-Mefty O, Mrak RE, et al. Cranial chordomas in children and adolescents. J Neurosurg 1996;84:584–91.
23. Coffin CM, Swanson PE, Wick MR, et al. Chordoma in childhood and adolescence. A clinicopathologic analysis of 12 cases. Arch Pathol Lab Med 1993;117:927–33.
24. Wold LE, Laws ER Jr. Cranial chordomas in children and young adults. J Neurosurg 1983;59:1043–7.
25. Gil Z, Patel SG, Cantu G, et al. Outcome of craniofacial surgery in children and adolescents with malignant tumors involving the skull base: an international collaborative study. Head Neck 2009;31:308–17.
26. Tsai EC, Santoreneos S, Rutka JT. Tumors of the skull base in children: review of tumor types and management strategies. Neurosurg Focus 2002;12:e1.
27. Laws ER Jr. Transsphenoidal microsurgery in the management of craniopharyngioma. J Neurosurg 1980;52:661–6.
28. Snyderman C, Kassam A, Carrau R, et al. Acquisition of surgical skills for endonasal skull base surgery: a training program. Laryngoscope 2007;117:699–705.
29. Kassam AB, Vescan AD, Carrau RL, et al. Expanded endonasal approach: vidian canal as a landmark to the petrous internal carotid artery. J Neurosurg 2008;108: 177–83.
30. Cavallo LM, Messina A, Cappabianca P, et al. Endoscopic endonasal surgery of the midline skull base: anatomical study and clinical considerations. Neurosurg Focus 2005;19:E2.
31. Cavallo LM, Messina A, Gardner P, et al. Extended endoscopic endonasal approach to the pterygopalatine fossa: anatomical study and clinical considerations. Neurosurg Focus 2005;19:E5.
32. Kassam AB, Snyderman C, Gardner P, et al. The expanded endonasal approach: a fully endoscopic transnasal approach and resection of the odontoid process: technical case report. Neurosurgery 2005;57:E213 [discussion: E213].
33. Zanation AM, Snyderman CH, Carrau RL, et al. Endoscopic endonasal surgery for petrous apex lesions. Laryngoscope 2009;119:19–25.
34. Kassam A, Snyderman CH, Carrau RL, et al. Endoneurosurgical hemostasis techniques: lessons learned from 400 cases. Neurosurg Focus 2005;19:E7.
35. Valentine R, Wormald PJ. Carotid artery injury after endonasal surgery. Otolaryngol Clin North Am 2011;44:1059–79.
36. Valentine R, Wormald PJ. Controlling the surgical field during a large endoscopic vascular injury. Laryngoscope 2011;121:562–6.

37. Gardner PA, Tormenti MJ, Pant H, et al. Carotid artery injury during endoscopic endonasal skull base surgery: incidence and outcomes. Neurosurgery 2013; 73:261–9 [discussion: 269–70].
38. Hadad G, Bassagasteguy L, Carrau RL, et al. A novel reconstructive technique after endoscopic expanded endonasal approaches: vascular pedicle nasoseptal flap. Laryngoscope 2006;116:1882–6.
39. Zanation AM, Carrau RL, Snyderman CH, et al. Nasoseptal flap reconstruction of high flow intraoperative cerebral spinal fluid leaks during endoscopic skull base surgery. Am J Rhinol Allergy 2009;23:518–21.
40. Shah RN, Surowitz JB, Patel MR, et al. Endoscopic pedicled nasoseptal flap reconstruction for pediatric skull base defects. Laryngoscope 2009;119:1067–75.
41. Fortes FS, Carrau RL, Snyderman CH, et al. The posterior pedicle inferior turbinate flap: a new vascularized flap for skull base reconstruction. Laryngoscope 2007;117:1329–32.
42. Suh JD, Chiu AG. Sphenopalatine-derived pedicled flaps. Adv Otorhinolaryngol 2013;74:56–63.
43. Patel MR, Shah RN, Snyderman CH, et al. Pericranial flap for endoscopic anterior skull-base reconstruction: clinical outcomes and radioanatomic analysis of preoperative planning. Neurosurgery 2010;66:506–12 [discussion: 512].
44. Patel MR, Taylor RJ, Hackman TG, et al. Beyond the nasoseptal flap: Outcomes and pearls with secondary flaps in endoscopic endonasal skull base reconstruction. Laryngoscope 2013;124(4):846–52.
45. Kim GG, Hang AX, Mitchell CA, et al. Pedicled extranasal flaps in skull base reconstruction. Adv Otorhinolaryngol 2013;74:71–80.
46. Kassam A, Carrau RL, Snyderman CH, et al. Evolution of reconstructive techniques following endoscopic expanded endonasal approaches. Neurosurg Focus 2005;19:E8.
47. Shah MV, Haines SJ. Pediatric skull, skull base, and meningeal tumors. Neurosurg Clin N Am 1992;3:893–924.
48. Zapata S, Kearns DB. Nasal dermoids. Curr Opin Otolaryngol Head Neck Surg 2006;14:406–11.
49. Pinheiro-Neto CD, Snyderman CH, Fernandez-Miranda J, et al. Endoscopic endonasal surgery for nasal dermoids. Otolaryngol Clin North Am 2011;44:981–7, ix.
50. Rahbar R, Shah P, Mulliken JB, et al. The presentation and management of nasal dermoid: a 30-year experience. Arch Otolaryngol Head Neck Surg 2003;129: 464–71.
51. Fornadley JA, Tami TA. The use of magnetic resonance imaging in the diagnosis of the nasal dermal sinus-cyst. Otolaryngol Head Neck Surg 1989;101:397–8.
52. Rohrich RJ, Lowe JB, Schwartz MR. The role of open rhinoplasty in the management of nasal dermoid cysts. Plast Reconstr Surg 1999;104:1459–66 [quiz: 1467; discussion: 1468].
53. Hedlund G. Congenital frontonasal masses: developmental anatomy, malformations, and MR imaging. Pediatr Radiol 2006;36:647–62 [quiz: 726–7].
54. Di Rocco F, Couloigner V, Dastoli P, et al. Treatment of anterior skull base defects by a transnasal endoscopic approach in children. J Neurosurg Pediatr 2010;6: 459–63.
55. Woodworth B, Schlosser RJ. Endoscopic repair of a congenital intranasal encephalocele in a 23 months old infant. Int J Pediatr Otorhinolaryngol 2005;69: 1007–9.
56. Jagannathan J, Dumont AS, Jane JA Jr, et al. Pediatric sellar tumors: diagnostic procedures and management. Neurosurg Focus 2005;18:E6.

57. Locatelli D, Massimi L, Rigante M, et al. Endoscopic endonasal transsphenoidal surgery for sellar tumors in children. Int J Pediatr Otorhinolaryngol 2010;74: 1298–302.

58. Rigante M, Massimi L, Parrilla C, et al. Endoscopic transsphenoidal approach versus microscopic approach in children. Int J Pediatr Otorhinolaryngol 2011; 75:1132–6.

59. Stamm AC, Vellutini E, Balsalobre L. Craniopharyngioma. Otolaryngol Clin North Am 2011;44:937–52, viii.

60. Fernandez-Miranda JC, Gardner PA, Snyderman CH, et al. Craniopharyngioma: a pathologic, clinical, and surgical review. Head Neck 2012;34:1036–44.

61. Gardner PA, Kassam AB, Snyderman CH, et al. Outcomes following endoscopic, expanded endonasal resection of suprasellar craniopharyngiomas: a case series. J Neurosurg 2008;109:6–16.

62. Koutourousiou M, Gardner PA, Fernandez-Miranda JC, et al. Endoscopic endonasal surgery for craniopharyngiomas: surgical outcome in 64 patients. J Neurosurg 2013;119:1194–207.

63. Byun WM, Kim OL, Kim D. MR imaging findings of Rathke's cleft cysts: significance of intracystic nodules. AJNR Am J Neuroradiol 2000;21:485–8.

64. Liu ZF, Wang DH, Sun XC, et al. The site of origin and expansive routes of juvenile nasopharyngeal angiofibroma (JNA). Int J Pediatr Otorhinolaryngol 2011;75: 1088–92.

65. Snyderman CH, Pant H, Carrau RL, et al. A new endoscopic staging system for angiofibromas. Arch Otolaryngol Head Neck Surg 2010;136:588–94.

66. Radkowski D, McGill T, Healy GB, et al. Angiofibroma. Changes in staging and treatment. Arch Otolaryngol Head Neck Surg 1996;122:122–9.

67. Zanation AM, Mitchell CA, Rose AS. Endoscopic skull base techniques for juvenile nasopharyngeal angiofibroma. Otolaryngol Clin North Am 2012;45:711–30, ix.

68. Jian BJ, Bloch OG, Yang I, et al. A comprehensive analysis of intracranial chordoma and survival: a systematic review. Br J Neurosurg 2011;25:446–53.

69. Schreiber A, Villaret AB, Maroldi R, et al. Fibrous dysplasia of the sinonasal tract and adjacent skull base. Curr Opin Otolaryngol Head Neck Surg 2012;20:45–52.

70. Amit M, Fliss DM, Gil Z. Fibrous dysplasia of the sphenoid and skull base. Otolaryngol Clin North Am 2011;44:891–902, vii–viii.

71. Tan YC, Yu CC, Chang CN, et al. Optic nerve compression in craniofacial fibrous dysplasia: the role and indications for decompression. Plast Reconstr Surg 2007; 120:1957–62.

72. Pletcher SD, Metson R. Endoscopic optic nerve decompression for nontraumatic optic neuropathy. Arch Otolaryngol Head Neck Surg 2007;133:780–3.

Pediatric Maxillary and Mandibular Tumors

Samuel J. Trosman, MD, Paul R. Krakovitz, MD*

KEYWORDS

- Maxilla • Mandible • Tumor • Odontogenic cyst • Osteomyelitis • Ameloblastoma
- Langerhans cell histiocytosis • Osteosarcoma

KEY POINTS

- Pediatric masses of the jaw can include both benign and malignant processes of both odontogenic and nonodontogenic origin, as well as infectious processes.
- High-resolution imaging with computed tomography and/or MRI can be suggestive, but often a definitive diagnosis requires tissue for histopathology.
- Treatment is usually surgical and must take into account the growth potential of the facial bones, the aggressiveness of the lesion, and the rate of recurrence.
- The clinical presentation of certain benign jaw lesions may suggest an underlying genetic disorder.

INTRODUCTION

Pediatric maxillary and mandibular tumors encompass a broad range of causes, histopathologies, and clinical behaviors. Although many benign lesions are asymptomatic and are discovered only on a routine dental radiograph, locally aggressive lesions and malignancies can cause pain, facial swelling, and trismus. The work-up is often challenging because many of the tumors have nonspecific radiographic findings; open or excisional biopsy is often necessary for a definitive diagnosis. Treatments range from simple enucleation to a large segmental resection and reconstruction. The clinician must be cognizant of both odontogenic and nonodontogenic processes that can be involved in order to prevent either an unnecessarily aggressive resection with resultant facial deformity or an overly conservative resection that leads to recurrence.

NONODONTOGENIC BENIGN TUMORS
Osteoma

Osteomas are slow-growing benign osteogenic tumors most commonly discovered in late adolescents and young adults. They are composed of well-differentiated lamellar

Head and Neck Institute, Cleveland Clinic Foundation, 9500 Euclid Avenue, Cleveland, OH 44195, USA
* Corresponding author.
E-mail address: krakovp@ccf.org

Otolaryngol Clin N Am 48 (2015) 101–119
http://dx.doi.org/10.1016/j.otc.2014.09.008
0030-6665/15/$ – see front matter © 2015 Elsevier Inc. All rights reserved.

Abbreviations	
BL	Burkitt lymphoma
CGCG	Central giant cell granuloma
CT	Computed tomography
ES	Ewing sarcoma
FD	Fibrous dysplasia
LCH	Langerhans cell histiocytosis
MRI	Magnetic resonance imaging
NBCCS	Nevoid basal cell carcinoma syndrome
OKC	Odontogenic keratocyst
PCO	Primary chronic osteomyelitis
PFD	Polyostotic fibrous dysplasia
PTCH	Patched
XRT	Radiotherapy

or compact bone.[1,2] Although small endosteal (derived from bone marrow) lesions are often asymptomatic, larger lesions can cause a progressive enlargement of the affected area with impingement on adjacent structures. Paranasal sinus osteomas are more common than mandibular osteomas, and most of these arise in the frontal or ethmoid sinuses.[3] Maxillary osteomas are rare, and can remain asymptomatic for long periods of time. Mandibular lesions are commonly found in the posterior body or mandibular condyle, with the latter causing a progressive shift in occlusion.[1] Treatment includes either watchful waiting for smaller or asymptomatic maxillary tumors or conservative surgical excision for symptomatic tumors.

In addition to the differential from more aggressive bone-forming tumors, the discovery of a craniofacial osteoma is significant because of the association with Gardner syndrome, which is a triad consisting of colonic polyps, multiple osteomas, and soft tissue tumors such as epidermoid cysts and desmoid tumors.[4] Gardner syndrome is an autosomal dominant disorder with near 100% penetrance caused by a genetic mutation at chromosome 5. Colonic polyps begin to manifest during puberty and have a high rate of malignant transformation. The onset of multiple osteomas during puberty should alert the clinician to the possibility of Gardner's syndrome.

Osteoblastoma

Osteoblastomas are benign neoplasms of osteoblasts. In the pediatric population they are usually discovered during adolescence. Osteoblastomas often present with pain and swelling that is not relieved with nonsteroidal antiinflammatory drugs. Craniofacial osteoblastomas most commonly involve the medullary bone of the posterior mandible, appearing as radiopaque or radiolucent lesions with patchy areas of mineralization.[1] Most cases are treated successfully by local excision or curettage; however, an aggressive variant of osteoblastoma with irregular histologic features has been described with a recurrence rate of up to 50%.[2]

Fibrous Dysplasia

Fibrous dysplasia (FD) is a nonneoplastic disease caused by the replacement of normal bony architecture by fibrous connective tissue in a loose, whorled pattern intermixed with irregular areas of bony trabeculae.[1,5] It is caused by a sporadic mutation in the GNAS1 gene on chromosome 20, resulting in abnormal osteoblast differentiation and irregular bone formation.[5] The clinical presentation is that of painless, slowly progressive swelling of the involved bones. FD can be divided into monostotic or polyostotic disease.

Monostotic FD accounts for approximately 80% of patients and usually presents during the second decade of life at periods of significant bone growth. Between 10% and 25% of cases involve the head and neck, and the maxilla is involved twice as often as the mandible.[5] Maxillary lesions are often not monostotic and can involve multiple contiguous facial bones; hence the term craniofacial FD. Lesions classically appear as ground-glass calcifications on radiographs and computed tomography (CT) resulting from disorganized bony trabeculae and are often poorly demarcated, blending into surrounding normal bone (**Fig. 1**).

Polyostotic FD (PFD) involves 2 or more bones; about 25% of patients have involvement of more than half of the skeleton.[5] PFD can be seen in patients with multiple café-au-lait spots, termed Jaffe-Lichtenstein syndrome. PFD can also be seen in McCune-Albright syndrome, a combination of PFD, café-au-lait spots, and one of various endocrinopathies. PFD in McCune-Albright syndrome often affects the craniofacial skeleton first, with 90% of lesions present by 3 to 4 years of age.[6,7] Irregular, jagged café-au-lait spots (compared with the smooth, regular spots seen in neurofibromatosis) are often present at or shortly after birth. Endocrinopathies that may be present include precocious puberty (most common), hyperthyroidism, phosphate wasting, and growth hormone and prolactin excess.[7]

Treatment of FD depends on the severity of symptoms, the sites of involvement, and the skeletal maturity of the patient. In many cases the disease stabilizes after the child reaches skeletal maturity, thus small lesions without significant functional or aesthetic deformity can be treated with watchful waiting. Medical treatment with bisphosphonates, especially in children with McCune-Albright syndrome, has been shown to improve bone pain associated with FD, although it may not affect the natural progress of the disease.[8] Surgical removal of maxillary and mandibular disease can entail radical resection and reconstruction with bone graft or free osteocutaneous flap, or can be delayed by managing malocclusion with orthodontic treatment until facial skeletal maturity is reached with subsequent orthognathic procedures.[9] Radiation is not a recommended treatment of FD.

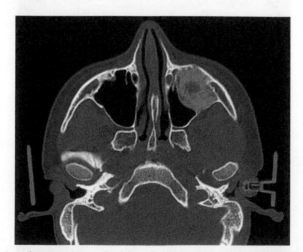

Fig. 1. FD involving the anterior wall of the maxillary sinus. Note the characteristic ground-glass opacity.

Juvenile Ossifying Fibroma

Juvenile ossifying fibromas are fibro-osseous lesions seen most commonly in the craniofacial skeleton in children aged 5 to 15 years.[10] There are 2 histopathologic subtypes:

1. Trabecular, occurring in younger children, with a predilection for the maxilla
2. Psammomatoid, which are more common and often seen in the orbitofrontal bones or paranasal sinuses,[11] although mandibular involvement of both subtypes has been seen

They present as either gradual or rapid painless expansions of the regions involved, with the potential to impinge on vital structures. Unlike the lesions of FD, they are typically well-circumscribed radiolucencies on radiograph and CT with expansion and possible perforation of overlying cortical bone.[11] Like FD, lesions can contain central calcifications, giving both a ground-glass appearance. Although treatment of slower-growing lesions may include conservative excision and/or curettage, a wide resection may be necessary for rapidly growing tumors, especially because they can present similarly to a malignancy.[10] There is also a much higher rate of recurrence than osteomas or FD, ranging from 30% to 60%.[12,13]

Central Giant Cell Granuloma

Central giant cell granulomas (CGCGs), formerly referred to as reparative granulomas, are benign tumors found in children, adolescents, and young adults. About 70% of CGCGs occur in the mandible, with a predilection for anterior portions of bone with possible expansion to the contralateral side.[1,14] Lesions are mostly asymptomatic, although more aggressive variants can present with localized swelling and pain. Radiographic findings are nonspecific because lesions may be unilocular or multilocular and can be confused with periapical cysts, ameloblastomas, and others (**Fig. 2**). Histopathologic examination is crucial for diagnosis, showing multinucleated giant cells in a background of loose cellular stroma containing spindle-shaped

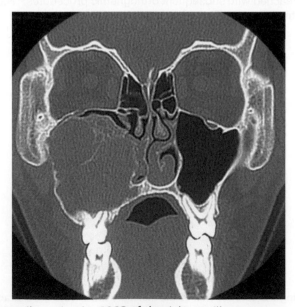

Fig. 2. Large, expansile, unilocular CGCG of the right maxilla.

mesenchymal cells.[1,15] CGCGs are histologically similar to brown tumors, thus hyperparathyroidism should be ruled out once discovered in children. CGCGs have been classified clinically into nonaggressive and aggressive lesions, with the rare aggressive subtype resulting in more rapid growth, pain, paresthesias, and a tendency to recur after surgical curettage.[14]

The treatment of CGCGs has classically been thorough surgical curettage; however, a recurrence rate of 11% to 49% has been reported,[16–20] with higher recurrence rates in aggressive subtypes and in younger patients. Radical resection is an option but can be disfiguring. Alternatives to surgery that have been investigated include calcitonin injections, intralesional steroid injection, and interferon alfa-2a. Intradermal and intranasal salmon calcitonin have been used with moderate success in younger patients when trying to avoid a large resection and in aggressive lesions as an adjunct to curettage.[21–24] Intralesional steroid injections have had a success rate of about 65% in limited cases, although there are few if any randomized controlled trials studying injections.[25] Interferon alfa-2a has recently been used in aggressive lesions to curtail rapid growth and possibly diminish the size of the tumors; however, preliminary evidence suggests that total remission may not be possible without additional surgery.[26]

Cherubism

Cherubism refers to a rare skeletal dysplasia caused by an autosomal dominant mutation in the SH3BP2 gene on chromosome 4. It presents clinically as bilateral cheek swelling caused by symmetric fibro-osseous lesions involving the posterior mandible.[1,27] The disease usually becomes clinically evident between the ages of 2 and 7 years. Lesions can expand to involve the orbital floor, causing characteristic upturned eyes with exposure of the inferior sclera. On radiography the lesions appear as multilocular, expansile radiolucencies that are usually bilateral and symmetric. Most cases of cherubism stabilize by puberty and regress thereafter, thus less severely affected children can be followed with watchful waiting. Lesions causing severe cosmetic deformity or functional compromise can be treated surgically, preferably after puberty during the quiescent phase.

NONODONTOGENIC CYSTS

Nonodontogenic cysts of the maxilla and mandible in children are uncommon compared with their odontogenic counterparts. These lesions are often clinically similar to odontogenic cysts, with the diagnosis only established by histopathologic examination at the time of surgery.

Simple bone cysts, also known as traumatic bone cysts or hemorrhagic bone cysts, are made of cavities within bone without a true epithelial lining. They are generally encountered during adolescence and are rare in children less than 5 years of age.[1] Nearly all cases in the head and neck involve the mandible. They are thought to arise out of trauma that causes intraosseous hemorrhage and resultant pseudocyst formation after reorganization. Surgical exploration for large or symptomatic lesions is warranted. The walls of the cavity are thin and shiny with minimal tissue obtained because of the lack of an epithelial structure. Curettage of the surrounding bone is often necessary to obtain a definitive diagnosis and to rule out more aggressive lesions.[1,28] Recurrences are uncommon.

Aneurysmal bone cysts are rare benign lesions consisting of intraosseous blood-filled spaces separated by fibrous connective tissue septae. The cause is unknown, although trauma may be an inciting event.[29] About 60% of lesions occur during the first 2 decades of life, and 3% of cases involve the head and neck, with most cases involving the mandible.[30] The usual presentation is rapid onset of pain and jaw swelling that may be mistaken for acute osteomyelitis.[29] MRI is helpful for diagnosis, showing characteristic trabeculations separating spaces filled with blood (**Fig. 3**).[29] Treatment of the lesion is surgical. Curettage may be difficult because of the vascularity of the cyst, thus enucleation or en bloc resection may be necessary for larger lesions.

LANGERHANS CELL HISTIOCYTOSIS

Langerhans cell histiocytosis (LCH) refers to a spectrum of diseases characterized by the proliferation of antigen-presenting dendritic histiocytes, or Langerhans cells.[31] More than 60% of cases are diagnosed in children less than 16 years old,[32] with up to 70% of cases involving the head and neck.[31] In children, the skull is the most common site involved, with the frontal bone being the most common bone affected. Only about 10% of cases involve the jaw,[31] which differs from adults in whom the mandible is the most common bone affected.

LCH is most commonly limited to a single organ system, especially in children between 5 and 16 years of age.[33] Previously termed eosinophilic granulomas, lesions present as monostotic or polyostotic radiolucencies that can give teeth a floating-in-air appearance on radiographs because of the underlying bone loss. Children present with jaw swelling, pain, loose teeth, and gingival recession that can often be misdiagnosed as periodontitis.[34]

Multisystem involvement in LCH is more commonly seen in children less than 3 years old.[31] Nearly any organ system can be involved with the characteristic lesions of LCH, including brain, lung, liver, bone marrow, and skin. Between 10% and 20% of patients with systemic involvement develop diabetes insipidus.[33]

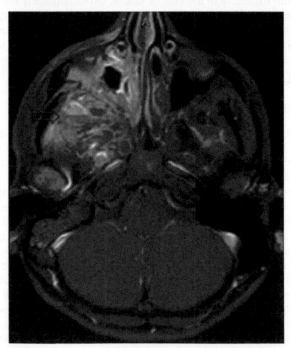

Fig. 3. Large aneurysmal bone cyst originating in the posterior maxilla extending to completely occupy the right masticator space. Note multiple blood-fluid levels (*red arrow*) and septations. A, anterior.

The treatment and prognosis in LCH depends on the extent of disease and sites of involvement. Isolated osseous lesions of the jaw have the best prognosis, with granulomas responding well to curettage or local excision.[31] Intralesional steroid injections have also been shown to be efficacious in some lesions.[35] Children with multisystem involvement require prolonged multiagent chemotherapy.[31]

OSTEOMYELITIS

Osteomyelitis of the craniofacial skeleton most commonly involves the mandible. Most cases are caused by spread of an odontogenic bacterial infection to cortical and cancellous bone. Chronic bacterial osteomyelitis is usually defined as an infection lasting longer than 4 weeks and is characterized by suppuration, sequestration of bone, and/or fistula formation. Imaging often shows sclerosis and periosteal thickening of bone with progressive lucencies over time (**Fig. 4**). Cases lasting longer than 1 month without a clear odontogenic cause are referred to as primary chronic osteomyelitis (PCO), characterized by insidious onset of pain, swelling, and trismus without purulent drainage or cervical lymphadenopathy.[36] Although PCO is characterized by a high recurrence rate after treatment, the clinical course tends toward eventual spontaneous remission.[37,38]

The treatment of bacterial osteomyelitis of the jaw often involves long-term parenteral antibiotics in addition to resection of any necrotic bone. Conservative approaches such as decortication can be attempted for milder cases; however, antibiotic-resistant cases with fistula formation may require marginal or segmental resection.

ODONTOGENIC CYSTS

Odontogenic cysts are common in the pediatric population. Although many odontogenic cysts are asymptomatic and found incidentally on radiographs, they can lead to bone destruction and displacement of teeth.[39] Odontogenic cysts arise from the

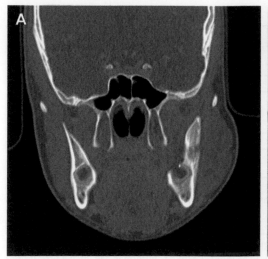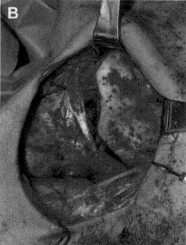

Fig. 4. (*A*) Coronal CT scan of chronic osteomyelitis involving the left mandible, with areas of lucency within the bone and periosteal thickening. (*B*) Intraoperative image of segmental mandibulectomy. The cortical bone has a characteristic moth-eaten appearance.

epithelium associated with tooth development and can occur in both the maxilla and the mandible. Compared with adults, children have a higher proportion of developmental cysts and fewer inflammatory cysts.[40,41] Although typically benign, malignant transformation of various odontogenic cysts has been reported. A summary of the most common clinically benign odontogenic cysts in children is shown in **Table 1**.

Keratocystic Odontogenic Tumors

Although odontogenic keratocysts (OKCs) are still classified as odontogenic cysts, they have been given the name keratocystic odontogenic tumors by the latest World Health Organization classification because of their characteristic histologic features and aggressive clinical behavior. OKC originates from cell rests in the dental lamina of either the maxilla or mandible.[42] They can be found at any age from infancy to adult, but within the pediatric population they most commonly occur during adolescence. The mandible is involved in more than 60% of cases, with a predilection for the posterior body and ascending ramus.[1]

Although small OKCs are usually asymptomatic, they can grow to be extremely large, causing pain, swelling, and drainage (**Fig. 5**). Unlike dentigerous and periapical cysts they tend not to cause obvious bone expansion within the medullary cavity, which can be helpful in making the diagnosis on radiographs; however, this finding is nonspecific. The definitive diagnosis of OKC is based on histopathologic examination, showing a thin fibrous capsule, an epithelial lining 4 to 8 cell layers in thickness, and a palisaded basal cell layer.[42]

Because the diagnosis of OKC is usually not confirmed until the cyst is studied on pathology, the treatment is similar to that of other odontogenic cysts, namely by enucleation and curettage. However, unlike other cysts, the recurrence rate is much higher, with certain studies showing a recurrence rate up to 60%.[43] Although the exact mechanism for recurrence is unknown, proposed mechanisms include incomplete removal of the cyst lining and odontogenic rests left behind after enucleation.[44] Strategies described for reducing recurrence rates include peripheral ossectomy, chemical cauterization of the cavity, and decompression with a drain.[1]

Table 1
Common clinically benign odontogenic cysts

	Dentigerous Cyst	Eruption Cyst	Periapical Cyst
Type of cyst	Developmental	Developmental	Inflammatory
Cause	Crown of an unerupted tooth	Separation of dental follicle during eruption	Dental pulp necrosis assoc. with nonvital tooth
Typical age (y)	>10	<10	All
Location	Third molars, maxillary canines	Incisors, first molars	All
Treatment	Marsupialization or extraction of tooth/ enucleation	None; if tooth does not erupt then simple excision	Root canal or tooth extraction with enucleation/ curettage

Data from Avelar RL, Antunes AA, Carvalho RW, et al. Odontogenic cysts: a clinicopathological study of 507 cases. J Oral Sci 2009;51(4):581–6; Manor E, Kachko L, Puterman MB, et al. Cystic lesions of the jaws - a clinicopathological study of 322 cases and review of the literature. Int J Med Sci 2012;9(1):20–6; and Neville BW, Damm DD, Allen CM, et al, editors. Oral and Maxillofacial Pathology. 3rd edition. St Louis (MO): Saunders Elsevier; 2009. p. 1–984.

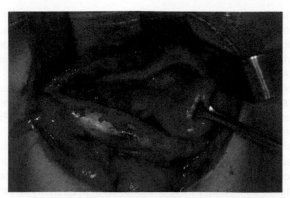

Fig. 5. Resection of a left posterior mandibular odontogenic keratocyst.

If children present with multiple or recurrent OKCs, they should be worked up for nevoid basal cell carcinoma syndrome (NBCCS), or Gorlin syndrome. NBCCS is an autosomal dominant syndrome caused by mutations in the Patched (PTCH) tumor suppressor gene. Although there are many clinical entities that manifest in NBCCS, most patients have multiple basal cell carcinomas. These carcinomas usually appear during puberty or later but have also been described during the first decade of life. OKCs are present in at least 75% of patients, are frequently multiple, and often occur during childhood and adolescence. Other common findings in NBCCS include palmar/plantar pits, calcification of the falx cerebri, enlarged head circumference accompanied by a mild hypertelorism, and rib anomalies.[1]

ODONTOGENIC TUMORS
Odontoma

Odontomas are by far the most common type of odontogenic tumor in children. They are considered to be hamartomatous malformations rather than true neoplasms and thus usually follow a benign course. They can be found in young children but are more typically discovered during adolescence on radiographs obtained for other reasons.

Odontomas consist primarily of enamel and dentin. They can be divided into compound odontomas, made up of collections of small toothlike structures, or complex odontomas, which consist of a calcified mass of enamel and dentin. These subtypes can be differentiated on imaging. When symptomatic, the most common clinical presentation is delayed eruption of permanent teeth and retained primary teeth.[45] Surgical excision is curative.

Ameloblastoma

Ameloblastoma is the most common clinically significant odontogenic tumor in both children and adults. Ameloblastomas arise from odontogenic epithelium, and can theoretically arise from rests of dental lamina, from basal cells of oral mucosa, or from the lining of a preexisting odontogenic cyst.[1] Ameloblastomas are rare before the age of 10 years and nearly all involve only the mandible.[46] There are 3 subtypes: solid/multicystic, unicystic, and peripheral. The peripheral subtype is extremely uncommon in pediatrics.

Solid or multicystic ameloblastomas account for two-thirds of cases in the pediatric population.[46] The typical presentation is painless jaw swelling or slow expansion of the jaw. Multicystic ameloblastomas appear radiographically as multilocular radiolucent lesions with a characteristic soap bubble or honeycomb configuration. Resorption of tooth roots and cortical bone expansion can also be seen. Solid ameloblastomas can be mistaken for a unilocular lesion based on radiographic findings. In one study in children, 57% of solid tumors presented as unilocular cysts on radiograph.[46] Definitive diagnosis is made by histopathologic examination.

Unicystic ameloblastomas account for one-third of pediatric cases. They present similarly to the solid/multicystic subtype, and radiographically appear as a single well-defined lucency that may be mistaken for an odontogenic cyst (**Fig. 6**). Definitive diagnosis requires histologic examination of the cyst.

Treatment of ameloblastoma in children depends on many factors, including the age of the child, the subtype of ameloblastoma, and whether the lesion represents a recurrence. For solid or multicystic tumors, recurrence rates of up to 75% have been found after enucleation and curettage, owing to the tumors' propensity to infiltrate bone.[1,47] Some clinicians advocate an aggressive marginal resection with up to 1 cm past the radiographic margin with a bone graft; however, this must be weighed against the resulting deformity of the jaw and the impact on jaw and lower facial growth. Preoperative incisional biopsy or intraoperative frozen sections can help confirm the diagnosis and subtype.

Unicystic ameloblastomas are thought to be less aggressive and have less risk of recurrence than solid/multicystic ameloblastomas after enucleation and curettage, with recurrence rates ranging from 10% to 25%.[47–50] Many clinicians have advocated a more aggressive approach for mural histologic variant tumors with extension into the fibrous cyst wall, because these lesions are more likely to have residual tumor remaining at the periphery. However, the diagnosis of unicystic ameloblastoma often is not made until histologic examination following enucleation and curettage of a presumed odontogenic cyst. Regardless of approach, close postoperative follow-up is necessary because more than 50% of recurrences occur within 5 years of treatment.[51] Recurrences are typically treated with a more aggressive surgical resection.

Malignant Ameloblastoma

A well-differentiated ameloblastoma can, rarely, give rise to distant metastases that are histologically identical to the primary craniofacial tumor. These tumors are referred to as malignant ameloblastomas. This type is in contrast with ameloblastic carcinoma, which is a disease primarily of middle-aged adults.[52]

Malignant ameloblastoma has been observed in patients aged 4 years and older.[1] About 80% of reported primary tumors originate in the mandible.[53] Metastasis occurs on average 10 to 20 years after the primary is discovered, and usually follows multiple recurrences.[53,54] The lungs are the most common site of metastasis, with 80% of

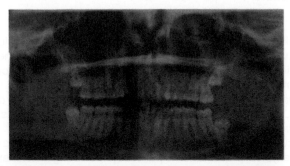

Fig. 6. Panoramic radiograph of a large left mandibular ameloblastoma.

cases showing lung involvement.[53] About 15% of cases have shown metastases to cervical lymph nodes.[54]

The prognosis for malignant ameloblastoma is poor. The primary treatment is surgical excision with adequate margins, including wedge resection of involved lung parenchyma and selective neck dissection for pulmonary and cervical lymph node involvement, respectively. Adjuvant chemotherapy and radiation have resulted in symptomatic improvement but have not shown any survival benefit.[53]

Other Odontogenic Tumors

Less common odontogenic tumors include ameloblastic fibroma, ameloblastic fibro-odontoma, and odontogenic myxoma (**Table 2**).

ODONTOGENIC MALIGNANCIES

Malignant transformation of odontogenic tumors is a rare occurrence. As discussed earlier, malignant ameloblastomas usually come from transformation of their benign counterparts, usually after several recurrences. The incidence is thought to be less than 1%.

Ameloblastic fibrosarcomas arise from ameloblastic fibromas or ameloblastic fibro-odontomas about 50% of the time.[1] They generally occur in adolescents and young adults, with 80% of known cases involving the mandible. In most cases only the mesenchymal portion shows malignant features histologically. They present as mandibular pain and swelling, with more rapid growth than would be expect in an ameloblastic fibroma. A radiolucent singular lesion with ill-defined margins on imaging is suggestive. Although locally aggressive, regional and distant metastases are uncommon. The treatment of choice is wide surgical excision. Postoperative radiation and chemotherapy have been used successfully in cases after incomplete excision.[57]

Table 2
Other odontogenic tumors

	Ameloblastic Fibroma	Ameloblastic Fibro-Odontoma	Odontogenic Myxoma
Tumor origin	Mixed: neoplastic epithelium and mesenchyme	Similar to ameloblastic fibroma, also contains enamel and dentin	Mesenchyme only
Age	Adolescence	Average 10 y	Mostly adolescents or young adults but also occurs during infancy
Site	Posterior mandible	Posterior mandible	Mandible > maxilla; central incisors in infants
Recurrence rate (%)	15–20	<5	5–25
Malignant transformation	Ameloblastic fibrosarcoma (from recurrent ameloblastic fibroma)	Ameloblastic fibrosarcoma (rare)	Rare

Data from Refs.[1,55,56]

NONODONTOGENIC MALIGNANCIES
Osteosarcoma

Osteosarcomas are the most common primary malignant tumors of bone in children.[58] However, involvement of the mandible or maxilla in the pediatric population is rare. The most common symptoms are localized pain and swelling; paresthesias, ocular symptoms, and loosening of teeth are also seen depending on infiltration of the tumor. On radiographs the tumors can appear radiodense or radiolucent with ill-defined borders (**Fig. 7**). Osteophytic bone production on the surface of the lesions can result in a classic sunburst appearance, although this is seen in a minority of lesions.[1]

Survival in children is better in osteosarcoma of the jaw compared with extremity osteosarcoma[58] because of the smaller risk of pulmonary and other distant metastases.[58,59] Several studies have shown that complete surgical resection is the strongest predictor of survival.[60–63] In addition, survival advantages have been shown for patients receiving both neoadjuvant and adjuvant chemotherapy.[64] Neoadjuvant therapy in particular may be an effective option to decrease tumor burden in children with initially unresectable disease. Adjuvant radiation has also been shown to improve local control and survival in patients with positive or uncertain margins[59] and in patients with incompletely resected high-grade tumors when combined with chemotherapy.[58]

Special mention should be made of osteosarcomas arising from bone previously subject to irradiation. Osteosarcoma is the most common postirradiation sarcoma, accounting for 50% of all cases,[1] with an incidence of about 0.03% to 0.8%.[65] The average latent period is about 14 years. The histopathology, appearance, and prognosis of these tumors seem to be similar to those of cases arising de novo.[66]

Rhabdomyosarcoma

Rhabdomyosarcoma is the most common pediatric soft tissue sarcoma involving the head and neck,[67] although it involves the mandible less than 5% of the time.[68] Early diagnosis and treatment are crucial, because rhabdomyosarcomas frequently recur and metastasize. The mainstay of treatment is complete surgical resection if feasible, often with adjuvant chemotherapy and radiation. Combination modality treatment has improved survival rates over the past few decades, with rates of more than 80% being reported in tumors following gross resection compared with less than 10% in older series.[69] However, the use of adjuvant radiation in the pediatric population runs a

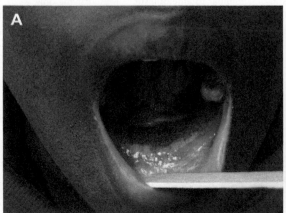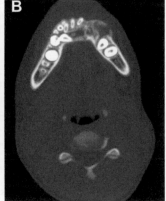

Fig. 7. (A) Osteosarcoma of the mandible resulting in a raised, firm lesion on the mandibular gingiva. (B) Axial CT shows the expansile mass with cortical breakthrough.

significant risk of late effects on vision, hearing, facial growth, and secondary malignancy.[70] Prudent lifelong follow-up should be performed. Some investigators have recommended avoidance of radiation when complete surgical resection can be performed.[70,71]

Ewing Sarcoma

Ewing sarcoma (ES) is the second most common primary malignant tumor of bone in childhood and adolescence.[72] Like osteosarcoma, ES occurs most commonly in long bones, with only 1% to 2% of cases involving the jaw or other craniofacial bones.[1] There is a predilection for the mandibular ramus, with very few documented cases involving the maxilla.[73] It presents as pain and localized swelling, commonly penetrating the bony cortex and resulting in a soft tissue mass overlying the mandible. Lesions cause irregular bone destruction with ill-defined margins on radiographs; the classic onion-skin periosteal reaction described in long bones is less commonly seen in the jaw.[1]

Histologic diagnosis of ES may be difficult, because it must be differentiated from other small blue cell tumors such as metastatic neuroblastoma and variants of osteosarcoma and rhabdomyosarcoma. In 85% to 90% of cases, tumor cells show a translocation between chromosomes 11 and 22 [t(11;22)(q24;q12)] which can be detected using fluorescent in situ hybridization or reverse transcriptase polymerase chain reaction.[1,72]

Although the prognosis for children with ES was previously extremely poor, multidisciplinary treatment has increased 5-year survival from 10% to 50% to 70% over the past 20 years.[74,75] Disease that is seemingly local has been shown to be associated with occult micrometastases that are not picked up at the time of primary surgery, thus neoadjuvant chemotherapy is often used even when the disease is resectable.[74] Adjuvant chemotherapy and radiation are also used because tumors tend to be sensitive to treatment.[72]

Burkitt Lymphoma

Although both Hodgkin and non-Hodgkin lymphoma are most typically seen in the head and neck involving cervical lymph nodes, the endemic form of Burkitt lymphoma (BL) characteristically affects the facial skeleton of African children aged from 2 to 9 years.[76] It is most common in eastern Africa, with an estimated incidence of 7.5 per 100,000 children.[76] Boys are affected nearly twice as often as girls. Nearly all cases of endemic BL are associated with Epstein-Barr virus, which is postulated to deregulate the c-MYC proto-oncogene, leading to its chromosomal translocation. Nearly 50% of cases involve the mandible and nearby facial bones, which is in contrast with the sporadic form of BL more commonly seen in the United States, which tends to involve abdominal viscera. Presenting signs include jaw swelling that eventually leads to increasing pain and loose teeth with associated cervical lymphadenopathy.[77] Treatment with multiagent chemotherapy has greatly increased survival rates.[78]

Metastatic Tumors to the Maxilla and Mandible

Metastatic disease of the jaw occurs much more frequently in adult cancers (eg, breast, lung, prostate) than in pediatric malignancies. Sarcomas arising in distant bone or soft tissues that are more common in a younger population rarely metastasize to the jaw compared with the carcinomas discussed earlier. There have been a handful of case reports of Wilms tumor presenting as a metastatic mandibular mass in children less than 5 years of age.[79–81] There have also been about 15 reported cases of neuroblastoma metastatic to the jaw, with nearly all cases involving the mandible. In cases

Table 3 Nonodontogenic malignancies				
	Osteosarcoma	Rhabdomyosarcoma	ES	BL	Metastasis
Neoplastic origin	Osteoid-producing mesenchyme	Muscle	Bone (cell unknown)	Lymphocytes	Variable
Cause	Sporadic, postirradiation	Sporadic	t(11;22) translocation	Epstein-Barr virus	Variable
Location	Alveolar ridge, mandibular ramus/condyle	Orbit, nasal cavity > mandible	Mandibular ramus	Mandible	Mandible
Treatment	Surgery ± neoadjuvant chemotherapy, adjuvant chemotherapy/XRT	Surgery ± chemotherapy/XRT	neoadjuvant chemotherapy, surgery ± adjuvant chemotherapy/XRT	Multiagent chemotherapy	Chemotherapy

Abbreviation: XRT, radiotherapy.

that present as an isolated mandibular mass, a primary location should be sought. Treatment of metastatic disease usually involves systemic chemotherapy.[82,83]

Table 3 summarizes the most common nonodontogenic malignancies of the maxilla and mandible.

SUMMARY

The variable presentations of pediatric maxillary and mandibular tumors can make diagnosis challenging for the clinician. The progression of swelling and the presence of pain are important prognostic factors. Imaging studies, including panoramic radiographs, CT scans, and MRI, are extremely helpful in suggesting a characteristic diagnosis and/or determining the extent of disease. Multidisciplinary involvement and communication is crucial in the diagnosis and treatment of these tumors.

REFERENCES

1. Neville BW, Damm DD, Allen CM, et al, editors. Oral and maxillofacial pathology. 3rd edition. St Louis (MO): Saunders Elsevier; 2009. p. 1–984.
2. White LM, Kandel R. Osteoid-producing tumors of bone. Semin Musculoskelet Radiol 2000;4(1):25–43.
3. Halawi AM, Maley JE, Robinson RA, et al. Craniofacial osteoma: clinical presentation and patterns of growth. Am J Rhinol Allergy 2013;27(2):128–33.
4. Cankaya AB, Erdem MA, Isler SC, et al. Oral and maxillofacial considerations in Gardner's syndrome. Int J Med Sci 2012;9(2):137–41.
5. Menon S, Venkatswamy S, Ramu V, et al. Craniofacial fibrous dysplasia: surgery and literature review. Ann Maxillofac Surg 2013;3(1):66–71.
6. Hart ES, Kelly MH, Brillante B, et al. Onset, progression, and plateau of skeletal lesions in fibrous dysplasia and the relationship to functional outcome. J Bone Miner Res 2007;22(9):1468–74.
7. Dumitrescu CE, Collins MT. McCune-Albright syndrome. Orphanet J Rare Dis 2008;3:12.
8. Glorieux FH, Rauch F. Medical therapy of children with fibrous dysplasia. J Bone Miner Res 2006;21(Suppl 2):P110–3.
9. Fattah A, Khechoyan D, Phillips JH, et al. Paediatric craniofacial fibrous dysplasia: the hospital for sick children experience and treatment philosophy. J Plast Reconstr Aesthet Surg 2013;66(10):1346–55.
10. Rinaggio J, Land M, Cleveland DB. Juvenile ossifying fibroma of the mandible. J Pediatr Surg 2003;38(4):648–50.
11. Tolentino ES, Centurion BS, Tjioe KC, et al. Psammomatoid juvenile ossifying fibroma: an analysis of 2 cases affecting the mandible with review of the literature. Oral Surg Oral Med Oral Pathol Oral Radiol 2012;113(6):e40–5.
12. Johnson LC, Yousefi M, Vinh TN, et al. Juvenile active ossifying fibroma. Its nature, dynamics and origin. Acta Otolaryngol Suppl 1991;488:1–40.
13. Waldron CA. Fibro-osseous lesions of the jaws. J Oral Maxillofac Surg 1993;51(8): 828–35.
14. Triantafillidou K, Venetis G, Karakinaris G, et al. Central giant cell granuloma of the jaws: a clinical study of 17 cases and a review of the literature. Ann Otol Rhinol Laryngol 2011;120(3):167–74.
15. Barnes L, Eveson JW, Reichart P, et al, editors. Pathology and genetics of head and neck tumours. WHO classification of tumours, vol. 9. Lyon (France): IARC Press; 2005.

16. Bataineh AB, Al-Khateeb T, Rawashdeh MA. The surgical treatment of central giant cell granuloma of the mandible. J Oral Maxillofac Surg 2002;60:756–61.
17. Whitaker SB, Waldron CA. Central giant cell lesions of the jaws. A clinical, radiologic, and histopathologic study. Oral Surg Oral Med Oral Pathol 1993;75:199–208.
18. De Lange J, van den Akker HP. Clinical and radiological features of central giant-cell lesions of the jaw. Oral Surg Oral Med Oral Pathol Oral Radiol Endod 2005; 99:464–70.
19. de Lange J, van den Akker HP, van den Berg H. Central giant cell granuloma of the jaw: a review of the literature with emphasis on therapy options. Oral Surg Oral Med Oral Pathol Oral Radiol Endod 2007;104:603–15.
20. Rawashdeh MA, Bataineh AB, Al-Khateeb T. Long-term clinical and radiological outcomes of surgical management of central giant cell granuloma of the maxilla. Int J Oral Maxillofac Surg 2006;35:60–6.
21. Flanagan AM, Nui B, Tinkler SM, et al. The multinucleate cells in giant cell granulomas of the jaw are osteoclasts. Cancer 1988;62:1139–45.
22. Chambers TJ, Fuller K, McSheehy PM, et al. The effects of calcium regulating hormones on bone resorption by isolated human osteoclastoma cells. J Pathol 1985; 145:297–305.
23. de Lange J, Rosenberg AJ, van den Akker HP, et al. Treatment of central giant cell granuloma of the jaw with calcitonin. Int J Oral Maxillofac Surg 1999;28:372–6.
24. Romero M, Romance A, Garcia-Recuero JI, et al. Orthopedic and orthodontic treatment in central giant cell granuloma treated with calcitonin. Cleft Palate Craniofac J 2011;48(5):519–25.
25. Marx RE, Stern DS. Oral and maxillofacial pathology, a rationale for diagnosis and treatment. 1st edition. Hanover Park (IL): Quintessence Publishing Company; 2003.
26. De Lange J, van den Akker HP, van den Berg H, et al. Limited regression of central giant cell granuloma by interferon alpha after failed calcitonin therapy: a report of 2 cases. Int J Oral Maxillofac Surg 2006;35(9):865–9.
27. Papadaki ME, Lietman SA, Levine MA, et al. Cherubism: best clinical practice. Orphanet J Rare Dis 2012;7(Suppl 1):S6.
28. Grecchi F, Zollino I, Candotto V, et al. A case report of haemorrhagic-aneurismal bone cyst of the mandible. Dent Res J (Isfahan) 2012;9(Suppl 2):S222–4.
29. Breuer C, Paul H, Zimmermann A, et al. Mandibular aneurysmal bone cyst in a child misdiagnosed as acute osteomyelitis: a case report and a review of the literature. Eur J Pediatr 2010;169(8):1037–40.
30. Motamedi MH, Navi F, Eshkevari PS, et al. Variable presentations of aneurysmal bone cysts of the jaws: 51 cases treated during a 30-year period. J Oral Maxillofac Surg 2008;66(10):2098–103.
31. Cochrane LA, Prince M, Clarke K. Langerhans' cell histiocytosis in the paediatric population: presentation and treatment of head and neck manifestations. J Otolaryngol 2003;32(1):33–7.
32. Malpas JS. Langerhans cell histiocytosis in adults. Hematol Oncol Clin North Am 1998;12(2):259–68.
33. Devaney KO, Putzi MJ, Ferlito A, et al. Head and neck Langerhans cell histiocytosis. Ann Otol Rhinol Laryngol 1997;106(6):526–32.
34. Li Z, Li ZB, Zhang W, et al. Eosinophilic granuloma of the jaws: an analysis of clinical and radiographic presentation. Oral Oncol 2006;42(6):574–80.
35. Putters TF, de Visscher JG, van Veen A, et al. Intralesional infiltration of corticosteroids in the treatment of localized Langerhans cell histiocytosis of the mandible. Int J Oral Maxillofac Surg 2005;34(5):571–5.

36. Theologie-Lygidakis N, Schoinohoriti O, Iatrou I. Surgical management of primary chronic osteomyelitis of the jaws in children: a prospective analysis of five cases and review of the literature. Oral Maxillofac Surg 2011;15(1):41–50.
37. Suei K, Tanimoto K, Miyaushi M, et al. Partial resection of the mandible for the treatment of diffuse sclerosing osteomyelitis: report of four cases. J Oral Maxillofac Surg 1997;55(4):410–5.
38. Bevin CR, Inwards CY, Keller EE. Surgical management of primary chronic osteomyelitis: a long-term retrospective analysis. J Oral Maxillofac Surg 2008;66(10): 2073–85.
39. Daley TD, Wysocki GP, Pringle GA. Relative incidence of odontogenic tumors and oral and jaw cysts in a Canadian population. Oral Surg Oral Med Oral Pathol 1994;77(3):276–80.
40. Manor E, Kachko L, Puterman MB, et al. Cystic lesions of the jaws - a clinicopathological study of 322 cases and review of the literature. Int J Med Sci 2012;9(1):20–6.
41. Avelar RL, Antunes AA, Carvalho RW, et al. Odontogenic cysts: a clinicopathological study of 507 cases. J Oral Sci 2009;51(4):581–6.
42. Nayak MT, Singh A, Singhvi A, et al. Odontogenic keratocyst: what is in the name? J Nat Sci Biol Med 2013;4(2):282–5.
43. Li TJ. The odontogenic keratocyst: a cyst, or a cystic neoplasm? J Dent Res 2011;90(2):133–42.
44. Brannon RB. The odontogenic keratocyst. A clinicopathologic study of 312 cases. Part II. Histologic features. Oral Surg Oral Med Oral Pathol 1977;43(2):233–55.
45. Kulkarni VK, Vanka A, Shashikiran ND. Compound odontoma associated with an unerupted rotated and dilacerated maxillary central incisor. Contemp Clin Dent 2011;2(3):218–21.
46. Zhang J, Gu Z, Jiang L, et al. Ameloblastoma in children and adolescents. Br J Oral Maxillofac Surg 2010;48(7):549–54.
47. Ord RA, Blanchaert RH, Nikitakis NG, et al. Ameloblastoma in children. J Oral Maxillofac Surg 2002;60(7):762–70.
48. Shteyer A, Lustmann J, Lewin-Epstein J. The mural ameloblastoma: a review of the literature. J Oral Surg 1978;36(11):866–72.
49. Leider AS, Eversole LR, Barkin ME. Cystic ameloblastoma. A clinicopathologic analysis. Oral Surg Oral Med Oral Pathol 1985;60(6):624–30.
50. Robinson L, Martinez MG. Unicystic ameloblastoma: a prognostically distinct entity. Cancer 1977;40(5):2278–85.
51. Huang IY, Lai ST, Chen CH, et al. Surgical management of ameloblastoma in children. Oral Surg Oral Med Oral Pathol Oral Radiol Endod 2007;104(4):478–85.
52. Yoon HJ, Hong SP, Lee JI, et al. Ameloblastic carcinoma: an analysis of 6 cases with review of the literature. Oral Surg Oral Med Oral Pathol Oral Radiol Endod 2009;108(6):904–13.
53. Van dam SD, Unni KK, Keller EE. Metastasizing (malignant) ameloblastoma: review of a unique histopathologic entity and report of Mayo Clinic experience. J Oral Maxillofac Surg 2010;68(12):2962–74.
54. Laughlin EH. Metastasizing ameloblastoma. Cancer 1989;64(3):776–80.
55. Buchner A, Vered M. Ameloblastic fibroma: a stage in the development of a hamartomatous odontoma or a true neoplasm? Critical analysis of 162 previously reported cases plus 10 new cases. Oral Surg Oral Med Oral Pathol Oral Radiol 2013;116(5):598–606.
56. Chen Y, Wang JM, Li TJ. Ameloblastic fibroma: a review of published studies with special reference to its nature and biological behavior. Oral Oncol 2007;43(10): 960–9.

57. Gilani SM, Raza A, Al-Khafaji BM. Ameloblastic fibrosarcoma: a rare malignant odontogenic tumor. Eur Ann Otorhinolaryngol Head Neck Dis 2014;131(1):53–6.
58. Huh WW, Holsinger FC, Levy A, et al. Osteosarcoma of the jaw in children and young adults. Head Neck 2012;34(7):981–4.
59. Guadagnolo BA, Zagars GK, Raymond AK, et al. Osteosarcoma of the jaw/craniofacial region: outcomes after multimodality treatment. Cancer 2009; 115(14):3262–70.
60. Granados-Garcia M, Luna-Ortiz K, Castillo-Oliva HA, et al. Free osseous and soft tissue surgical margins as prognostic factors in mandibular osteosarcoma. Oral Oncol 2006;42(2):172–6.
61. Patel SG, Meyers P, Huvos AG, et al. Improved outcomes in patients with osteogenic sarcoma of the head and neck. Cancer 2002;95(7):1495–503.
62. Daw NC, Mahmoud HH, Meyer WH, et al. Bone sarcomas of the head and neck in children: the St Jude Children's Research Hospital experience. Cancer 2000; 88(9):2172–80.
63. Jasnau S, Meyer U, Potratz J, et al. Craniofacial osteosarcoma experience of the Cooperative German-Austrian-Swiss Osteosarcoma Study Group. Oral Oncol 2008;44(3):286–94.
64. Smeele LE, Kostense PJ, van der Waal I, et al. Effect of chemotherapy on survival of craniofacial osteosarcoma: a systematic review of 201 patients. J Clin Oncol 1997;15(1):363–7.
65. Mark RJ, Poen J, Tran LM, et al. Postirradiation sarcomas. A single-institution study and review of the literature. Cancer 1994;73(10):2653–62.
66. Mark RJ, Bailet JW, Poen J, et al. Postirradiation sarcoma of the head and neck. Cancer 1993;72(3):887–93.
67. Bras J, Batsakis JG, Luna MA. Rhabdomyosarcoma of the oral soft tissues. Oral Surg Oral Med Oral Pathol 1987;64(5):585–96.
68. Williams TP, Vincent SD. Embryonal rhabdomyosarcoma of the mandible. J Oral Maxillofac Surg 1987;45(5):441–3.
69. Lazzaro B, Schwartz D, Lewis J, et al. Rhabdomyosarcoma involving the oral cavity, mandible, and roots of the third molar: a clinical-pathologic correlation and review of literature. J Oral Maxillofac Surg 1990;48(1):72–7.
70. Yamaguchi S, Nagasawa H, Suzuki T, et al. Sarcomas of the oral and maxillofacial region: a review of 32 cases in 25 years. Clin Oral Investig 2004;8(2):52–5.
71. Rao BN, Santana VM, Fleming ID, et al. Management and prognosis of head and neck sarcomas. Am J Surg 1989;158(4):373–7.
72. Shibasaki M, Iwai T, Maegawa J, et al. Mandibular Ewing sarcoma with chromosomal translocation t(21;22)(q22;q12). J Craniofac Surg 2013;24(4):1469–72.
73. Karimi A, Shirinbak I, Beshkar M, et al. Ewing sarcoma of the jaws. J Craniofac Surg 2011;22(5):1657–60.
74. Gradoni P, Giordano D, Oretti G, et al. The role of surgery in children with head and neck rhabdomyosarcoma and Ewing's sarcoma. Surg Oncol 2010;19(4): e103–9.
75. Whaley JT, Indelicato DJ, Morris CG, et al. Ewing tumors of the head and neck. Am J Clin Oncol 2010;33(4):321–6.
76. Orem J, Mbidde EK, Lambert B, et al. Burkitt's lymphoma in Africa, a review of the epidemiology and etiology. Afr Health Sci 2007;7(3):166–75.
77. Patton LL, McMillan CW, Webster WP. American Burkitt's lymphoma: a 10-year review and case study. Oral Surg Oral Med Oral Pathol 1990;69(3):307–16.
78. Ngoma T, Adde M, Durosinmi M, et al. Treatment of Burkitt lymphoma in equatorial Africa using a simple three-drug combination followed by a salvage regimen

for patients with persistent or recurrent disease. Br J Haematol 2012;158(6): 749–62.

79. Jia J, Chen XM, Sun ZJ, et al. Mandibular metastasis of nephroblastoma: a rare case. Int J Oral Maxillofac Surg 2006;35(12):1160–1.
80. Doykos JD. Wilms' tumor metastiatic to mandible and oral mucosa. Report of a case. Oral Surg Oral Med Oral Pathol 1969;27(2):220–4.
81. Favia GF, Lacaita MG, Laforgia N. Nephroblastoma. A clinical anatomical study of a case with mandibular metastases. Minerva Stomatol 1986;35(4):361–4.
82. Manor E, Kapelushnik J, Joshua BZ, et al. Metastatic neuroblastoma of the mandible: a cytogenetic and molecular genetic study. Eur Arch Otorhinolaryngol 2012;269(8):1967–71.
83. Cohn SL, Pearson AD, London WB, et al. The International Neuroblastoma Risk Group (INRG) classification system: an INRG task force report. J Clin Oncol 2009;27(2):289–97.

Pediatric Teratoma and Dermoid Cysts

Josée Paradis, MD, MSc, FRCSC[a], Peter J. Koltai, MD[b],*

KEYWORDS

- Pediatric • Teratoma • Dermoid cysts • Head & neck

KEY POINTS

- Teratomas and dermoid cysts are germ cell neoplasms that can occur in the cervical and craniofacial regions.
- Presentation of these neoplasms varies in degree of severity, from cosmetic deformities to airway distress requiring emergent intervention.
- Nasal lesions (particularly if suspicious for a nasal dermoid) require imaging before biopsy to assess for intracranial extension.
- Treatment consists of airway management if respiratory distress is present, and early surgical intervention.
- Postoperative follow-up is required to monitor for recurrence.

TERATOMAS

Epidemiology

The word "teratoma" is derived from "teraton," a Greek word meaning "a monster," highlighting what the ancients thought about these maldevelopments.[1] The incidence of teratomas is 1:4000 births.[2] No sex predilection for teratomas in the head and neck region has been observed.[3] The etiology of teratomas is not fully understood; however, they likely occur in part when individual pluripotent cells fail to complete migration and continue dividing in an aberrant location, typically along the midline.[4] Teratomas have been found to occur in isolation or in association with other anomalies. Examples of previously reported comorbidities include central nervous system lesions, Klinefelters, Trisomy 13, Trisomy 21, congenital heart defect, Beckwith-Wiedemann syndrome, and cleft lip and palate.[1]

Disclosures: J. Paradis has nothing to disclose; Acclarent - Scientific advisory board, Medtronic - Royalty agreement (P.J. Koltai).
[a] Department of Otolaryngology, Head & Neck Surgery, Division of Pediatric Otolarynoglogy, University of Western Ontario, 800 Commissioners Road East, London, Ontario N6A 5W9, Canada; [b] Division of Pediatric Otolaryngology, Lucile Packard Children's Hospital, Stanford University School of Medicine, 801 Welch Road, Stanford, CA 94305-5739, USA
* Corresponding author.
E-mail address: koltai@stanford.edu

Otolaryngol Clin N Am 48 (2015) 121–136
http://dx.doi.org/10.1016/j.otc.2014.09.009
0030-6665/15/$ – see front matter © 2015 Elsevier Inc. All rights reserved.

Abbreviations	
AFP	Alpha-fetoprotein
CT	Computed tomography
EXIT	Ex utero intrapartum treatment

Classification

Teratomas are classified by the anatomic location in which they occur. General anatomic classifications include the following:

- Gonadal: teratomas involving testis or ovaries
- Extragonadal: teratomas located in regions such as sacrococcygeal, mediastinal, gastric, retroperitoneal, intracranial, cervical, and craniofacial.[1]

The sacrococcygeal region is the overall most common location. This article focuses on cervical and craniofacial teratomas.

Teratomas in the head and neck region account for approximately 2% to 5% of all germ cell neoplasms, with cervical teratomas being the most common. The incidence of cervical teratomas is estimated to be between 1:20,000 and 1:40,000 live births and are often identified on a prenatal ultrasound.[5] Cervical teratomas may extend into the mediastinum or displace the trachea, causing pulmonary hypoplasia.[1] As a result, there is an increased risk of respiratory-related morbidity and mortality and perinatal fetal interventions, such as an EXIT (ex utero intrapartum treatment) procedure may be required (refer to the article by Walz and Schroeder, elsewhere in this issue for further detail). If untreated, cervical teratomas have an estimated mortality rate of 80% to 100%.

Craniofacial teratomas have occurred in the orbit, pharynx, oropharynx, middle ear, sinonasal tract, and palate. A palatal teratoma is named an epignathus, and is the most common craniofacial teratoma in newborns (**Fig. 1**). These teratomas can present with fetal polyhydramnios due to impaired fetal swallowing and are often identified antenatally. Once identified, an EXIT procedure should be seriously considered. An epignathus is typically attached to the palate via a stalk. After initial resection and establishment of the airway, further imaging is necessary to determine persistence of teratoma within the infratemporal fossa and parapharynx, as demonstrated in **Figs. 1** and **3**.

Histology

Teratomas are composed of all 3 embryonic layers: endoderm, mesoderm, and ectoderm. They are further classified as being either mature or immature. Mature teratomas are the most common histologic type in children and contain only mature elements, such as skin, hair, fat, tissue, cartilage, bone, and glands.[1,6] Immature teratomas contain immature elements, such as neuroepithelial tissue and immature mesenchyme.[7] Microscopic foci of a yolk sac tumor, an immature element, have been found to be a predictor of recurrence after resection.[1] Congenital cervical teratomas have an estimated 5% risk of malignancy, with risk increasing with advanced age of diagnosis.[3,8]

Tumor Markers

Alpha-fetoprotein (AFP) is normally elevated in neonates and decreases in the postnatal period. Persistently high AFP may be suggestive of a teratoma. Additionally,

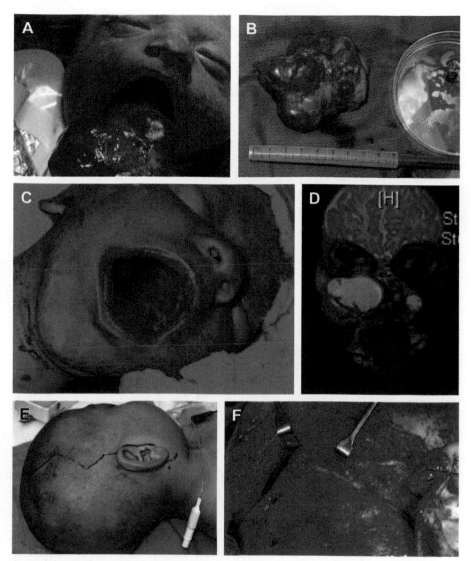

Fig. 1. (*A*) An infant with an epignathus. The teratoma was identified prenatally and an exit procedure was planned. The epignathus was attached to right palate by a small stalk. This was easily excised by removing the stalk's attachment point. The patient was successfully intubated orally post resection. (*B*) Resected epignathus. Stalk is seen on the left side of the specimen. (*C*) Palatal defect post resection of epignathus. (*D*) Two years later, a persistent teratoma was identified in the right infratemporal fossa. (*E*) Approach to the persistent teratoma in right infratemporal fossa. Demarcation of a hemicoronal stealth incision. (*F*) Exposure of zygoma (preplating) with hemicoronal incision. (*G*) Preplating of zygoma before removal. (*H*) Plated zygoma removed allowing access to the infratemporal fossa. (*I*) Elevation of temporalis muscle. (*J*) Exposure of 2 teratomas within the infratemporal fossa, deep to temporalis muscle (as seen retracted). (*K*) Reconstruction. Plated zygoma and temporalis muscle sewn to native position. (*L*) Postoperative MRI demonstrating complete resection of teratoma.

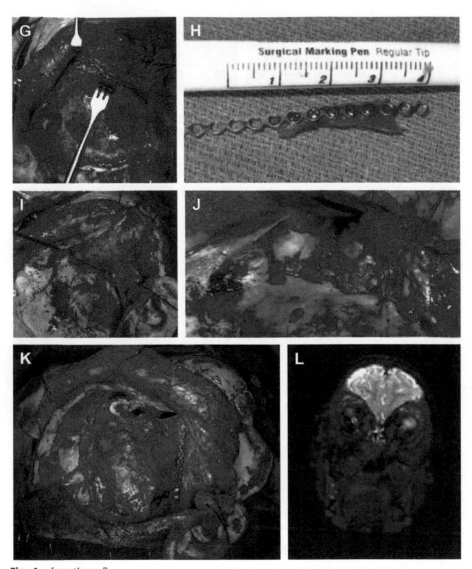

Fig. 1. (*continued*)

postoperative half-life of AFP is 6 days; therefore, AFP can be used to monitor for residual disease or recurrence.[1]

Genetics

There is inconclusive evidence of a genetic link for teratomas. In children, however, deletions on chromosomes 1 and 6 have been observed. In adults, deletions on chromosome 12 have been seen.[1]

Presentation and Diagnosis of Teratomas

Teratomas present in the antenatal, perinatal, or postnatal periods. Polyhydramnios is observed in approximately 0.41% of pregnancies, and when present, is associated with a congenital malformation 20% of the time. Among cervical teratomas, 18% to 20% present with polyhydramnios due to impaired fetal swallowing.[9] Prenatal ultrasounds can aid in the identification of teratomas. If a suspicion of a teratoma arises in the prenatal period, a fetal MRI can provide further information regarding the relationship between the teratoma and the airway, the degree of airway compression, and its proximity to great vessels. Identifying fetal teratomas in the prenatal period provides the opportunity to establish a birthing plan (ie, cesarean delivery vs vaginal birth) as well as any life-saving airway interventions, such as an EXIT procedure (discussed in the article by Walz and Schroeder, elsewhere in this issue). Teratomas diagnosed in the postnatal period typically manifest as a firm mass in any of the regions previously discussed.

Lesions suspicious for a teratoma in the nasal cavity or nasopharynx require imaging, such as a computed tomography (CT) scan or MRI, so as to rule out an encephalocele or intracranial connections before biopsy or surgical resection.[3] **Fig. 2** depicts a nasopharyngeal teratoma extending into oropharynx (**Fig. 2A–B**).

Management of Teratomas

The primary goal in treating infants with teratomas is to minimize respiratory distress in the neonatal period by providing respiratory and airway support when necessary. The secondary goal is early surgical excision, which decreases the risk of sequelae, such as infection leading to sepsis, ulcerations, coagulopathies, and hemodynamic disturbances.[10] **Fig. 3** demonstrates a cervical teratoma, the surgical approach, and post resection defect (**Fig. 3A–G**). Furthermore, early surgical intervention decreases the risk of malignant transformation.[9] Teratomas are generally well-defined lesions; however, they have been observed to infiltrate nearby tissue, requiring resection of local structures.[9] Overall, the surgery risk of mortality is estimated to be as high as 15%.[11]

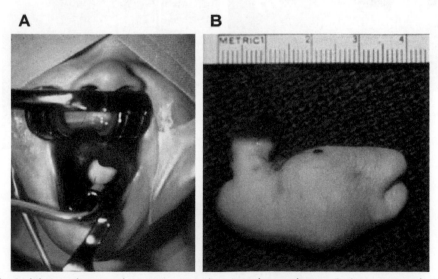

Fig. 2. (*A*) Nasopharyngeal teratoma extending into the oropharynx. Patient presented with respiratory distress at birth. (*B*) Resected nasopharyngeal teratoma. Stalk was attached to the right tonsil. The 2 mounds on the right side of the specimen were protruding in and obstructing the choana.

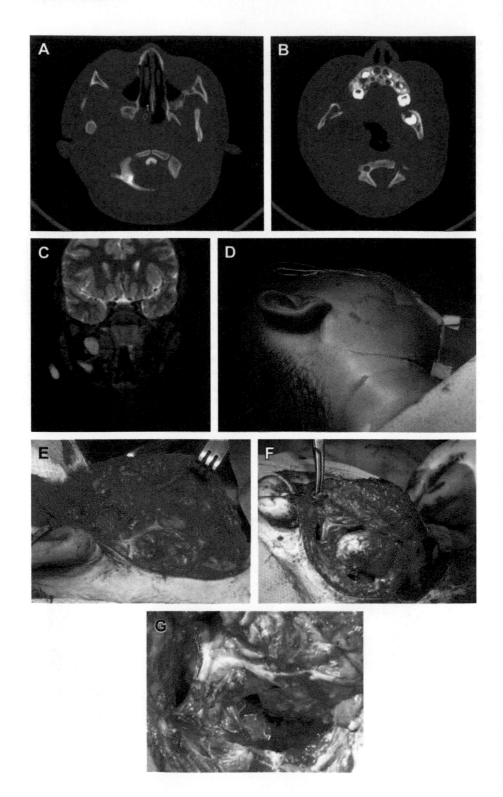

Postoperative Care

Postoperatively, airway support is often required, either from direct airway involvement, or from injuries to airway-related structures, such as injury to the recurrent laryngeal or vagus nerves. Intensive care admission should be arranged. Specific postoperative monitoring is dependent on the extent of surgical resection and the structures and organs involved; for example, neuro vitals, ophthalmologic evaluations, or endocrine monitoring (eg, calcium and/or thyroid function).

Long-term patient follow-up needs to be established to review the final pathology report and to monitor for postoperative complications, healing, recurrence, and malignant transformation.

DERMOID CYSTS
Epidemiology

Dermoid cysts are benign cutaneous tumors. Congenital dermoids are present at birth, but only 40% are noted then. Approximately 70% of dermoid cysts are diagnosed before the age of 5 years.[12] In general, dermoid cysts grow slowly during the first few years of life, and remain relatively unchanged thereafter.[13] Although some investigators report no gender predilection, others report a slight female preponderance.[12,13]

Presentation of Dermoid Cysts

Typically, dermoid cysts present as a firm mass that do not transilluminate or pulsate. Further, they do not change in size with crying or jugular vein compression.

Although dermoid cysts can occur anywhere on the body, they most frequently present in the head and neck region, and most commonly at embryologic fusion lines, such as the lateral third of the eyebrow (**Fig. 4**, **Figs. 5–8**), midline of the neck (**Fig. 9**), or nasolabial fold.[13] Nasal dermoid cysts are the most frequent midline congenital nasal malformation.[14] They can present with a cutaneous pit secreting sebaceous material and may become intermittently infected. A hair protruding from the pit is pathognomonic of a nasal dermoid cyst (**Fig. 10**).

Histology and Pathogenesis

Dermoid cysts are formed by entrapped ectoderm and mesoderm, typically along embryonic fusion planes. They may contain mature skin appendages on their outer wall. Their lumens are lined by stratified squamous epithelium and may be filled with keratin and hair.

Diagnosis of Dermoid Cysts

The workup of a dermoid cyst is dependent on its location. A suspected dermoid cyst on the scalp rarely requires further investigation and can proceed to surgical excision.

◄

Fig. 3. A 4-year-old girl delivered in Mexico with an epignathus. The epignathus was resected. Patient presented with a recurrent teratoma involving the nasopharynx, ipsilateral parapharyngeal space, and ipsilateral cervical neck. (*A*) Axial CT scan. Recurrent teratoma involving the nasopharynx. (*B*) Axial CT. Recurrent teratoma involving the cervical neck extending into ipsilateral parapharyngeal space. (*C*) MRI: coronal view. Recurrent teratoma involving the cervical neck and parapharyngeal space. (*D*) Parotidectomy incision extended into a neck incision within a skin crease. (*E*) Parotidectomy approach. Facial nerve was nicely dissected. (*F*) Cervical teratoma extending into the parapharyngeal space after dissection and mobilization of the facial nerve. (*G*) Postsurgical resection of cervical teratoma.

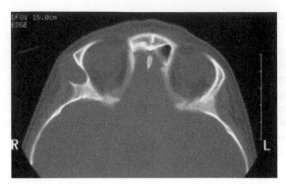

Fig. 4. Axial CT image showing a dermoid involving right lateral and superior orbital rim.

However, a midline dermoid cyst, particularly in the nasal region, requires imaging before surgical intervention to determine dysraphism or intracranial extension. A CT scan will demonstrate bony changes suggestive, but not diagnostic of, intracranial extension, whereas an MRI can determine intracranial involvement.

Complications of Untreated Dermoid Cysts

When left untreated, a dermoid cyst may become infected and drain. An infected dermoid cyst can lead to osteomyelitis, meningitis, and cerebral abscess.[13] Other reported complications include bony erosion, intracranial extension, and eyelid displacement.

Treatment of Dermoid Cysts

Aspiration or biopsy should be avoided when a dermoid cyst is suspected, as they increase the risk of introducing infection, particularly when occurring on the nose. Small dermoid cysts can be observed and do not require immediate surgical excision; however, they are often excised when first noted, or shortly thereafter to avoid complications.

Surgical approaches

Surgical excision is completed with meticulous dissection and inclusion of the capture site and periosteum when it is attached to a bone. The treatment goal is complete excision without disruption of the cyst wall. In the event of cyst wall rupture, all surrounding adjacent tissue should be carefully dissected. It is possible for a cyst to be adherent to vital surrounding tissue, and if so, incomplete excision is acceptable. Close monitoring for recurrence is required in all cases, but in particular for those with incomplete resection. Complications of surgical excision include, but are not limited to, edema, bruising and scarring, and recurrence.

CONGENITAL NASAL DERMOIDS

The prevalence of a congenital midline nasal dermoid cyst is estimated at 1:30,000 live births in the United States, and are more common in Asian individuals (1:6000 live births).[15] Nasal dermoids are the most common congenital midline nasal mass, and make up approximately 10% of all facial dermoids. They typically occur sporadically, and although rare, some familial cases have been reported.

Embryology

Knowledge of the embryology of the nose is necessary to understand the formation of nasal dermoids. During the eighth and ninth weeks of gestation, the nasal and frontal

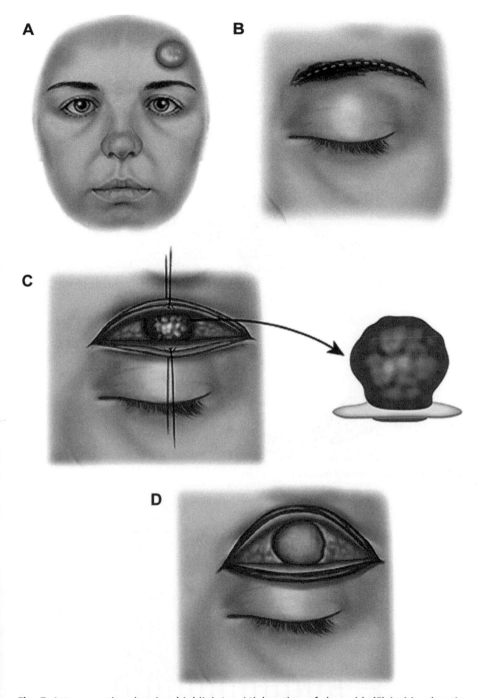

Fig. 5. Intraoperative drawing highlighting (*A*) location of dermoid, (*B*) incision location camouflaged in superior brow line, (*C*) dissection exposing dermoid/excised dermoid including a cuff of periosteum, and (*D*) excision defect.

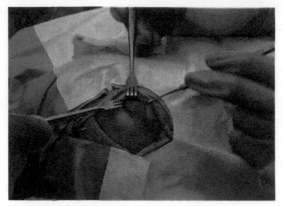

Fig. 6. Dissection exposing the dermoid.

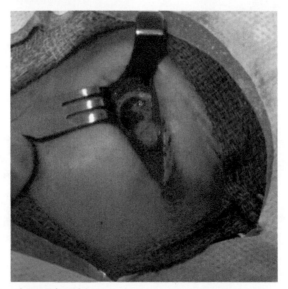

Fig. 7. Defect after dermoid excision.

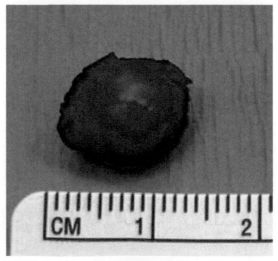

Fig. 8. Excised dermoid including cuff of periosteum.

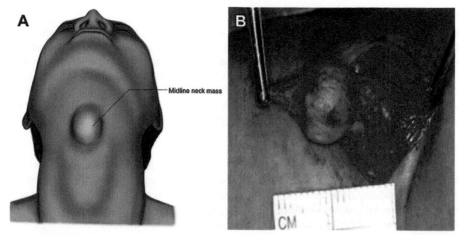

Fig. 9. (*A*) Preoperative drawing of midline neck mass. (*B*) Intraoperative photos of cervical midline dermoid.

bones develop but remain separated by a space called the fonticulus nasofrontalis. Another space is formed between the nasal bones and the deeper cartilaginous capsule called the prenasal space. Once the frontal and nasal bones fuse, the nasofrontalis space is closed and the foramen cecum is formed. Once formed, a projection of the dura diverticulum extends from the foramen cecum to the skin of the tip of the nose. As the prenasal space closes, the dura normally retracts into the cranium and is separated from the skin. The dura then normally obliterates severing the neuroectodermal connection. A congenital nasal dermoid occurs when the process occurs incompletely or aberrantly.

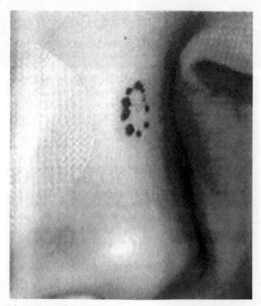

Fig. 10. Nasal dermoid with pathognomonic hair protruding from pit.

Presentation of Congenital Dermoid Cysts

Congenital nasal dermoid cysts can present as a cyst, sinus, or fistula anywhere along the midline from the glabella to columella.[16] A pit with a protruding hair is pathognomonic of a congenital nasal dermoid (see **Fig. 4**). Nasal dermoids can present along the external nose, intranasal deep to nasal bones, or even as a nasopharyngeal mass resulting in airway obstruction. It may extend intracranially, with up to 30% of these communicating with the dura. Dural communication has not been correlated with a particular type of presentation.[15] The nasal root and/or nasal bridge also may be broadened.

Radiology

Imaging is required when a congenital nasal dermoid is suspected. A CT scan is ideal for bony anatomy, and can be useful for image-guided surgery and for determining extent of skull base defects. An enlarged foramen cecum or bifid crista galli is suggestive of intracranial involvement but is not diagnostic (**Fig. 11**A, B). An absent foramen cecum and normal crista galli makes intracranial extension unlikely.

An MRI is optimal for determining soft tissue boundaries and intracranial extension. High-intensity signal on T1-weighted images surrounding the crista galli in a newborn can be suggestive of an intracranial dermoid, as the crista galli in infants are unossified and do not contain marrow fat (see **Fig. 11**C).[17]

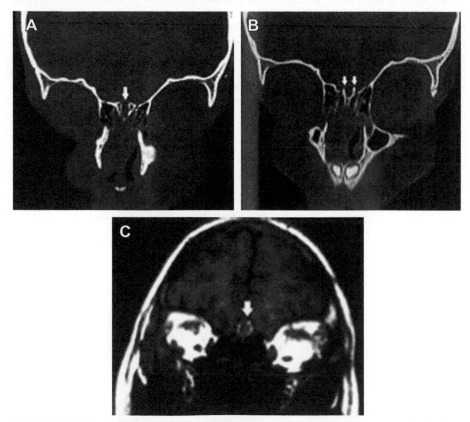

Fig. 11. (*A*) CT image showing widened foreman cecum suggestive of intracranial extension. (*B*) CT image showing bifid crista galli suggestive of intracranial extension. (*C*) MRI T1-weighted image demonstrating an intracranial dermoid.

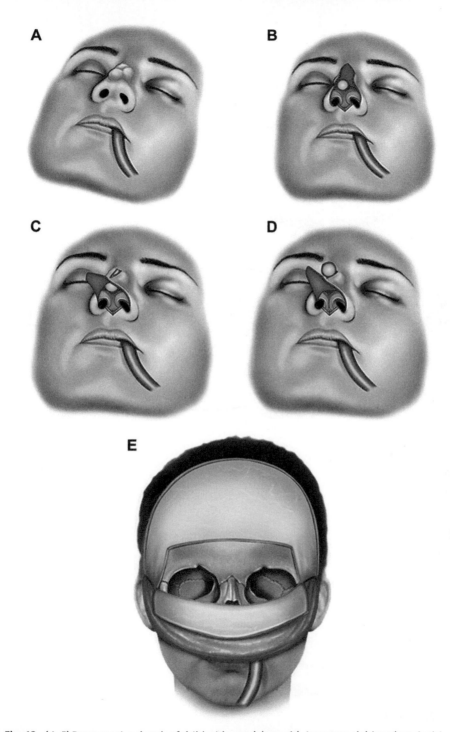

Fig. 12. (*A, B*) Preoperative sketch of child with nasal dermoid. An external rhinoplasty incisions used to approach the nasal dermoid. (*C, D*) Vertical rhinotomy incisions for additional exposure. (*E*) Subcranial approach: Craniofacial exposure with elevation and preservation of pericranial flaps. (*F*) Subcranial approach: Nasal bone removed en block with dermoid and frontal osteotomy performed. (*G, H*) Subcranial approach: Removal of nasal dermoid tract along with frontal table bone. Flaps are replaced and secured with resorbable plates and screws.

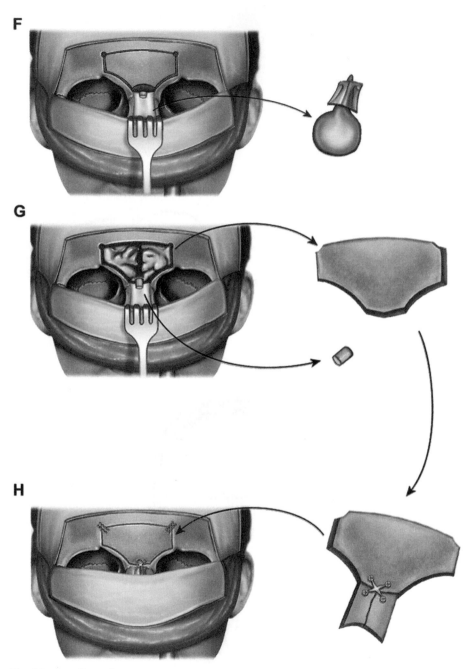

Fig. 12. (*continued*)

Treatment of Congenital Dermoid Cysts

Treatment of a congenital dermoid cyst is a surgical. Collaboration between otolaryngology and neurosurgery is ideal when intracranial extension is present. Surgery can be delayed until age 1 year; however, surgery is recommended sooner if there are signs of complications, such as infection, deformity, rapid growth, or airway obstruction.[15]

Pollock criteria for surgical approach
Pollock[18] established 4 criteria for surgical approach for congenital nasal dermoids.

1. First, the chosen surgical approach should allow for optimal exposure, allowing for the possibility of both medial and lateral osteotomies if necessary.
2. Second, the approach must allow for repair of the cribriform defects and/or repair of a cerebrospinal fluid leak.
3. Third, the approach must facilitate reconstruction of the nasal dorsum if required.
4. Last, the approach should have an acceptable scar and cosmetic outcome. In addition to these criteria, Leung et al proposes a fifth: an approach to consider ease of intracranial access with minimal brain retraction.[15]

Extracranial dermoids and approaches
Excision of an extracranial nasal dermoid most likely requires an external excision. Examples of external incisions include vertical midline rhinotomy, lateral rhinotomy, and external rhinoplasty (**Fig. 12A–B**).[19]

Intracranial dermoids and approaches
Surgical removal of a nasal dermoid with an intracranial extension often necessitates an external incision, as described previously, in combination with a bicoronal incision with subpericranial flap elevation. A craniotomy may be needed for intracranial extension or for large skull base defects. The anterior bifrontal craniotomy has been the standard approach used. A bicoronal incision is made and subpericranial flaps are elevated. A frontal bone flap is created allowing access into the cranium. Frontal lobes are then retracted to access the anterior skull base as the frontal bar is left intact. Complications of this approach include brain edema and injury to the olfactory filament due to brain retraction.

Alternatively, a subcranial approach can be used to eliminate the need for brain retraction. In this approach, the nasal bones are removed en bloc and a limited inferior midline bifrontal craniotomy is performed with osteotomies completed superiorly across the frontal bones, inferiorly across the nasofrontal suture, and posteriorly separating the nasal septum and crista galli (see **Fig. 12C–H**). The subcranial approach provides excellent exposure to the floor of the anterior cranial fossa and has been shown to have minimal effect on long-term facial skeleton growth when used in the pediatric population.[20]

REFERENCES

1. Lakhoo K. Neonatal teratomas. Early Hum Dev 2010;86:643–7.
2. Coppit GL, Perkins JA, Manning S. Nasopharyngeal teratomas and dermoids: a review of the literature and case series. Int J Pediatr Otorhinolaryngol 2000;52: 219–27.
3. Huth ME, Heimgartner S, Schnyder I, et al. Teratoma of the nasal septum in a neonate: an endoscopic approach. J Pediatr Surg 2008;43:2102–5.
4. Woodward P, Sohaey R, Kennedy A, et al. From the archives of the AFIP–a comprehensive review of fetal tumors with pathologic correlation. Radiographics 2005;25:215–42.
5. Rosenfield CR, Coln CD, Duenholter JH. Fetal cervical teratoma as a cause of polyhydramnios. Pediatrics 1979;64:176–9.

6. Wakhlu A, Wakhlu AK. Head and neck teratomas in children. Pediatr Surg Int 2000;16:333–7.
7. Cukurova I, Gumussoy M, Yaz A, et al. A benign teratoma presenting as an obstruction of the nasal cavity: a case report. J Med Case Rep 2012;6:147–51.
8. Byard RW, Jimenez CL, Carpenter BF, et al. Congenital teratomas of the neck and nasopharynx: a clinical and pathological study of 18 cases. J Paediatr Child Health 1990;26:12–6.
9. Shine NP, Sader C, Gollow I, et al. Congenital cervical teratomas: diagnostic, management, and postoperative variability. Auris Nasus Larynx 2006;33:107–11.
10. Rothschild MA, Catalano R, Urken M, et al. Evaluation and management of congenital cervical teratoma. Case report and review. Arch Otolaryngol Head Neck Surg 1994;120(4):444–9.
11. Gundry SR, Wesley JR, Klein MD, et al. Cervical teratomas in the newborn. J Pediatr Surg 1983;18:382–6.
12. Pollard ZF, Harley RD, Calhoun J. Dermoid cysts in children. Pediatrics 1976;57: 379–82.
13. Orozco-Covarrubias L, Lara-Carpio R, Saez-De-Ocariz M, et al. Dermoid cysts: a report of 75 pediatric patients. Pediatr Dermatol 2013;30(6):706–11.
14. Hughes GB, Sharpino G, Hunt W, et al. Management of the congenital midline nasal mass–a review. Head Neck Surg 1980;2:222–33.
15. Leung MK, Krakovitz PR, Kotlai PJ. Chapter 30: congenital sinonasal disorders. In: Kennedy DW, Hwang PH, editors. Rhinology: diseases of the nose, sinuses, skull base. Thieme Medical Publishers, Inc. 333 Seventh Ave. New York, NY 10001.
16. Pensler JM, Bauer B, Naidich TP. Craniofacial dermoids. Plast Reconstr Surg 1988;82(6):953–8.
17. Szeremeta W, Parikh TD, Widelitiz JS. Congenital nasal malformation. Otolaryngol Clin North Am 2007;40:97–112.
18. Pollock RA. Surgical approaches to the nasal dermoid cyst. Ann Plast Surg 1983; 10(6):498–501.
19. Koltai PJ, Hoehn J, Bailey CM. The external rhinoplasty approach for rhinologic surgery in children. Arch Otolaryngol Head Neck Surg 1992;118(4):401–5.
20. Shlomi B, Chaushu S, Gil Z, et al. Effects of the subcranial approach on facial growth and development. Otolaryngol Head Neck Surg 2007;136(1):27–32.

Pediatric Inflammatory Adenopathy

Edward B. Penn Jr, MD*, Steven L. Goudy, MD

KEYWORDS

- Pediatric lymphadenopathy • Cervical lymphadenopathy
- Chronic granulomatous disease • Chédiak-Higashi syndrome • Cat-scratch disease

KEY POINTS

- The differential diagnosis in pediatric lymphadenopathy includes bacterial, viral, fungal, and idiopathic causes.
- A systematic approach to patient evaluation must be used because the differential diagnosis, presentation, and work up must consider infectious, immunologic, neoplastic, and idiopathic disorders.
- A thorough history and physical are vital to determining the diagnosis and ruling out a malignant process.

INTRODUCTION

Pediatric cervical adenopathy is a frequently encountered clinical concern that often presents to an otolaryngologist. A systematic approach to the evaluation of these patients must be used because the differential diagnosis, presentation, and work up must consider infectious, immunologic, neoplastic, and idiopathic disorders (**Fig. 1**). The assessment and diagnosis hinge on a thorough physical examination, the decision for laboratory data, and necessary imaging. A complete history, including recent travel, ethnicity, and other social dynamics, may influence exposure to different pathogens. A detailed history, physical examination, laboratory assessment, and appropriate radiologic examinations can often identify the disease process before the need for surgical intervention.

BACTERIAL

Bacterial Cervical Lymphadenitis

Recent reports have identified an increased incidence of pediatric deep neck infections. The increase in methicillin-resistant *Staphylococcus aureus* (MRSA) has played

Department of Otolaryngology, Monroe Carell Jr Children's Hospital, Vanderbilt University, 2200 Children's Way, DOT 7, Nashville, TN 37232, USA
* Corresponding author.
E-mail address: edward.b.penn@vanderbilt.edu

Otolaryngol Clin N Am 48 (2015) 137–151
http://dx.doi.org/10.1016/j.otc.2014.09.010
0030-6665/15/$ – see front matter © 2015 Elsevier Inc. All rights reserved.

Abbreviations	
CGD	Chronic granulomatous disease
CHS	Chédiak-Higashi syndrome
CSD	Cat-scratch disease
CXR	Chest radiograph
EBV	Epstein-Barr virus
FNA	Fine-needle aspiration
HAART	Highly active antiretroviral therapy
IM	Infectious mononucleosis
MRSA	Methicillin-resistant *Staphylococcus aureus*
NTM	Nontuberculous mycobacteria
PCR	Polymerase chain reaction
PPD	Purified protein derivative
US	Ultrasound

a role in the increasing prevalence of this disease. *S aureus* is cultured from pediatric neck abscesses in up to 60% of the cases; 22% to 29% are MRSA.[1-4] Although reactive lymphadenopathy is commonly in response to upper respiratory illnesses, the duration and severity of these infections is usually short lived.

Clinical presentation

Presentation typically involves neck mass, fever, cervical lymphadenopathy, poor oral intake, and neck stiffness.[5] Coticchia and colleagues[5] found that children younger than 4 years with bacterial cervical lymphadenitis had a higher incidence of agitation, cough, drooling, lethargy, palatal or pharyngeal swelling, respiratory distress, retractions, rhinorrhea, and stridor than children older than 4 years.

Diagnosis

Diagnosis can be made clinically, although is usually supported by imaging that includes ultrasound (US) or CT. Imaging modalities may aid in revealing characteristics

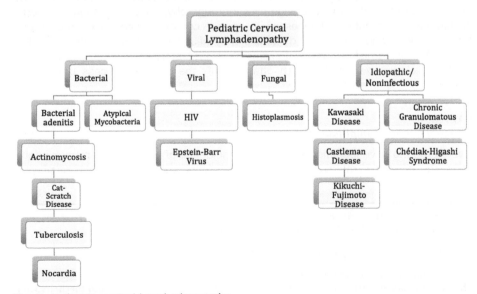

Fig. 1. Pediatric cervical lymphadenopathy.

consistent with an infected congenital anomaly such as a branchial cleft cyst or a thyroglossal duct cyst. Common pathogens include streptococcus and staphylococcus species, which can account for up to 80% of cultures.[2]

Management

Up to 90% to 100% of community-acquired MRSA is sensitive to clindamycin and trimethoprim-sulfamethoxazole. Nosocomial strains of MRSA may have a resistance to these 2 antibiotics at a rate of up to 10% to 20% and is universally resistant to erythromycin.[3] Treatment involves broad-spectrum (with gram-positive and gram-negative coverage) oral or intravenous antibiotics with surgical intervention reserved for those with frank abscess formation seen on imaging or failure of medical management. Increasing antibiotic resistance plays a role in empiric antibiotic therapy because up to 18% of methicillin-sensitive *S aureus* is resistant to clindamycin.[2] Cabrera and colleagues[6] retrospectively reviewed 89 children with head and neck infections and the most common bacteria isolated was group B streptococcus. Age seems to be a determining factor in the bacterial type because children less than age 1 year are more likely to have *S aureus* as the infecting organism.[5]

Infection progression

Often, when these infections progress to suppuration, surgical intervention is required because complications of this this process can include

- Airway obstruction
- Internal jugular vein thrombosis
- Neurologic defects
- Carotid blowout
- Death

Adenitis may spread and seed adjacent deep cervical spaces such as the retropharyngeal space, parapharyngeal space, or submandibular space. The retropharyngeal space lies posterior to the buccopharyngeal fascia and may be synonymous with the prevertebral space. A transoral approach is used for incision and drainage of this area. The parapharyngeal space lies lateral to the buccopharyngeal fascia and medial to the pterygoid muscle and parotid gland and may be approached via a transoral or external transcervical approach. The submandibular space, which runs from the hyoid bone to the mandible, is also approached via an external transcervical approach.

Actinomycosis

Actinomycosis is a progressive granulomatous infection characterized by abscesses, draining sinuses, and fibrosis of tissues.[7,8] The pathogens are fermentative organisms, including *Actinomyces*, *Propionibacterium*, and *Bifidobacterium*.[7,9] Gram-positive, diphtheroid *Actinomyces* species produces most of the infections. The most commonly affected site is the cervicofacial location.[7,8] Many sites may become affected by the infection, including thorax, pelvis, and central nervous system, which can lead to spinal cord compression. Actinomycosis is a fastidious bacteria, evident because it requires enriched culture media at 37°C to grow and must be aided by 6% to 10% ambient carbon dioxide. Growth can be detected between 3 and 21 days. Of note, *Nocardia* and *Actinomyces* are clinically indistinguishable on gram stain although *Nocardia* is aerobic and partially acid-fast.[7] These organisms live as endosaprophytes in dental caries, tonsillar crypts, and in the gingiva with no environmental reservoir.[7,10] Patients presenting with poor dental hygiene along with extensive cervical lymphadenopathy should be evaluated for *Actinomycosis*.[9]

Clinical presentation

Presentation of an *Actinomycosis* infection can occur at any age. In the pediatric population it occurs with dental caries and lymphadenopathy at the angle of the mandible or in the submandibular region. Acutely, this can present as cellulitic change in the overlying skin with edema and pain. The chronic form of the disease can present as chronic inflammation and induration, and progress to multiple abscesses with draining sinus tracts, of which 25% contain sulfur granules.[7] Presentation can include low-grade fever and enlargement of locoregional cervical lymph nodes but can also become more extensive and include osteomyelitis.

Diagnosis

Diagnosis is based on culture results of incisional or excisional biopsy, or fine-needle aspiration (FNA) samples with multiple biopsies at different levels recommended to enhance possibly of diagnosis.[7] CT or MRI can be used to evaluate this area with the common findings of an enhancing soft tissue mass with an low attenuating center with adjacent soft tissue inflammation.[11] An actinomycosis infection in a child indicates the need for evaluation for an underlying immunologic deficiency such as chronic granulomatous disease (CGD).[9]

Management

The treatment choice is penicillin G (50–75 mg/kg/d intravenously in 4 daily divided doses) for 4 to 6 weeks. This may be followed by oral penicillin V (30–60 mg/kg/d administered in 4 divided doses) for 2 to 12 months. Tetracycline can be used for patients who are allergic to penicillin; however, it can cause dental staining. Duration of therapy depends on disease burden, sites of infection, and radiologic and clinical response to therapy. Medical therapy alone may be adequate for treatment but adjuvant surgical debridement may also be indicated.[7,9] Surgical therapy, although not curative alone, is indicated for curettage of bone, resection of necrotic tissue, excision of sinus tracts, and drainage of soft tissue abscesses.[7]

Cat-Scratch Disease

The frequent occurrence of cat-scratch disease (CSD) with associated cervical lymphadenopathy makes this one of the most common causes of infectious cervical lymphadenopathy. The incidence of this in the Unites States is 9.3 per 100,000.[12,13] The pathogen is the gram-negative bacteria *Bartonella henselae*. Kittens are the reservoir for this bacterium. Infections typically involve children and adolescents younger than 18 years old with boys and girls equally affected.[12] After a scratch or bite, the typical presentation usually begins as erythema, papules, or pustules occurring at the scratch line with adenopathy in the affected region 2 to 3 weeks after the incident and may remain up to 6 months in 20% of patients.[12,14]

Clinical presentation

Patients may present with general malaise, headache, and fever; however, the most common clinical manifestations range from painless lymphadenopathy not involving the overlying skin to large cervical abscesses.[12,13,15,16] After upper-extremity adenopathy, head and neck presentation is the second most common site. Cervical and submandibular nodes make up most of the sites affected, followed by preauricular or parotid involvement.[15,17]

Diagnosis

Diagnosis is based on biopsy or serologic testing. Previously, diagnosis was clinical and based on history of contact with a kitten, positive CSD skin test, regional lymphadenopathy in which other causes have been ruled out, and an excisional lymph node biopsy with histopathologic findings of CSD.[12,18] Warthin-Starry silver staining is used to visualize pleomorphic bacilli in the walls of blood vessels and in microabscesses. Bacilli may stain positive by Warthin-Starry staining early in the disease process but is rarely detected later in the disease.[13,14] On excisional biopsy in the early stage of the disease, reactive lymphoid hyperplasia develops, whereas later in the course of the disease granuloma formation and microabscesses may form.[12] Serologic testing consists of IgG and IgM antibodies, with IgM antibodies the most sensitive. If negative, polymerase chain reaction (PCR) detection of *Bartonella* DNA is used on biopsy material.[13] Both granulomas and abscesses may be found in the same specimen. The resultant lymphadenopathy enlarges and may not resolve for 2 or 3 months.[17]

Management
Treatment is usually supportive but definitive diagnosis must be ascertained before observation. Signs of systemic disease, which may be seen in immune-compromised hosts, can include endocarditis, osteolytic lesions, and meningoencephalitis. Systemic symptoms warrant treatment consisting of ciprofloxacin, erythromycin, rifampin, or gentamycin.[13,15]

Nocardia

Nocardia is found in soil around the world and commonly presents as neck adenopathy in immunocompromised individuals; it can be associated with disseminated disease.[9]

Diagnosis
Diagnosis remains difficult unless there is a high level of suspicion for this process as the primary symptom is a painless neck mass. The organism is very slow growing and biopsy must be obtained to obtain tissue for diagnosis. *Nocardia* infections diagnosed in children require further work-up for an underlying immunodeficiency.

Management
The treatment choices for *Nocardia* infections are: trimethoprim-sulfamethoxazole, imipenem, amikacin, and linezolid.[9] Boiron and colleagues[19] reviewed nocardial infections from 1987 to 1990 and determined that recent treatment with corticosteroids represented a significant factor for increased mortality from these infections.

Nontuberculous Mycobacteria

Nontuberculous mycobacteria (NTM) infection also commonly presents with cervical lymphadenopathy in children. These ubiquitous organisms are seen in the soil but can also be found in water, milk, and domestic animals.[20] Organisms that cause NTM typically include *Mycobacterium intracellulare* complex, *M scrofulaceum*, and *M kansasii*.

Clinical presentation
The typical presentation is a painless neck mass seen in an immunocompetent child that has been unresponsive to standard antibiotics.[21] This can be associated with skin discoloration, including erythema or a violaceous discoloration, and, less often, fistula formation.[21] This occurs most often in female patients and children younger than 5 years old.[20,21] These lesions are slow growing but a late complication is fistulization and drainage. Infection commonly involves the submandibular and cervical area and upper cervical area and often presents with parotid involvement (**Figs. 2** and **3**).[21]

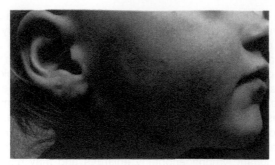

Fig. 2. Atypical mycobacteria infection with associated skin involvement.

Diagnosis

Diagnosis is based on purified protein derivative (PPD) intradermal testing or on cultured tissue and PCR testing for mycobacterial RNA from biopsy (excisional or FNA). Imaging usually involves US, CT, or MRI. Findings on these studies are nonspecific but can consist of solid hypoechoic masses that can appear hypodense on CT.[21] Histopathologic results reveal chronic granulomatous inflammation with areas of caseous necrosis.[21]

Management

Treatment usually involves an oral antibiotic regimen consisting of rifampin and clarithromycin. If this fails, surgical excision or curettage can be used as an alternative approach to reduce the burden of disease. If surgical excision is planned, the technique involves removing that total mass en bloc with any involved skin or adjacent tissue, closing the skin to prevent fistula formation.[21] When adherence to facial nerve is encountered or tissue involvement is extensive, a wait-and-see approach can be considered with adjuvant oral antimycobacterial antibiotics.[21] Recent studies have suggested that observation, with or without antibiotic therapy, often can lead to resolution of 6 months to 1 year.[22] Some investigators have postulated that the depth of cervical disease helps determine outcome, whereas disease deeper to the sternocleidomastoid muscle was more likely to require no intervention and resolve without morbidity.[23]

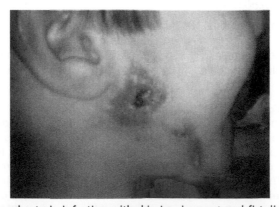

Fig. 3. Atypical mycobacteria infection with skin involvement and fistulization.

Tuberculosis Lymphadenitis

Tuberculosis is a chronic air-borne infectious disease caused by *M tuberculosis*. Nearly 2 billion people are affected by this disease globally.[12] High-risk groups include the immunocompromised, elderly, healthcare workers, and immigrants.

Clinical presentation
Individuals infected typically have pulmonary hilar and cervical lymphadenopathy that is commonly bilateral. This typically indicates hematogenous spread from pulmonary disease. Cervical lymphadenopathy can be part of the primary infection or secondary (organ) tuberculosis.[12] Early-phase lymphadenitis is characterized by a nontender, firm lymph node, which develops caseous necrosis and softens into an abscess.

Diagnosis
Screening for this disease process is based on a positive PPD. Other diagnostic tests may include chest radiograph (CXR) and excisional biopsy or FNA of cervical lymph node with PCR testing. Ziehl-Neelsen staining of obtained tissue occasionally shows short rod-shaped bacteria in the coagulation necrosis.[12] Histology is characterized by central caseous necrosis surrounded by an epithelioid cell layer and sporadic Langerhans giant cells.[12]

Management
Healing occurs with calcification of the affected node. Treatment consists of isolation of a patient with active disease along with a multidrug antitubercular regimen. Incision and drainage of cervical lymphadenopathy should be avoided because there is concern for fistulization.

VIRAL
Human Immunodeficiency Virus

Human immunodeficiency virus (HIV) is transmitted through inoculation of infected body fluid. This retrovirus affects CD4+ cells, is internalized, and results in a decreased number of T-helper cells. Up to 60% to 75% of HIV infected pediatric patients have head and neck manifestations.[24] Secondary to the increased risk of infection, they are prone to otolaryngologic manifestations of this disease, which include[25,26]

- Cervical lymphadenopathy
- Acute otitis media
- Oral candidiasis
- Parotid hypertrophy
- Chronic serous otitis media

Age of patients with head and neck symptom presentation ranges from 2 months to 6 years and 55% of children will develop their first otolaryngologic sign before the age of 3 years and 98% before the age of 9 years.[24,26]

HIV is typically transmitted vertically from mother to child during pregnancy, labor and delivery, and breast-feeding, although the rate of transmission has reduced dramatically due to the use of highly active antiretroviral therapy (HAART).[24] The progression of HIV occurs due to the progressive deterioration of the host's cell-mediated immune system and leads to opportunistic infections.[27] Common bacterial infections during HIV-related immunosuppression include[24]

- *Mycobacterium*
- *Pneumocystis*

- *Cytomegalovirus*
- Epstein-Barr virus (EBV)
- Toxoplasmosis
- CSD

Clinical presentation
Many patients may present with typical head and neck infections that commonly affect children, including sinusitis, otitis media, adenoid hypertrophy, and cervical lymphadenopathy.

Diagnosis
Diagnosis of HIV occurs by antibody detection using ELISA and Western blot, PCR of viral genes, and CD4+ count. Worldwide, there are more than 2 million HIV-positive children with over 90% of the new infections occurring in Sub-Saharan Africa.

Management
Treatment includes identification of underlying disease process and treatment with HAART, which acts on different aspects of the viral cycle.[24]

Epstein-Barr Virus

EBV is commonly associated with Infectious mononucleosis (IM). In industrialized countries and higher socioeconomic groups, half of the population has experienced a primary EBV infection between 1 to 5 years old.[28] The incidence of IM in the United States is 500 per 100,000 per year.[29] Transmission is usually through infected saliva.[28,29] IM is characterized by[28,29]

- Pharyngitis
- Fever
- Fatigue
- Generalized lymphadenopathy
- Cervical lymphadenopathy (one of the most common presenting symptoms)
- Association with splenomegaly in up to 65%

IM as a result of EBV infection has also been associated with palatal petechia, palpebral edema, and a transient and morbilliform skin rash that can be associated with penicillin or beta lactam administration. The pharyngotonsillitis may be exudative. Splenic rupture can occur in 0.5% to 1% and upper airway obstruction can occur due to reactive lymphoid hyperplasia, which is treated with corticosteroids.[29]

Diagnosis
Diagnosis can be achieved via monospot testing to assess the amount of circulating heterophile antibodies (IgM). A positive monospot test has a sensitivity of 85% and a specificity of 94%.[28,29] Testing can be done for antibodies to the virus including: IgM and IgG against viral capsid antigen. IgM appears on presentation of the virus and disappears in 4 to 8 weeks, whereas IgG levels are detected at the time of or shortly after presentation and persist at low levels throughout life.[28] Additional laboratory work may reveal lymphocytosis, atypical lymphocytes on peripheral smear in up to 83.3%, and elevated liver enzymes.[28] Imaging is not commonly needed because diagnosis is usually confirmed by laboratory work up. Imaging may be reserved for assessment of oropharyngeal compromise and to evaluate for a peritonsillar abscess, which in some cases can be bilateral.[30]

Management

Treatment is largely supportive; acetaminophen or nonsteroidal anti-inflammatory medications for fever, odynophagia, and aggressive hydration. Avoidance of exertion is suggested due to the risk of splenic rupture, although bed rest is unnecessary. Recommendations for return to sports or strenuous activity include waiting for a minimum of 3 weeks after the onset of symptoms or until the patient is afebrile, until the clinical symptoms and findings have resolved, or until the patient feels well enough to play.[29,31] Antiviral treatment has been shown to decrease viral shedding in saliva during treatment with rebound after discontinuation, whereas corticosteroid use has not proven effective in treatment or clearing of the virus.[29] The virus has also been implicated in some cases of histiocytic necrotizing lymphadenitis, a self-limiting process characterized by fever and cervical lymphadenopathy.[32]

FUNGAL
Histoplasmosis

Histoplasmosis infection represents a fungal opportunistic infection from the pathogen *Histoplasma capsulatum*. It is caused by inhalation of chicken dropping or bat guano with fungal spores from this organism. This infection is especially prevalent in the Mississippi Valley and northeastern United States because 75% of the population is asymptomatic carriers.[33] This is of particular concern in the elderly and the immunocompromised, as well as the pediatric population. Acute disseminated disease is most commonly found in children and is fatal unless treated quickly. A flu-like syndrome can initially manifest accompanying cervical lymphadenitis. This infection can spread through a hematogenous route that can affect the following sites in decreasing order[33]:

- Tongue
- Palate
- Buccal mucosa
- Larynx

Diagnosis

Evaluation with CXR, CT, and/or MRI often reveals cervical or supraclavicular lymphadenitis with a mediastinal mass (**Fig. 4**).[34] The diagnosis is confirmed by a fungal culture and antigen and antibody detection. Fungal testing of a peripheral blood smear in disseminated disease may also be performed. Hematoxylin-eosin staining reveals a granulomatous process (**Fig. 5**).

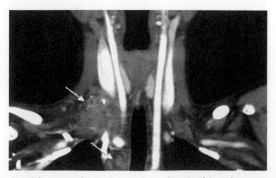

Fig. 4. Histoplasmosis with supraclavicular and mediastinal involvement (*white arrows*).

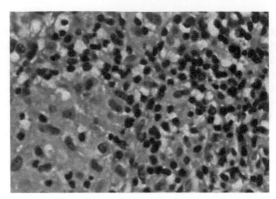

Fig. 5. Histoplasmosis. Hematoxylin-eosin stain of granulomatous inflammation of excised lymph node, 200×.

Management

Treatment consists of the appropriate antifungal, such as azoles or amphotericin B. Gomori methenamine stains reveal intracellular or extracellular yeast forms (**Fig. 6**). Biopsy, debridement, and excision of the cervical disease may aid in diagnosis, whereas antifungal medication is the mainstay to treat the mediastinal disease.

IDIOPATHIC OR NONINFECTIOUS
Chronic Granulomatous Disease

CGD is a primary immunodeficiency disorder, affecting 1 in 1 million individuals, which is characterized by recurrent infections and granuloma formations, usually involving the skin, lungs, and soft tissues, in addition to the reticuloendothelial system.[9,24] This disorder is usually X-linked but can be autosomal recessive and is due to a disorder of NADPH oxidase complex. There is a failure to generate superoxide, hydrogen peroxide, and hypochlorite, which are all crucial in respiratory burst in leukocytes. This results in recurrent bacterial and fungal infections, including recurrent pneumonias and skin and soft tissue infections, including cervical lymphadenopathy.[24] These recurrent infections typically involve catalase positive organisms that can include S *aureus*, *Serratia marcescens*, *Burkholderia cepacia*, *Nocardia* spp, and *Aspergillus*.[9,24]

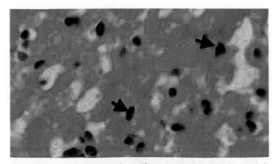

Fig. 6. Histoplasmosis. Gomori methenamine silver stain highlighting the yeast forms, 400× (*black arrows*).

Clinical presentation

Pediatric patients can present with a painless, slowly progressive cervicofacial mass or as an acute, painful, fluctuant cervical mass. Disseminated involvement can include pulmonary, ocular, and skin lesions.[9]

Management

Treatment involves aggressive management with antibiotics and frequently involves surgical incision and drainage. If *Nocardia* is the associated pathogen, treatment consists of aggressive antibiotics as well as surgical intervention and, although controversial, interferon-gamma as prophylaxis against disseminated *Nocardia* infections in children with CGD.[9]

Chédiak-Higashi Syndrome

Chédiak-Higashi syndrome (CHS) is a rare immune deficiency disorder associated with a defect in neutrophil function. About 50% to 85% of patients eventually enter an accelerated phase, manifested by fever, lymphadenopathy, anemia, jaundice, neutropenia, thrombocytopenia, and widespread lymphohistiocytic organ infiltrates.[35] CHS stems from a deficiency in the LYST gene that impairs fusion of intravesicular vesicles and affects chemotaxis, degranulation, and granule-mediated killing of bacteria.[24] Infections are recurrent and are typically from staphylococcus and beta hemolytic streptococci and can affect cervical lymph nodes and cause generalized lymphadenopathy.

Clinical presentation

Patients are clinically characterized by oculocutaneous albinism, photophobia, silver gray hypopigmented hair, and recurrent pyogenic infections, particularly the skin, respiratory tract, and gastrointestinal tract.[36] Symptoms typically develop soon after birth or in children younger than 4 years old.[36] Other clinical manifestations include peripheral neuropathy, platelet defects, and mental retardation.[24]

Diagnosis

Diagnosis of CHS can be confirmed by finding characteristic giant cytoplasmic granules in lymph nodes and in all the granule-containing cells of the body, particularly in white blood cells of the blood and the bone marrow but also on FNA or excisional lymph node biopsy.[35,36] Disease can advance to involvement of the spleen, liver, and bone marrow, and lead to pancytopenia and death, although bone marrow transplantation can be attempted. As many as 80% of patients will die within the first decade of life.[24,36]

Castleman Disease

Castleman disease is a rare lymphoproliferative disorder that commonly occurs in the mediastinum but can occur in the neck, abdomen, and axilla. Presentation is typically a slowly enlarging painless neck mass in a child as young as 2 months and as old as 132 months.[37] The incidence is 1 per 100,000 with a peak incidence in the fourth decade of life. Only 29 cases in pediatric patients have been reported in the literature.[38] The current classification of the disease is based on histology with three subtypes[38,39]:

1. Hyaline vascular type
2. Plasma cell type
3. Mixed type

The most common subtype is hyaline vascular subtype, which is unicentric with a low rate or recurrence after surgical excision.[37–39] Plasma cell type is more commonly multicentric, associated with systemic symptoms, and treatment includes steroids, chemoradiation, or immunotherapy.[37] The most common location for cervical Castleman disease is level V followed by level II or III. US, CT and/or MRI can be used to assess the lesion. CT usually reveals a homogenous mass that is isointense to soft tissue, whereas MRI reveals a hyperintense T2-weighted signal and homogeneous isointense to hyperintense T1-weighted signal.[37] The most common US characteristics include oval or elliptical hypoechogenic hyperemic mass.[37] The role of FNA is limited because it is rarely diagnostic; however, it can rule out lymphoma or other aggressive processes.[38] No specific laboratory abnormalities are specific for this disease.

Diagnosis and management

Diagnosis and treatment is surgical excision and should be completed to rule out other malignancies. The prognosis for pediatric patients is favorable with no other treatment indicated, as opposed to multicentric disease in adults, which has been treated with chemotherapy and radiation.[38,39] No pediatric cases in the literature have had recurrence at a mean follow-up of 31 months.[37]

Kawasaki Disease

Kawasaki disease is an acute systemic inflammatory disease, also known as mucocutaneous lymph node syndrome, due to multisystem vasculitis in small and medium-sized vessels. This disease affects children between 6 months and 5 years of age with a male to female patient ratio of 1.5 to 1, and is the leading cause of acquired pediatric heart disease.[40] The highest incidence is in Asian ethnic groups affecting 17 to 20.8 per 100,000 children younger than 5 years old.

Diagnosis

There is no specific laboratory test to diagnose this disease process and diagnosis remains based on the following clinical criteria:

- Fever for at least 5 days or more
- At least 4 of the following 5 signs: (1) conjunctival injection, (2) edema and erythema of the distal extremities with periungual desquamation of the fingers and toes, (3) erythema of the lips and oral mucosa, (4) strawberry tongue, and (5) oropharyngeal mucosal injection or unilateral cervical lymphadenopathy.[41,42]

The lymphadenopathy occurs in 50% to 60% of patients and, on palpation, is firm and nonfluctuant.[41] In 12% of patients, cervical adenopathy is the initial presenting symptom.[43] Locations commonly include upper and middle jugular; posterior nodes are also involved.[41] On CT, lymphadenopathy appears to be unilateral with perinodal infiltration that has been associated with a retropharyngeal or peritonsillar hypodensity, as well as tonsillar hypertrophy.[44] Lymphadenopathy does not respond to oral antibiotics in the course of this disease.[41] Laboratory tests often find elevated C-reactive protein, platelet count (thrombocytosis), eosinophilia, and erythrocyte sedimentation rate.

Atypical clinical presentations

Atypical presentations of Kawasaki disease in the literature include presentations with a peritonsillar abscess, retropharyngeal abscess, or exudative tonsillitis with cervical lymphadenopathy.[40,42,43,45]

The importance of early diagnosis and treatment is due to the feared cardiac complications that result in a mortality of 2% in affected populations[42] Perivasculitis of the coronary arteries may result in aneurysm formation, obstruction, thrombosis, and myocardial infarctions.[42]

Management

Treatment consists of high-dose aspirin until fever resolves and is used for its anti-inflammatory factors and platelet-inhibiting effect. Intravenous immunoglobulin is used and has been shown to decrease the incidence of coronary aneurysms from 17% to 4 %. Cardiac evaluation, including an ECG and echocardiogram, as well as referral to a pediatric cardiologist, must be made promptly to identify and follow cardiac sequelae. The head and neck symptoms typically are self-limiting and do not require any additional treatment or follow-up.[43]

Kikuchi-Fujimoto Disease

Kikuchi-Fujimoto disease as a disease of unknown cause and is characterized by painful lymphadenopathy, fever, and weight loss that can be mistaken for a malignancy.[46,47] The cause of this disease remains unknown, although cytomegalovirus, human herpes virus 6, and parvovirus B19 are implicated.

Diagnosis

Diagnosis is based on excisional lymph node biopsy and must be performed to rule out malignancy. Pathologic features in biopsied lymph nodes show intensive proliferation of activated lymphocytes mottled by necrotic foci in which polymorphonuclear leukocytes are characteristically absent.[47] Differences separating Kikuchi disease from lymphoma include rapidly enlarging, firm, painful, and mobile lymphadenopathy.[46] In the United States, 13 cases have been reported to date.[46]

Management

Empiric antibiotic therapy has been used to treat most cases of Kikuchi disease with no success. Although treatment of this disease is supportive because symptoms seem to resolve after several months, Feder and colleagues[46] reviewed several case series which revealed up to of 4 of 169 patients with suspected Kikuchi developed systemic lupus erythematosus later in life.

REFERENCES

1. Neff L, Newland JG, Sykes KJ, et al. Microbiology and antimicrobial treatment of pediatric cervical lymphadenitis requiring surgical intervention. Int J Pediatr Otorhinolaryngol 2013;77(5):817–20.
2. Guss J, Kazahaya K. Antibiotic-resistant *Staphylococcus aureus* in community-acquired pediatric neck abscesses. Int J Pediatr Otorhinolaryngol 2007;71(6):943–8.
3. Inman JC, Rowe M, Ghostine M, et al. Pediatric neck abscesses: changing organisms and empiric therapies. Laryngoscope 2008;118(12):2111–4.
4. Novis SJ, Pritchett C, Thorne M, et al. Pediatric deep space neck infections in U.S. children, 2000–2009. Int J Pediatr Otorhinolaryngol 2014;78(5):832–6.
5. Coticchia JM, Getnick G, Yun R, et al. Age-, site-, and time-specific differences in pediatric deep neck abscesses. Arch Otolaryngol Head Neck Surg 2004;130(2): 201–7.
6. Cabrera CE, Deutsch ES, Eppes S, et al. Increased incidence of head and neck abscesses in children. Otolaryngol Head Neck Surg 2007;136(2):176–81.
7. Oostman O, Smego RA. Cervicofacial actinomycosis: diagnosis and management. Curr Infect Dis Rep 2005;7(3):170–4.
8. Hung PC, Wang HS, Chiu CH, et al. Cervical spinal cord compression in a child with cervicofacial actinomycosis. Brain Dev 2014;36(7):634–6.
9. Bassiri-Jahromi S, Doostkam A. Actinomyces and *Nocardia* infections in chronic granulomatous disease. J Glob Infect Dis 2011;3(4):348–52.

10. Kutluhan A, Salviz M, Yalciner G, et al. The role of the *Actinomyces* in obstructive tonsillar hypertrophy and recurrent tonsillitis in pediatric population. Int J Pediatr Otorhinolaryngol 2011;75(3):391–4.
11. Park JK, Lee HK, Ha HK, et al. Cervicofacial actinomycosis: CT and MR imaging findings in seven patients. AJNR Am J Neuroradiol 2003;24(3):331–5.
12. Asano S. Granulomatous lymphadenitis. J Clin Exp Hematop 2012;52(1):1–16.
13. Ridder GJ, Boedeker CC, Technau-Ihling K, et al. Role of cat-scratch disease in lymphadenopathy in the head and neck. Clin Infect Dis 2002;35(6):643–9.
14. McEwan J, Basha S, Rogers S, et al. An unusual presentation of cat-scratch disease. J Laryngol Otol 2001;115(10):826–8.
15. Petrogiannopoulos C, Valla K, Mikelis A, et al. Parotid mass due to cat scratch disease. Int J Clin Pract 2006;60(12):1679–80.
16. Carithers HA. Cat-scratch disease. An overview based on a study of 1,200 patients. Am J Dis Child 1985;139(11):1124–33.
17. Chiu AG, Hecht D, Prendville S, et al. Atypical presentations of cat scratch disease in the head and neck. Otolaryngol Head Neck Surg 2001;125(4):414–6.
18. Bergmans AM, Groothedde JW, Schellekens, et al. Etiology of cat scratch disease: comparison of polymerase chain reaction detection of *Bartonella* (formerly *Rochalimaea*) and *Afipia felis* DNA with serology and skin tests. J Infect Dis 1995; 171(4):916–23.
19. Boiron P, Provost F, Chevrier, et al. Review of nocardial infections in France 1987 to 1990. Eur J Clin Microbiol Infect Dis 1992;11(8):709–14.
20. Luong A, McClay JE, Jafri HS, et al. Antibiotic therapy for nontuberculous mycobacterial cervicofacial lymphadenitis. Laryngoscope 2005;115(10):1746–51.
21. Rahal A, Abela A, Arcand PH, et al. Nontuberculous mycobacterial adenitis of the head and neck in children: experience from a tertiary care pediatric center. Laryngoscope 2001;111(10):1791–6.
22. Amir J. Non-tuberculous mycobacterial lymphadenitis in children: diagnosis and management. Isr Med Assoc J 2010;12(1):49–52.
23. Harris RL, Modayil P, Adam J, et al. Cervicofacial nontuberculous *mycobacterium* lymphadenitis in children: is surgery always necessary? Int J Pediatr Otorhinolaryngol 2009;73(9):1297–301.
24. De Vincentiis GC, Sitzia E, Bottero S, et al. Otolaryngologic manifestations of pediatric immunodeficiency. Int J Pediatr Otorhinolaryngol 2009;73(Suppl 1): S42–8.
25. Chow JH, Stern JC, Kaul A, et al. Head and neck manifestations of the acquired immunodeficiency syndrome in children. Ear Nose Throat J 1990;69(6):416–9, 422–3.
26. Gondim LA, Zonta RF, Fortkamp E, et al. Otorhinolaryngological manifestations in children with human immunodeficiency virus infection. Int J Pediatr Otorhinolaryngol 2000;54(2–3):97–102.
27. Taipale A, Pelkonen, Taipale M, et al. Otorhinolaryngological findings and hearing in HIV-positive and HIV-negative children in a developing country. Eur Arch Otorhinolaryngol 2011;268(10):1527–32.
28. Abdel-Aziz M, El-Hoshy H, Rashed M, et al. *Epstein-Barr* virus infection as a cause of cervical lymphadenopathy in children. Int J Pediatr Otorhinolaryngol 2011;75(4):564–7.
29. Luzuriaga K, Sullivan JL. Infectious mononucleosis. N Engl J Med 2010;362(21): 1993–2000.
30. Alpert G, Fleisher GR. Complications of infection with *Epstein-Barr* virus during childhood: a study of children admitted to the hospital. Pediatr Infect Dis 1984; 3(4):304–7.

31. Putukian M, O'Connor FG, Stricker P, et al. Mononucleosis and athletic participation: an evidence-based subject review. Clin J Sport Med 2008;18(4):309–15.
32. Seo JH, Lee JS, Lee EJ, et al. Comparison of clinical features and EBV expression in histiocytic necrotizing lymphadenitis of children and adults. Int J Pediatr Otorhinolaryngol 2014;78(5):748–52.
33. Pignataro L, Torretta S, Capaccio P, et al. Unusual otolaryngological manifestations of certain systemic bacterial and fungal infections in children. Int J Pediatr Otorhinolaryngol 2009;73(Suppl 1):S33–7.
34. McGraw EP, Kane JM, Kleiman MB, et al. Cervical abscess and mediastinal adenopathy: an unusual presentation of childhood histoplasmosis. Pediatr Radiol 2002;32(12):862–4.
35. Nargund AR, Madhumathi DS, Premalatha CS, et al. Accelerated phase of chediak higashi syndrome mimicking lymphoma–a case report. J Pediatr Hematol Oncol 2010;32(6):e223–6.
36. Patne SC, Kumar S, Bagri NK, et al. Chédiak-higashi syndrome: a case report. Indian J Hematol Blood Transfus 2013;29(2):80–3.
37. Rabinowitz MR, Levi J, Conard K, et al. Castleman disease in the pediatric neck: a literature review. Otolaryngol Head Neck Surg 2013;148(6):1028–36.
38. Zawawi F, Varshney R, Haegert DG, et al. Castleman's Disease: a rare finding in a pediatric neck. Int J Pediatr Otorhinolaryngol 2014;78(2):370–2.
39. Puram SV, Hasserjian RP, Faquin WC, et al. Castleman disease presenting in the neck: report of a case and review of the literature. Am J Otolaryngol 2013;34(3):239–44.
40. Yap CY, Lin LH, Wang NK. An atypical presentation of Kawasaki disease: a 10-year-old boy with acute exudative tonsillitis and bilateral cervical lymphadenitis. Clinics (Sao Paulo) 2012;67(6):689–92.
41. Bayers S, Shulman ST, Paller AS. Kawasaki disease: part I. Diagnosis, clinical features, and pathogenesis. J Am Acad Dermatol 2013;69(4):501.e1–11 [quiz: 511–2].
42. Homicz MR, Carvalho D, Kearns DB, et al. An atypical presentation of Kawasaki disease resembling a retropharyngeal abscess. Int J Pediatr Otorhinolaryngol 2000;54(1):45–9.
43. Yoskovitch A, Tewfik TL, Duffy CM, et al. Head and neck manifestations of Kawasaki disease. Int J Pediatr Otorhinolaryngol 2000;52(2):123–9.
44. Kato H, Kanematsu M, Kato Z, et al. Computed tomographic findings of Kawasaki disease with cervical lymphadenopathy. J Comput Assist Tomogr 2012;36(1):138–42.
45. Langley EW, Kirse DK, Barnes CE, et al. Retropharyngeal edema: an unusual manifestation of Kawasaki disease. J Emerg Med 2010;39(2):181–5.
46. Feder HM Jr, Liu J, Rezuke WN. Kikuchi disease in Connecticut. J Pediatr 2014;164(1):196–200.e1.
47. Fujimori T, Shioda K, Sussman EB, et al. Subacute necrotizing lymphadenitis–a clinicopathologic study. Acta Pathol Jpn 1981;31(5):791–7.

Disorders and Tumors of the Salivary Glands in Children

Paul Lennon, MB BCh, FRCS (ORL HNS)[a], V. Michelle Silvera, MD[b],
Antonio Perez-Atayde, MD[c], Michael J. Cunningham, MD[d],
Reza Rahbar, DMD, MD[d],*

KEYWORDS

- Pediatric ear/nose/throat • Salivary glands • Pediatric tumors head and neck
- Hemangioma

KEY POINTS

- Salivary gland neoplasms are rare in children.
- An asymptomatic swelling in the periauricular region is the most common presenting complaint in older children.
- Approximately 50% of salivary gland lesions are malignant, dictating a thorough diagnostic evaluation by a head and neck surgeon.
- Surgical excision is the primary treatment of lesions.
- Histopathologic findings determine prognosis.

INTRODUCTION

Disorders of the salivary glands can be broadly divided into neoplastic and nonneoplastic disease. Further divisions can be made, as salivary gland lesions are associated with a wide spectrum of etiology (**Table 1**). The age of the patient narrows the potential diagnoses, with vascular lesion often presenting at birth or within the first year of life,[1] whereas solid tumors, with notable exceptions, are more likely to occur in older children.[2,3] Inflammatory disease usually has a relatively rapid onset in contrast to neoplastic or congenital processes, which have more insidious onsets.[4]

[a] Department of Otolaryngology, Head and Neck Surgery, St. James's Hospital, James's Street, Dublin 8, Ireland; [b] Boston Children's Hospital, Department of Radiology 300 Longwood Avenue Main Building, 2nd Floor, Boston, MA 02115, USA; [c] Boston Children's Hospital, Department of Pathology, 300 Longwood Avenue, Bader, 1st Floor, Boston, MA 02115, USA; [d] Boston Children's Hospital, Department of Otolaryngology & Communication Enhancement, 333 Longwood Avenue, 3rd Floor, Boston, MA 02115, USA
* Corresponding author.
E-mail address: Reza.rahbar@childrens.harvard.edu

Otolaryngol Clin N Am 48 (2015) 153–173
http://dx.doi.org/10.1016/j.otc.2014.09.011
0030-6665/15/$ – see front matter © 2015 Elsevier Inc. All rights reserved.

Table 1 Differential diagnosis	
Nonneoplastic lesions	
Congenital/developmental	First branchial arch anomalies
Inflammatory and infection	Acute bacterial sialadenitis Viral: mumps, cytomegalovirus, Coxsackie A or B, or parainfluenza virus Human immunodeficiency virus (HIV)-associated salivary glands Recurrent parotitis in children (RPC)
Granulomatous disease	Mycobacterial disease Actinomycosis Sarcoidosis
Necrotizing sialometaplasia	
Autoimmune	Sjögren syndrome
Cysts	Ranula Mucocele
Neoplastic tumors	
Benign epithelial	Pleomorphic adenoma
Benign mesenchymal	Hemangioma Lymphangioma
Malignant-epithelial	Mucoepidermoid carcinoma Acinic cell carcinoma Adenoid cystic carcinoma Sialoblastoma
Mesenchymal	Rhabdomyosarcoma

Tenderness of the affected area is most often associated with inflammatory disease. Persistent, firm, painless, well-circumscribed lesions should be thoroughly investigated with imaging such as ultrasonography, computed tomography (CT), and MRI, and occasionally with fine-needle aspiration in older children.[5] In a large review of 9993 salivary gland lesions, 430 were in children, accounting for 4.3% of the total.[6] Of the lesions in children, 262 were nonneoplastic and 168 others were considered tumors. This review discusses neoplastic lesions of the salivary glands in children, and malignant epithelial tumors in particular.

NEOPLASTIC TUMORS
Benign Epithelial Tumors

Pleomorphic adenoma
Pleomorphic adenomas (PAs) account for approximately half of all epithelial tumors of the salivary glands and more than 90% of benign salivary gland epithelial tumors.[2,6–20] Composite analysis of several studies reveals that most (62%; range 56%–77%) PAs occur in the parotid gland, with the submandibular gland (26%; range 11%–40%) and the minor salivary glands (12%; range 0%–21%) being less frequent sites of origin.[6,8,9,16,18,21–23] The female to male ratio is approximately 1.4:1.[22] The typical presentation of a PA is a slow-growing, painless, and firm mass with an average duration of symptoms of approximately 12 months.[17,22] On ultrasonography, CT, and MRI, PAs are most commonly well defined. On CT, small calcifications can be seen and on MRI, PAs are typically very bright on T2-weighted images and show homogeneous or heterogeneous enhancement (**Fig. 1**). On gross inspection, PAs are well circumscribed

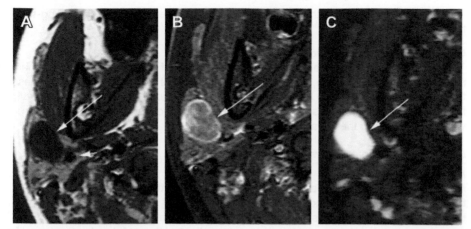

Fig. 1. Parotid pleomorphic adenoma, Imaging. (*A*) The lesion (*long arrow*) is low in signal intensity relative to the parotid gland on this axial T1-weighted image, and is located within the superficial portion of the gland, lateral to the right retromandibular vein (*short arrow*). (*B*) Axial T1-weighted postgadolinium fat-saturation image shows heterogeneous enhancement of the tumor (*arrow*). (*C*) The tumor (*arrow*) is very bright on the axial fast spin-echo inversion recovery (FSEIR) image.

and lobulated with a smooth surface. Classic histologic features include epithelial/myoepithelial cells in a myxochondroid matrix (**Fig. 2**).[24] The relative amounts of cellular and stromal tissue have no bearing on the aggressiveness of the tumor.[25] The preferred treatment of parotid PAs involves superficial parotidectomy or total parotidectomy, depending on lesion location.[22] This approach yields local control rates in excess of 95%.[26] By contrast, the risk of tumor recurrence following lesion enucleation approaches 43%.[27] Although PAs are benign neoplasms, there is potential for malignant transformation. The average incidence of carcinoma ex pleomorphic adenoma is estimated to be 6.2%.[28] The risk of malignant degeneration in an untreated patient seems to be related, in part, to how long the lesion has been present, increasing from approximately 1.5% in the first 5 years to 9.5% for PAs present for longer than 15 years.[29] Carcinomas ex pleomorphic adenoma are rare in children, with only 4 cases identified in the composite review of retrospective series.[15,21,30] Long life expectancy, combined with documented recurrences up to 30 years after

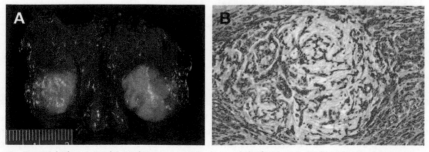

Fig. 2. Parotid Pleomorphic Adenoma, Pathology. (*A*) The irregularly spherical tumor is well demarcated from the surrounding soft tissue and has a white-gray cut surface with mucoid areas. (*B*) Histopathologically the tumor consists of glandular and tubular structures and focally prominent myxoid stroma (Hematoxylin & eosin).

initial resection, increases the recurrence risk in children, with resultant long-term follow-up being mandatory.[24]

Other benign epithelial tumors

The remaining benign epithelial tumors consist mostly of Warthin tumors and others such as lymphoepitheliomas, myoepitheliomas, and basal cell adenomas.[2,15,16] These tumors are exceedingly rare in the pediatric setting, so adult guidelines are generally followed. Treatment involves surgical resection, usually consisting of parotidectomy with preservation of the facial nerve.

Benign Mesenchymal Tumors

Hemangioma

Approximately 30% of hemangiomas are present at birth and the rest arise shortly thereafter.[1] Hemangiomas account for 90% of all salivary tumors in children younger than 1 year.[31] In some series they account for approximately half of all pediatric salivary gland tumors.[9] Hemangiomas undergo a distinct pattern of development, proliferating rapidly during the first 1 to 2 months of life. Often a second growth spurt occurs between 4 and 6 months of age, followed by a slower course of involution, which is generally complete by the first decade of life. With regard to salivary gland hemangiomas, 80% arise in the parotid glands, 18% arise in the submandibular glands, and 2% arise in the minor salivary glands.[32]

Clinical presentation Hemangiomas present as soft, unilateral masses, with or without a bluish discoloration of the skin. Doppler sonography, CT, and MRI can be used to characterize infantile hemangiomas. All imaging modalities show a lobulated, solid, hypervascular mass (**Fig. 3**).[33] Histologically, hemangiomas are unencapsulated aggregates of closely packed, thin-walled capillaries, usually with endothelial lining. Blood-filled vessels are separated by scant connective tissue (**Fig. 4**). Treatment is not required unless the lesion is complicated by ulceration or infection, or causes

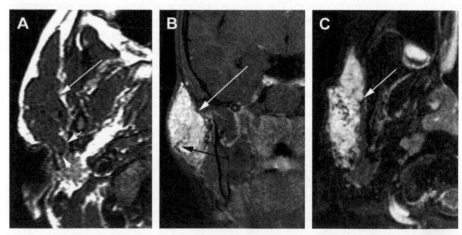

Fig. 3. Parotid hemangioma, Imaging. (*A*) Axial T1-weighted image shows a well-circumscribed, macrolobulated mass (*long arrow*) within the superficial portion of the right parotid gland. Note the sharp demarcation between the tumor and the adjacent unaffected parotid parenchyma (*short arrow*). (*B*) Coronal T1-weighted postgadolinium fat-saturation image shows intense enhancement of the tumor (*white arrow*). Note the small, serpiginous signal voids (*black arrow*) within this lesion representing vessels. (*C*) The axial FSEIR image also shows the mass to be well circumscribed, macrolobulated, and bright in signal (*arrow*).

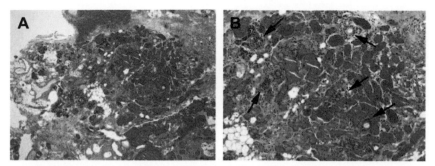

Fig. 4. Parotid Hemangioma, Pathology. (*A*) The parotid gland and surrounding soft tissue are profusely infiltrated by small vascular structures, which are engorged with blood (Hematoxylin & eosin). (*B*) Hemangioma at higher magnification separating glands and ducts of the parotid gland (*arrows*) (Hematoxylin & eosin).

compression of the airway,[33] which occurs more often with segmental hemangiomas.[1] Management choices include sclerotherapy, surgery (parotidectomy), and, more recently, oral propranolol.[34,35]

Lymphatic malformations Lymphatic malformations (LMs) are congenital anomalies of the lymphatic system, 90% of which are detected by age 2 years.[33] LMs often present suddenly as a palpable mass related to intralesional hemorrhage or infection. On MRI, LMs are well circumscribed, multicystic, predominantly bright on T2-weighted images, and often show fluid-fluid levels within the cystic components (**Fig. 5**). Pathologically, LM is a complex of multiple cysts lined with lymphatic vascular endothelium (**Fig. 6**). Unlike hemangiomas of infancy, LMs do not undergo spontaneous regression.[4] Treatment options consist of sclerotherapy with agents such as OK-432, doxycycline, ethanol, or sodium tetradecyl sulfate 3% for macrocystic lesions, surgery, or combinations of both.[36]

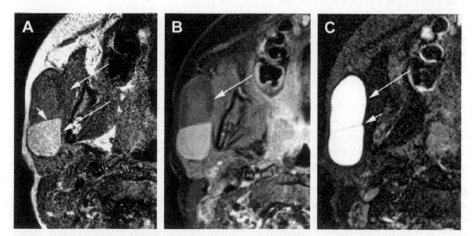

Fig. 5. Parotid lymphatic malformation, Imaging. (*A*) Axial T1-weighted image shows 2 compartments within this cystic lesion (*long arrows*). The posterior cystic component (*short arrow*) is bright, reflecting a higher proteinaceous content than the anterior portion of the lesion. (*B*) Axial T1-weighted postgadolinium fat-saturation image shows no enhancement of the contents or walls of the lesion (*arrow*). (*C*) The lesion is very bright (*long arrow*) on the axial FSEIR image, and an internal septation (*short arrow*) is well visualized.

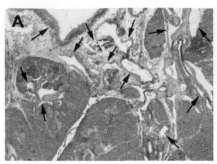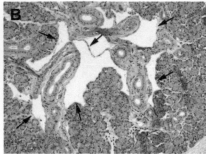

Fig. 6. Parotid Lymphatic Malformation, Pathology. (A) Malformed lymphatic vessels, some with a cystic appearance, are present within the parotid gland and surrounding soft tissue (*arrows*) (Hematoxylin & eosin). (B) The walls of the lymphatic vessels are characteristically thin and are lined by flattened lymphothelium (*arrows*) (Hematoxylin & eosin).

Malignant Epithelial Tumors

Overview

Malignancies of the salivary glands in children and adolescents are exceedingly rare, with an estimated annual incidence of 0.08 per 100,000.[37] Most information on salivary gland neoplasms is derived from retrospective studies conducted at tertiary care oncologic institutions.[2,7–21,30,38–41] Approximately 50% of major salivary gland tumors in children are malignant, which is more than twice the proportion reported in the adult population.[2,12,23] The most common anatomic site for malignant salivary gland tumors in children is the parotid gland.[11] In one large clinical series[23]:

- 82% of 315 pediatric epithelial salivary gland malignancies arose within the parotid gland
- 11% arose within minor salivary glands
- 7% arose within the submandibular gland
- Less than 1% arose within the sublingual gland

Mucoepidermoid carcinoma is by far the most common type of malignant salivary gland tumor in children, accounting for more than 60%. Acinic cell carcinoma (11%) and adenocarcinoma (10%) are also relatively common, whereas adenoid cystic carcinoma (9%), carcinoma ex pleomorphic adenoma (1%) and squamous cell carcinoma (<1%) are comparatively rare.[23]

Epidemiology Most malignant salivary gland tumors occur in older children and adolescents. One epidemiology study reported an average age of 13.4 years at diagnosis.[3] Benign salivary gland neoplasms, on the other hand, present at a slightly older age (15 years on average). There is a near equal distribution of malignant salivary gland tumors between the sexes.[23]

Clinical presentation Most commonly, a salivary gland neoplasm presents as a firm mass. As an estimated 50% of these tumors are malignant, a thorough diagnostic evaluation is critical.[42] The average duration a mass is present before clinical presentation is 8 to 12 months.[2,17,21] Parotid gland tumors are usually asymptomatic; rarely adenoid cystic and acinar cell carcinomas are painful.[19,40] Bimanual palpation of submandibular and sublingual masses may reveal fixation of the mass to surrounding structures. The incidence of facial nerve paresis at presentation approaches 4%.[7,13,14,16,18,39,40] Lymphatic metastases are documented at presentation in 3.5% of children.[2,9,11,39]

Diagnosis of salivary gland tumors Malignant tumors of the minor salivary glands can be challenging to diagnose because of their site-dependent presentation. For example, minor salivary gland malignancies of the hard palate can mimic bone lesions,[43] and those of laryngeal origin may produce airway obstruction, dysphagia, and hoarseness. More than 50% of minor salivary gland malignancies are located within the oral cavity in the pediatric population.[44]

Imaging Ultrasonography is helpful in distinguishing solid from cystic masses in the salivary glands. In addition, this imaging modality is noninvasive, does not use ionizing radiation, and can often be performed without sedation.[45] Once it has been determined that a parotid or submandibular lesion is solid, more detailed assessment with CT or MRI is recommended.[12] Sedation and radiation considerations may dictate which procedure is initially chosen because in younger children, MRI more commonly requires sedation but does not expose the child to radiation. CT is useful in assessing the size of the lesion, identifying tumor calcifications, defining osseous involvement, and demonstrating lymph node metastases.[46] MRI allows for detailed soft-tissue characterization of the tumor and provides important information in regard to tumor margins, the extent of depth of the lesion, and the pattern of tumoral infiltration into the adjacent parenchyma,[47] and may identify perineural spread.[48] Imaging features strongly suggestive of parotid malignancy are poorly defined tumoral margins with infiltration into the parapharyngeal space and surrounding musculature (see **Fig. 1**; **Figs. 7–10**).[49] Fine-needle aspiration cytology is a diagnostic tool that has a reliable sensitivity and specificity in adults.[50] Although its use in children has some advocates,[51] the role of fine-needle aspiration is controversial,[52] and often requires sedation or general anesthesia in younger children.[13] When undertaken, accuracy can be as low as 33%.[39]

Staging pediatric salivary gland malignancies For major salivary gland malignancies, the adult TNM staging system is used.[53] For minor salivary gland malignancies the

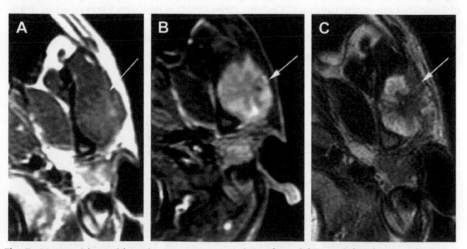

Fig. 7. Mucoepidermoid carcinoma, Imaging. (*A*) On the axial T1-weighted image the lesion (*arrow*) is slightly hyperintense relative to the parotid gland and masticator muscle, and difficult to discern. (*B*) Axial T1-weighted postgadolinium fat-saturation image shows heterogeneous enhancement of the tumor within the superficial portion of the left parotid gland (*arrow*). (*C*) Axial FSEIR image shows the heterogeneous composition of the tumor (*arrow*).

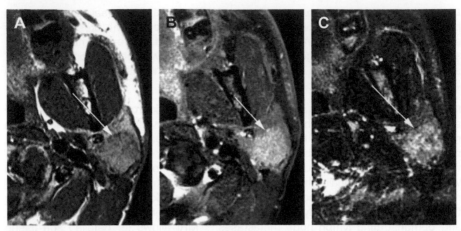

Fig. 8. Acinic cell carcinoma, Imaging. (*A*) The tumor (*arrow*) is hypointense relative to the parotid gland on the axial T1-weighted image. (*B*) Axial T1-weighted postgadolinium fat-saturation image shows relatively homogeneous enhancement of the tumor (*arrow*) with indistinct margins. (*C*) Tumor (*arrow*) is heterogeneous in signal intensity on the axial FSEIR image.

staging system for squamous cell carcinomas, which is tumor-site dependent, is used. Children are often diagnosed at an earlier stage than adults.[37] There is no single grading system for salivary gland cancers. Certain cancers are considered low grade (eg, basal cell adenocarcinoma and acinic cell adenocarcinoma) and others high grade (eg, squamous cell carcinoma and undifferentiated carcinoma).[53] Salivary gland malignancies can also be stratified into low-risk and high-risk tumors, with low-risk tumors being those that do not require treatment beyond excision.[54] The caveat is that high-grade versions of "intrinsically" low-grade tumors exist, as do low-grade versions of typically high-grade tumors.[54] Cellular differentiation has also been used to grade

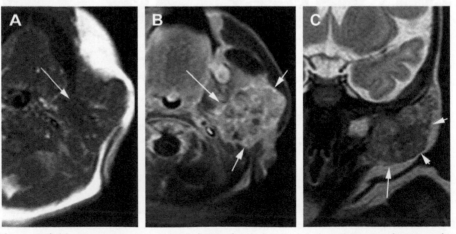

Fig. 9. Sialoblastoma, Imaging. (*A*) The lesion (*arrow*) is slightly hypointense relative to the parotid gland on the axial T1-weighted image. (*B*) Axial T1-weighted postgadolinium fat-saturation image shows heterogeneous enhancement of the tumor (*arrows*). (*C*) Tumor (*arrows*) is relatively hypointense on the coronal T2-weighted image, suggesting a high nucleus to cytoplasmic ratio.

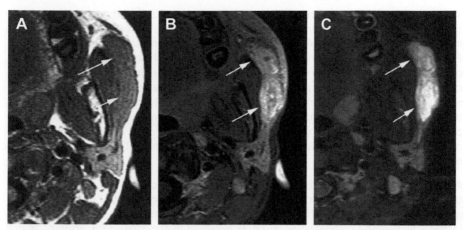

Fig. 10. Rhabdomyosarcoma, Imaging. (*A*) Axial T1-weighted image shows tumor (*arrows*) arising from accessory parotid tissue. (*B*) Axial T1-weighted postgadolinium fat-saturation image shows heterogeneous enhancement of the circumscribed mass (*arrows*). (*C*) Axial FSEIR image shows tumor (*arrows*) to be hyperintense relative to the parotid gland and masseter muscle.

salivary gland malignancies into well differentiated, moderately differentiated, poorly differentiated, undifferentiated, and anaplastic categories. Using this system, a significantly higher percentage of tumors in children (88%) are reported to be well differentiated or moderately differentiated in comparison with adults (49%).[37]

Treatment of pediatric salivary gland neoplasms The treatment of choice for most salivary gland neoplasms is complete removal of tumor with adequate margins.[38] For submandibular tumors, complete excision of the gland is recommended.[55] Parotidectomy is considered a safer and more definitive procedure than tumor enucleation, as the latter results in higher rates of recurrence and facial nerve dysfunction. Total parotidectomy is recommended for tumors with deep lobe involvement, suspected or confirmed high-grade tumors, or tumors with aggressive malignant potential such as those with facial nerve involvement, multiple intraparotid masses, or cervical metastasis.[38,55] Definitive surgery allows for very good local control, with rates approaching 97% in some series.[39,56]

Resection of the facial nerve is currently only recommended when there is gross anatomic or histopathologic evidence of neural invasion at the time of the surgery.[55] When resection of the facial nerve is necessary, immediate reanimation by means of primary anastomosis or free nerve graft is advocated.[57] Indications for neck dissection in adults with malignant salivary gland tumors include tumors larger than 3 cm, high-grade tumors, facial paralysis, extraglandular extension, and perilymphatic invasion.[58] In children, some clinicians recommend simultaneous neck dissection at the time of primary tumor excision only when cervical nodal metastases are clinically detected.[12,15,18,19] The clinical picture in children can be further complicated by lymph node hyperplasia, which is common, particularly in younger children, and may be mistaken for metastatic disease.[55]

Postsurgical paresis/paralysis Permanent facial nerve paresis or paralysis after surgery for benign parotid tumors in adults ranges from 3% to 5%,[59,60] whereas transient facial nerve dysfunction ranges from 46% to 65%.[59,60] These figures are notably higher when tumor enucleation rather than formal parotidectomy is undertaken.[61]

The risk of facial weakness may be greater in children than in adults, with one study reporting 10 of 21 cases having some facial nerve palsy.[18] This risk is also higher in infants than it is in older children and in those undergoing total parotidectomy.[14,62] Frey syndrome is characterized by hyperhidrosis and flushing of the lateral cervicofacial skin. These symptoms are due to abnormal skin innervation by the auriculotemporal nerve, which carries parasympathetic fibers that communicate with the sympathetic nervous system. Formal evaluation via a starch iodine test can reveal the presence of this syndrome in most postparotidectomy patients.[63] In children, reports of Frey syndrome range from 0% to 47%.[13,14,17,19,64] Children are typically managed expectantly.[64] In adults, injection of botulinum toxin type A is the treatment of choice.[63]

Postoperative radiation therapy for salivary gland malignancies Postoperative radiation therapy has been shown to improve local and regional control of salivary gland malignancies in patients of all ages.[65] The principal indications for radiotherapy include: high-grade malignancies, such as adenoid cystic carcinoma, squamous cell carcinoma, carcinoma ex pleomorphic adenoma, and undifferentiated carcinomas; gross or histopathologic evidence of perineural invasion or soft-tissue extension of tumor; multiple-level cervical lymph node metastases; and incomplete primary lesion resection.[18,19,38] Children receive adjuvant radiation therapy less frequently than adults, owing to the higher risk of postradiotherapy complications (51% vs 27%)[8,37] such as facial growth retardation[66] and secondary malignant neoplasms.[39,56,67,68] Intensity-modulated radiation therapy or proton beam therapy should be used in children whenever possible.[69]

Chemotherapy is generally reserved for patients with progressive local or metastatic disease that is not amenable to surgery or radiation therapy.[38]

Tumor recurrence Tumor recurrence is reported in 7% to 20% of patients.[19,70] Local and regional recurrence is more likely to occur in patients with positive margins, regardless of tumor grade. The 5-year overall survival for children with malignancies of the major salivary glands approaches 95%, in comparison with 59% for adults.[37] Most tumors in younger patients are low-grade lesions, and these have an inherently better prognosis.[71,72] Childhood salivary gland malignancies of the same stage and grade have outcomes similar to those of their adult counterparts.[14,15,19] When tumor grades are examined in patients of all ages, 5-year survival rates range from 92% to 100% in cases of low-grade tumors, 62% to 92% for intermediate-grade tumors, and 0% to 43% for high-grade tumors.[19,71–73] Poor prognostic factors include distant spread at diagnosis, development of second malignancies, male sex, high-grade tumors, large tumor size (>2.5 cm), perineural invasion, lymph node metastasis, soft-tissue extension, macroscopic residual disease, and pathologic diagnoses other than mucoepidermoid or acinar cell carcinoma.[37,41,65]

Mucoepidermoid carcinoma

Mucoepidermoid carcinoma (MEC) is the most common primary salivary gland malignancy in adults and children.[37] MEC accounts for approximately 30% of all epithelial carcinomas in patients of all ages, and represents up to 60% of all pediatric salivary gland malignancies.[6] Macroscopically, MECs are firm, smooth, often cystic masses, which are tan, white, or pink in color with well-defined borders or infiltrative edges.[74] Microscopically they are composed of epidermoid cells, mucous secreting cells, and intermediate cells (**Fig. 11**). Several quantitative point-scoring grading schemes exist for MECs,[75] including the Armed Forces Institute of Pathology grading system, the modified Healey system,[76] and the Brandwein system.[75] These systems assess

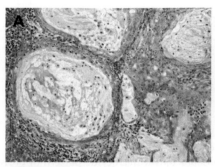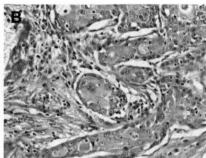

Fig. 11. Mucoepidermoid Carcinoma, Pathology. (*A*) Cystic structures are lined by mucous cells and contain mucin and mucinophages. Squamous epithelium is seen between arrowheads (Hematoxylin & eosin). (*B*) Islands and trabecules of well-differentiated squamous epithelium (Hematoxylin & eosin).

characteristics such as intracystic components, the presence of neural invasion or necrosis, mitotic rate, and cellular anaplasia to stratify tumors into low, intermediate, or high grades.[53] Most MECs in children are low grade, with relative frequencies of low (76%), intermediate (14%), and high (10%) grade.[23]

Metastasis of mucoepidermoid carcinomas With regard to low-grade MECs, lymphatic metastatic spread is observed in fewer than 5% of cases, whereas in cases of high-grade MEC lymph node metastases occur in up to 80%.[77] Low-grade MEC is generally treatable by surgical resection of primary tumor alone, whereas high-grade MEC requires ipsilateral neck dissection and adjuvant radiation therapy.[78] The overall 5-year survival rate for MEC ranges from 92% to 100% for low-grade tumors, 62% to 92% for intermediate-grade tumors, and 0% to 43% for high-grade tumors.[54]

Acinic cell carcinoma
Acinic cell carcinomas (ACC) make up approximately 10% of all malignant salivary gland tumors, accounting for 9% to 17% of parotid, 1% to 4% of submandibular, and 1% to 3% of minor salivary gland malignancies.[79–81]

Clinical presentation Pain may be a feature in up to one-third of patients. Unlike other salivary gland malignancies, pain does not necessarily portend a poor prognosis.[82] Most ACCs (88%) present locally.[83] Facial nerve palsy may occur in up to 10% of patients.[84] Cervical chain metastases are the most common, followed by metastases to lungs and bone.[82] Macroscopically most ACCs are well-circumscribed, solitary nodules, but some are ill defined. The cut surface of these lesions appears lobular and tumors are tan to red in color. Tumors vary from firm to soft, and solid to cystic.[74] Histologically 4 patterns of ACCs have been described, namely solid, microcystic, papillary-cystic, and follicular patterns. Different patterns may occur in a single lesion (**Fig. 12**).[85]

Staging of acinic cell carcinomas Because of the indolent nature of these tumors, ACCs were initially classified as benign. Recognition of tumor recurrences and metastases led these tumors to be recategorized as carcinomas.[86] ACCs were initially considered tumors with low malignant potential; however, many studies have found an unusually high rate of lymph node metastases and tumor recurrence in comparison with other low-risk tumors.[54] Grading systems are not widely used, as the histologic features of these tumors do not necessarily correlate with the clinical course.[87] Tumor

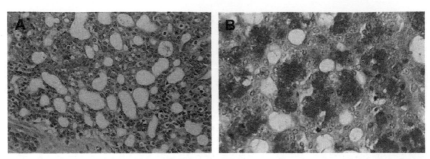

Fig. 12. Acinic Cell Carcinoma, Pathology. (*A*) Characteristic microcystic pattern of growth with lining cells devoid of a specific orientation around the spaces (Hematoxylin & eosin). (*B*) The cytoplasm of acinic cells is often basophilic and granular, owing to the presence of cytoplasmic zymogen granules (Hematoxylin & eosin).

staging is often a better predictor of prognosis in ACCs, with large tumor size, involvement of the deep lobe of the parotid gland, local invasion, metastases at presentation, and incomplete resection most predictive of tumor recurrence and a poor outcome.[74,88] Rates of local control according to stage (I, II, and III) are 85%, 63%, and 43%, respectively.[89]

Treatment of acinic cell carcinomas Elective neck dissection has not been shown to provide any survival benefit.[90] Radiotherapy is recommended in recurrent tumors, for those tumors with equivocal or positive margins, when there is evidence of tumor spillage, when nodal metastases or extraglandular extension is present, and for tumors greater than 4 cm in size.[83]

Tumor recurrence and metastasis First recurrences and metastases most commonly occur within 5 years of initial therapy (82%)[82]; however, similarly to adenoid cystic carcinomas (AdCCs), delayed local recurrences can be seen.[40] In all age groups, ACCs have the longest tumor-free interval of all salivary gland malignancies and also the best prognosis, with a 10-year relative survival rate of 85% to 88%.[81]

Adenoid cystic carcinoma
AdCCs account for 20% to 30% of all malignant salivary gland tumors in adults and 8.8% of malignant salivary gland tumors in children.[23] Most AdCCs in adults arise in minor salivary (36%) or submandibular (27%) glands.[91,92] In children, almost all reported adenoid cystic carcinomas were located within the parotid gland.[93,94] AdCCs present as slow-growing masses, but because of its proclivity for perineural invasion, pain and numbness are reported in 40% of children.[40,91] The presence of these symptoms correlate strongly with perineural invasion (43%–51%).[95] Large tumors (T3 and T4) have been shown to have a much higher incidence of perineural invasion (60%) in comparison with smaller (T1 and T2) tumors (23.5%).

Clinical presentation and prognosis A variety of other presenting complaints can be associated with AdCCs, including ulceration, nasal obstruction, hoarseness, and dysphagia, owing to the varied location of these tumors.[96] Up to 10% of patients may present with distant metastases, predominantly in the lungs.[91]

The gross appearance of AdCC is typically a firm, light tan, well defined, but nonencapsulated mass that invariably infiltrates surrounding normal tissues.[74] These solid tumors rarely display obvious cystic spaces on the cut surface. Microscopically they have been described as biphasic, composed of ducts and basal/myoepithelial cells with small basaloid cells surrounding cystic spaces.[40] These cells are arranged into 3 prognostically significant patterns: cribriform, tubular, and solid.[53,54] Any solid component imparts a poor prognosis, and the current World Health Organization classification system refers to these tumors by their predominant pattern.[54] Other prognostic factors include age older than 45 years, rapid progression of disease, paresthesias, tumor size, lymph node involvement, distant metastases, solid histologic type, and presence of residual tumor.[97]

Treatment of adenoid cystic carcinoma In adults, multimodality therapy, specifically surgery followed by radiation, is considered the standard of care for AdCCs. Postoperative radiotherapy has been shown to improve the 5-year local recurrence rate and disease-free survival rate in comparison with surgery alone.[92] The benefits of radiotherapy must be weighed against potential long-term side effects. The typical clinical course is slow but relentless tumor growth. The 5-year survival rate is favorable, at approximately 75% to 80%, but the 15-year survival rate is poor, estimated at 35%.[95,98] In the largest series of pediatric AdCC involving 5 children, only 1 of 5 patients was alive with no evidence of disease 7 years after presentation; the other 4 patients were followed for a longer period, and all 4 died of their disease between 11 and 28 years after presentation.[40] Lifelong follow-up of AdCC patients is clearly required.

Sialoblastoma
Sialoblastoma Is an extremely rare tumor, with less than 50 cases reported in the literature.[99] Initially considered to be a benign salivary gland tumor,[100] reports of aggressive behavior with rapid growth, recurrences, metastases,[101] and tumor-related mortality[101,102] led sialoblastoma to be categorized as a malignancy.[74,103]

Sialoblastomas are usually diagnosed on antenatal ultrasonography,[104] at birth, or shortly thereafter.[104] There are, however, reported cases of sialoblastoma diagnosed in children as late as age 5 years.[105] Approximately 75% of sialoblastomas arise from the parotid gland,[74,106] with the remainder originating in the submandibular gland,[107] ectopic salivary gland tissue,[108] and minor salivary glands.[109] The male to female ratio is 2:1.[74] Most patients present with an asymptomatic mass in the parotid or submandibular region, but massive tumors with skin necrosis[110] and facial nerve palsy are also described.[111] On MRI, these tumors typically show heterogeneous enhancement and may contain foci of hemorrhage (see **Fig. 9**).[110] Incisional biopsy of massive lesions is necessary to rule out other malignancies such as rhabdomyosarcoma (**Fig. 13**).[74] Characteristically, sialoblastomas are composed of numerous small, individual, and solid hypercellular islands of primitive basaloid epithelial cells with scant cytoplasm,

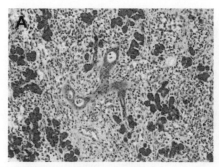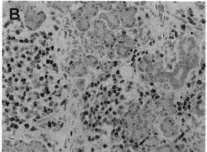

Fig. 13. Embryonal rhabdomyosarcoma, Pathology. (*A*) Embryonal rhabdomyosarcoma infiltrating the salivary gland. Tumor cells are small, spindled, and patternless (Hematoxylin & eosin). (*B*) Nuclear immunoreactivity for myogenin in a variable proportion of tumor cells is characteristic.

round to oval nuclei, single or few nucleoli, and a relatively fine chromatin pattern, separated by fibrous or fibromyxomatous stroma.[74,99] Sialoblastomas express S-100 and vimentin, smooth muscle actin, and p63 diffusely. Cytokeratin classically accentuates the ductal structures (**Fig. 14**).[112]

Surgical excision with tumor-free margins is the desired therapy. Massive tumors, however, are often unresectable and require some form of neoadjuvant therapy. Treatment with brachytherapy and chemotherapy has been reported, with successful outcomes.[106,108,113] Local recurrence (38%) is a common feature,[106] and recurrences have been successfully treated with further surgical excision,[101] chemotherapy,[104] radiotherapy, or a combination of these treatment modalities.[101,108] As a result, the overall prognosis is relatively good.[74,106] Two of the reported deaths in the literature occurred in neonates before any diagnosis or treatment, and were considered to be due to unrelated causes.[101,114] The third mortality involved a patient who initially presented with a parotid mass at 1 year of age, but was not diagnosed until the age of 4 years; this patient had extensive surgery but tumor recurred within 15 months, and the patient subsequently failed chemotherapy and further surgery.[102]

Mesenchymal Tumors

Rhabdomyosarcoma

Rhabdomyosarcomas of the salivary glands are exceptionally rare, and in one large study of adults and children with salivary gland tumors only 1 case of rhabdomyosarcoma in 600 patients was reported.[115] However, in another series of primary salivary gland malignancies in children, more than half of the tumors were rhabdomyosarcomas.[11] The investigators of that report acknowledged that the rhabdomyosarcomas may have arisen from periparotid tissues with subsequent extension into the parotid gland, as controversy exists whether "parotid sarcomas" originate in the gland itself or invade it secondarily.[116] Overall, the incidence of rhabdomyosarcomas in children is likely to be closer to 2% to 3%.[6]

Rhabdomyosarcomas of the parotid gland generally present as a swelling at the angle of the mandible, rapidly increasing in size.[117] The tumor presents at a younger age than other malignant salivary gland neoplasms, with 70% occurring between the ages of 1 and 9 years. The mean duration of symptoms before presentation is approximately 5 weeks.[116] Pain and facial paralysis are common presenting signs (24%),[116] reflecting the aggressive behavior of these tumors and the degree of tumor extension.[118] However, it must be noted that pain or nerve palsies often do not occur with rhabdomyosarcoma of the parotid gland, and further diagnostic evaluation of a

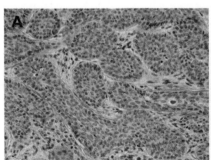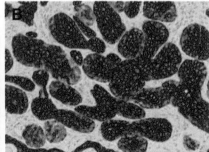

Fig. 14. Sialoblastoma, Pathology. (*A*) The tumor is composed of microlobules of basaloid cells surrounded by a well-developed basal lamina (Hematoxylin & eosin). (*B*) Tumor cells are highlighted by CK19 immunohistochemistry.

parotid mass in a child should proceed without delay. MRI is the imaging modality of choice (see **Fig. 10**). A delay in diagnosis may decrease the chance for complete resection. Most patients present with locally invasive or metastatic disease. The primary tumor is therefore often unresectable at diagnosis, with less than 5% of surgeries attaining clear margins.[116] Parotidectomy is recommended for early tumors. Otherwise, a biopsy should be performed followed by chemotherapy with 3 drugs, including an alkylating agent in patients with advanced-stage tumors and radiotherapy to the primary and metastatic tumor sites.[116] Whereas several small case series report extremely poor prognoses,[11,118] a larger series reported a 5-year overall survival rate of 84% with a median follow-up duration of 7 years.[116]

Other mesenchymal tumors
Fibrosarcoma,[27] reticulum cell sarcoma, spindle cell sarcoma,[40] fibrous histiocytoma, neurosarcoma, and osteosarcoma[119] of the salivary glands have all been reported in children. However, each entity is extremely rare, which limits the ability to make standardized treatment recommendations. One study did find that the prognosis correlated with the size of the neoplasm, type of sarcoma, and histologic grade, and that salivary gland sarcomas behave in an identical fashion to their soft-tissue counterparts.[119] Given the rarity of these tumors, it is important that management options are considered in a multidisciplinary fashion.

SUMMARY

Salivary gland neoplasms are rare in children. In infants most tumors are benign hemangiomas, with some notable exceptions such as sialoblastomas. An asymptomatic swelling in the periauricular region is the most common presenting complaint in older children. Approximately 50% of theses lesions are malignant, which dictates a thorough diagnostic evaluation by a head and neck surgeon. Surgical excision is the primary treatment modality. Prognosis is primarily determined by histopathologic findings.

REFERENCES

1. Waner M, North PE, Scherer KA, et al. The nonrandom distribution of facial hemangiomas. Arch Dermatol 2003;139(7):869–75.
2. da Cruz Perez DE, Pires FR, Alves FA, et al. Salivary gland tumors in children and adolescents: a clinicopathologic and immunohistochemical study of fifty-three cases. Int J Pediatr Otorhinolaryngol 2004;68(7):895–902.
3. Shapiro NL, Bhattacharyya N. Clinical characteristics and survival for major salivary gland malignancies in children. Otolaryngol Head Neck Surg 2006;134(4):631–4.
4. Koch BL, Myer CM 3rd. Presentation and diagnosis of unilateral maxillary swelling in children. Am J Otolaryngol 1999;20(2):106–29.
5. Jaryszak EM, Shah RK, Bauman NM, et al. Unexpected pathologies in pediatric parotid lesions: management paradigms revisited. Int J Pediatr Otorhinolaryngol 2011;75(4):558–63.
6. Krolls SO, Trodahl JN, Boyers RC. Salivary gland lesions in children. A survey of 430 cases. Cancer 1972;30(2):459–69.
7. Castro EB, Huvos AG, Strong EW, et al. Tumors of the major salivary glands in children. Cancer 1972;29(2):312–7.
8. Shikhani AH, Johns ME. Tumors of the major salivary glands in children. Head Neck Surg 1988;10(4):257–63.

9. Lack EE, Upton MP. Histopathologic review of salivary gland tumors in childhood. Arch Otolaryngol Head Neck Surg 1988;114(8):898–906.
10. Fonseca I, Martins AG, Soares J. Epithelial salivary gland tumors of children and adolescents in southern Portugal. A clinicopathologic study of twenty-four cases. Oral Surg Oral Med Oral Pathol 1991;72(6):696–701.
11. Rogers DA, Rao BN, Bowman L, et al. Primary malignancy of the salivary gland in children. J Pediatr Surg 1994;29(1):44–7.
12. Kessler A, Handler SD. Salivary gland neoplasms in children: a 10-year survey at the Children's Hospital of Philadelphia. Int J Pediatr Otorhinolaryngol 1994; 29(3):195–202.
13. Bull PD. Salivary gland neoplasia in childhood. Int J Pediatr Otorhinolaryngol 1999;49(Suppl 1):S235–8.
14. Orvidas LJ, Kasperbauer JL, Lewis JE, et al. Pediatric parotid masses. Arch Otolaryngol Head Neck Surg 2000;126(2):177–84.
15. Ribeiro Kde C, Kowalski LP, Saba LM, et al. Epithelial salivary glands neoplasms in children and adolescents: a forty-four-year experience. Med Pediatr Oncol 2002;39(6):594–600.
16. Yu GY, Li ZL, Ma DQ, et al. Diagnosis and treatment of epithelial salivary gland tumours in children and adolescents. Br J Oral Maxillofac Surg 2002;40(5):389–92.
17. Ethunandan M, Ethunandan A, Macpherson D, et al. Parotid neoplasms in children: experience of diagnosis and management in a district general hospital. Int J Oral Maxillofac Surg 2003;32(4):373–7.
18. Callender DL, Frankenthaler RA, Luna MA, et al. Salivary gland neoplasms in children. Arch Otolaryngol Head Neck Surg 1992;118(5):472–6.
19. Guzzo M, Ferrari A, Marcon I, et al. Salivary gland neoplasms in children: the experience of the Istituto Nazionale Tumori of Milan. Pediatr Blood Cancer 2006;47(6):806–10.
20. Ellies M, Schaffranietz F, Arglebe C, et al. Tumors of the salivary glands in childhood and adolescence. J Oral Maxillofac Surg 2006;64(7):1049–58.
21. Ogata H, Ebihara S, Mukai K. Salivary gland neoplasms in children. Jpn J Clin Oncol 1994;24(2):88–93.
22. Fu H, Wang J, Wang L, et al. Pleomorphic adenoma of the salivary glands in children and adolescents. J Pediatr Surg 2012;47(4):715–9.
23. Lennon P, Cunningham MJ. Salivary gland tumors. In: Rahbar R, editor. Pediatric head and neck tumors: A-Z guide to presentation and multimodality management. Boston: Springer Verlag; 2014. p. 311–27.
24. Rodriguez KH, Vargas S, Robson C, et al. Pleomorphic adenoma of the parotid gland in children. Int J Pediatr Otorhinolaryngol 2007;71(11):1717–23.
25. Michaels L, Hellquist HB. Ear, nose and throat histopathology. 2nd edition. New York: Springer; 2001.
26. Leverstein H, van der Wal JE, Tiwari RM, et al. Surgical management of 246 previously untreated pleomorphic adenomas of the parotid gland. Br J Surg 1997; 84(3):399–403.
27. Krolls SO, Boyers RC. Mixed tumors of salivary glands. Long-term follow-up. Cancer 1972;30(1):276–81.
28. Gnepp DR. Malignant mixed tumors of the salivary glands: a review. Pathol Annu 1993;28(Pt 1):279–328.
29. Seifert G. Histopathology of malignant salivary gland tumours. Eur J Cancer B Oral Oncol 1992;28B(1):49–56.
30. Dahlqvist A, Ostberg Y. Malignant salivary gland tumours in children. Acta Otolaryngol 1982;94(1–2):175–9.

31. Som PM, Brandwein-Gensler MS. Anatomy and pathology of the salivary glands. In: Som PM, Curtin HD, editors. Head and neck imaging. St Louis (MO): Elsevier Mosby; 2011. p. 2449–610.
32. Mehta D, Willging JP. Pediatric salivary gland lesions. Semin Pediatr Surg 2006; 15(2):76–84.
33. Boyd ZT, Goud AR, Lowe LH, et al. Pediatric salivary gland imaging. Pediatr Radiol 2009;39(7):710–22.
34. Leaute-Labreze C, Dumas de la Roque E, Hubiche T, et al. Propranolol for severe hemangiomas of infancy. N Engl J Med 2008;358(24):2649–51.
35. Weiss I, O TM, Lipari BA, et al. Current treatment of parotid hemangiomas. Laryngoscope 2011;121(8):1642–50.
36. Oosthuizen JC, Burns P, Russell JD. Lymphatic malformations: a proposed management algorithm. Int J Pediatr Otorhinolaryngol 2010;74(4):398–403.
37. Sultan I, Rodriguez-Galindo C, Al-Sharabati S, et al. Salivary gland carcinomas in children and adolescents: a population-based study, with comparison to adult cases. Head Neck 2011;33(10):1476–81.
38. Rahbar R, Grimmer JF, Vargas SO, et al. Mucoepidermoid carcinoma of the parotid gland in children: a 10-year experience. Arch Otolaryngol Head Neck Surg 2006;132(4):375–80.
39. Vedrine PO, Coffinet L, Temam S, et al. Mucoepidermoid carcinoma of salivary glands in the pediatric age group: 18 clinical cases, including 11 second malignant neoplasms. Head Neck 2006;28(9):827–33.
40. Baker SR, Malone B. Salivary gland malignancies in children. Cancer 1985; 55(8):1730–6.
41. Byers RM, Piorkowski R, Luna MA. Malignant parotid tumors in patients under 20 years of age. Arch Otolaryngol 1984;110(4):232–5.
42. Schuller DE, McCabe BF. The firm salivary mass in children. Laryngoscope 1977;87(11):1891–8.
43. Moraes P, Pereira C, Almeida O, et al. Paediatric intraoral mucoepidermoid carcinoma mimicking a bone lesion. Int J Paediatr Dent 2007;17(2):151–4.
44. Galer C, Santillan AA, Chelius D, et al. Minor salivary gland malignancies in the pediatric population. Head Neck 2012;34:1648–51.
45. Oldham KT, Aiken JA. Pediatric head and neck. In: Mulholland MW, Lillemoe KD, Doherty GM, et al, editors. Greenfield's surgery: scientific principles & practice. 5h edition. Philadelphia: Lippincott Williams & Wilkins; 2010.
46. Yuh WT, Sato Y, Loes DJ, et al. Magnetic resonance imaging and computed tomography in pediatric head and neck masses. Ann Otol Rhinol Laryngol 1991; 100(1):54–62.
47. Yousem DM, Kraut MA, Chalian AA. Major salivary gland imaging. Radiology 2000;216(1):19–29.
48. Parker GD, Harnsberger HR. Clinical-radiologic issues in perineural tumor spread of malignant diseases of the extracranial head and neck. Radiographics 1991;11(3):383–99.
49. Freling NJ, Molenaar WM, Vermey A, et al. Malignant parotid tumors: clinical use of MR imaging and histologic correlation. Radiology 1992;185(3):691–6.
50. Colella G, Cannavale R, Flamminio F, et al. Fine-needle aspiration cytology of salivary gland lesions: a systematic review. J Oral Maxillofac Surg 2010;68(9): 2146–53.
51. Liu ES, Bernstein JM, Sculerati N, et al. Fine needle aspiration biopsy of pediatric head and neck masses. Int J Pediatr Otorhinolaryngol 2001;60(2): 135–40.

52. Cho HW, Kim J, Choi J, et al. Sonographically guided fine-needle aspiration biopsy of major salivary gland masses: a review of 245 cases. AJR Am J Roentgenol 2011;196(5):1160–3.
53. Zarbo RJ. Salivary gland neoplasia: a review for the practicing pathologist. Mod Pathol 2002;15(3):298–323.
54. Seethala RR. An update on grading of salivary gland carcinomas. Head Neck Pathol 2009;3(1):69–77.
55. Cunningham MJ. Salivary gland surgery. In: Bluestone CD, editor. Surgical atlas of pediatric otolaryngology. Hamilton (Canada): BC Decker Inc; 2002.
56. Verma J, Teh BS, Paulino AC. Characteristics and outcome of radiation and chemotherapy-related mucoepidermoid carcinoma of the salivary glands. Pediatr Blood Cancer 2011;57(7):1137–41.
57. Revenaugh PC, Knott PD, Scharpf J, et al. Simultaneous anterolateral thigh flap and temporalis tendon transfer to optimize facial form and function after radical parotidectomy. Arch Facial Plast Surg 2012;14(2):104–9.
58. Medina JE. Neck dissection in the treatment of cancer of major salivary glands. Otolaryngol Clin North Am 1998;31(5):815–22.
59. Mehle ME, Kraus DH, Wood BG, et al. Facial nerve morbidity following parotid surgery for benign disease: the Cleveland Clinic Foundation experience. Laryngoscope 1993;103(4 Pt 1):386–8.
60. Laccourreye H, Laccourreye O, Cauchois R, et al. Total conservative parotidectomy for primary benign pleomorphic adenoma of the parotid gland: a 25-year experience with 229 patients. Laryngoscope 1994;104(12):1487–94.
61. Donovan DT, Conley JJ. Capsular significance in parotid tumor surgery: reality and myths of lateral lobectomy. Laryngoscope 1984;94(3):324–9.
62. Witt RL. The significance of the margin in parotid surgery for pleomorphic adenoma. Laryngoscope 2002;112(12):2141–54.
63. Kyrmizakis DE, Pangalos A, Papadakis CE, et al. The use of botulinum toxin type A in the treatment of Frey and crocodile tears syndromes. J Oral Maxillofac Surg 2004;62(7):840–4.
64. Xie CM, Kubba H. Parotidectomy in children: indications and complications. J Laryngol Otol 2010;124(12):1289–93.
65. Weber RS, Byers RM, Petit B, et al. Submandibular gland tumors. Adverse histologic factors and therapeutic implications. Arch Otolaryngol Head Neck Surg 1990;116(9):1055–60.
66. Denys D, Kaste SC, Kun LE, et al. The effects of radiation on craniofacial skeletal growth: a quantitative study. Int J Pediatr Otorhinolaryngol 1998;45(1):7–13.
67. Kaste SC, Hedlund G, Pratt CB. Malignant parotid tumors in patients previously treated for childhood cancer: clinical and imaging findings in eight cases. AJR Am J Roentgenol 1994;162(3):655–9.
68. Loy TS, McLaughlin R, Odom LF, et al. Mucoepidermoid carcinoma of the parotid as a second malignant neoplasm in children. Cancer 1989;64(10):2174–7.
69. Schoenfeld JD, Sher DJ, Norris CM Jr, et al. Salivary gland tumors treated with adjuvant intensity-modulated radiotherapy with or without concurrent chemotherapy. Int J Radiat Oncol Biol Phys 2012;82(1):308–14.
70. Auclair PL, Goode RK, Ellis GL. Mucoepidermoid carcinoma of intraoral salivary glands. Evaluation and application of grading criteria in 143 cases. Cancer 1992;69(8):2021–30.
71. Clode AL, Fonseca I, Santos JR, et al. Mucoepidermoid carcinoma of the salivary glands: a reappraisal of the influence of tumor differentiation on prognosis. J Surg Oncol 1991;46(2):100–6.

72. Nascimento AG, Amaral LP, Prado LA, et al. Mucoepidermoid carcinoma of salivary glands: a clinicopathologic study of 46 cases. Head Neck Surg 1986;8(6): 409–17.
73. Spiro RH, Armstrong J, Harrison L, et al. Carcinoma of major salivary glands. Recent trends. Arch Otolaryngol Head Neck Surg 1989;115(3):316–21.
74. Eveson JW, Kusafuka K, Stenman G, et al. Tumours of the salivary glands. In: Barnes L, Eveson JW, Reichart P, et al, editors. World Health Organization classification of tumours, pathology and genetics of head and neck tumours. Lyon (France): IARC Press; 2005. p. 209–81.
75. Brandwein MS, Ferlito A, Bradley PJ, et al. Diagnosis and classification of salivary neoplasms: pathologic challenges and relevance to clinical outcomes. Acta Otolaryngol 2002;122(7):758–64.
76. Batsakis JG, Luna MA. Histopathologic grading of salivary gland neoplasms: I. Mucoepidermoid carcinomas. Ann Otol Rhinol Laryngol 1990;99(10 Pt 1): 835–8.
77. Moll R, Ramaswamy A. The pathology of lymphogenic metastatic spread. In: Werner JA, Davis RK, editors. Metastases in head and neck cancer. Berlin: Springer; 2005. p. 75.
78. Aro K, Leivo I, Makitie AA. Management and outcome of patients with mucoepidermoid carcinoma of major salivary gland origin: a single institution's 30-year experience. Laryngoscope 2008;118(2):258–62.
79. Bjorndal K, Krogdahl A, Therkildsen MH, et al. Salivary gland carcinoma in Denmark 1990-2005: a national study of incidence, site and histology. Results of the Danish Head and Neck Cancer Group (DAHANCA). Oral Oncol 2011; 47(7):677–82.
80. Eveson JW, Cawson RA. Salivary gland tumours. A review of 2410 cases with particular reference to histological types, site, age and sex distribution. J Pathol 1985;146(1):51–8.
81. Wahlberg P, Anderson H, Biorklund A, et al. Carcinoma of the parotid and submandibular glands–a study of survival in 2465 patients. Oral Oncol 2002;38(7): 706–13.
82. Ellis GL, Corio RL. Acinic cell adenocarcinoma. A clinicopathologic analysis of 294 cases. Cancer 1983;52(3):542–9.
83. Hoffman HT, Karnell LH, Robinson RA, et al. National Cancer Data Base report on cancer of the head and neck: acinic cell carcinoma. Head Neck 1999;21(4): 297–309.
84. Laskawi R, Rodel R, Zirk A, et al. Retrospective analysis of 35 patients with acinic cell carcinoma of the parotid gland. J Oral Maxillofac Surg 1998;56(4):440–3.
85. Schwarz S, Zenk J, Muller M, et al. The many faces of acinic cell carcinomas of the salivary glands: a study of 40 cases relating histological and immunohistological subtypes to clinical parameters and prognosis. Histopathology 2012;61: 395–408.
86. Guimaraes DS, Amaral AP, Prado LF, et al. Acinic cell carcinoma of salivary glands: 16 cases with clinicopathologic correlation. J Oral Pathol Med 1989; 18(7):396–9.
87. Suzzi MV, Alessi A, Bertarelli C, et al. Prognostic relevance of cell proliferation in major salivary gland carcinomas. Acta Otorhinolaryngol Ital 2005;25(3):161–8.
88. Timon CI, Dardick I. The importance of dedifferentiation in recurrent acinic cell carcinoma. J Laryngol Otol 2001;115(8):639–44.
89. Spiro RH, Huvos AG, Strong EW. Acinic cell carcinoma of salivary origin. A clinicopathologic study of 67 cases. Cancer 1978;41(3):924–35.

90. Zbaren P, Schupbach J, Nuyens M, et al. Carcinoma of the parotid gland. Am J Surg 2003;186(1):57–62.
91. Sur RK, Donde B, Levin V, et al. Adenoid cystic carcinoma of the salivary glands: a review of 10 years. Laryngoscope 1997;107(9):1276–80.
92. Shen C, Xu T, Huang C, et al. Treatment outcomes and prognostic features in adenoid cystic carcinoma originated from the head and neck. Oral Oncol 2012;48(5):445–9.
93. Thavaraj V, Sridhar MR, Sethi A, et al. Adenoid cystic carcinoma of the lacrimal gland. Indian J Pediatr 2003;70(9):751–3.
94. Ustundag E, Iseri M, Aydin O, et al. Adenoid cystic carcinoma of the tongue. J Laryngol Otol 2000;114(6):477–80.
95. Fordice J, Kershaw C, El-Naggar A, et al. Adenoid cystic carcinoma of the head and neck: predictors of morbidity and mortality. Arch Otolaryngol Head Neck Surg 1999;125(2):149–52.
96. Nascimento AG, Amaral AL, Prado LA, et al. Adenoid cystic carcinoma of salivary glands. A study of 61 cases with clinicopathologic correlation. Cancer 1986;57(2):312–9.
97. da Cruz Perez DE, de Abreu Alves F, Nobuko Nishimoto I, et al. Prognostic factors in head and neck adenoid cystic carcinoma. Oral Oncol 2006;42(2):139–46.
98. Spiro RH, Huvos AG. Stage means more than grade in adenoid cystic carcinoma. Am J Surg 1992;164(6):623–8.
99. Ellis GL. What's new in the AFIP fascicle on salivary gland tumors: a few highlights from the 4th Series Atlas. Head Neck Pathol 2009;3(3):225–30.
100. Ellis GL, Auclair PL. Tumors of the salivary glands. Atlas of tumor pathology. 3 edition. Washington, DC: Armed Forces Institute of Pathology; 1996.
101. Williams SB, Ellis GL, Warnock GR. Sialoblastoma: a clinicopathologic and immunohistochemical study of 7 cases. Ann Diagn Pathol 2006;10(6):320–6.
102. Tatlidede S, Karsidag S, Ugurlu K, et al. Sialoblastoma: a congenital epithelial tumor of the salivary gland. J Pediatr Surg 2006;41(7):1322–5.
103. Ellis GL, Auclair PL. Tumors of the salivary glands. AFIP atlas of tumor pathology. 4th edition. Silver Spring (MD): ARP Press; 2008.
104. Siddiqi SH, Solomon MP, Haller JO. Sialoblastoma and hepatoblastoma in a neonate. Pediatr Radiol 2000;30(5):349–51.
105. Alvarez-Mendoza A, Calderon-Elvir C, Carrasco-Daza D. Diagnostic and therapeutic approach to sialoblastoma: report of a case. J Pediatr Surg 1999;34(12):1875–7.
106. Prigent M, Teissier N, Peuchmaur M, et al. Sialoblastoma of salivary glands in children: chemotherapy should be discussed as an alternative to mutilating surgery. Int J Pediatr Otorhinolaryngol 2010;74(8):942–5.
107. Vidyadhar M, Amanda C, Thuan Q, et al. Sialoblastoma. J Pediatr Surg 2008; 43(10):e11–3.
108. Shet T, Ramadwar M, Sharma S, et al. An eyelid sialoblastoma-like tumor with a sarcomatoid myoepithelial component. Pediatr Dev Pathol 2007;10(4): 309–14.
109. Saffari Y, Blei F, Warren SM, et al. Congenital minor salivary gland sialoblastoma: a case report and review of the literature. Fetal Pediatr Pathol 2011;30(1):32–9.
110. Yekeler E, Dursun M, Gun F, et al. Sialoblastoma: MRI findings. Pediatr Radiol 2004;34(12):1005–7.
111. Simpson PR, Rutledge JC, Schaefer SD, et al. Congenital hybrid basal cell adenoma–adenoid cystic carcinoma of the salivary gland. Pediatr Pathol 1986; 6(2–3):199–208.

112. Brandwein M, Al-Naeif NS, Manwani D, et al. Sialoblastoma: clinicopathological/immunohistochemical study. Am J Surg Pathol 1999;23(3):342–8.
113. Shan XF, Cai ZG, Zhang JG, et al. Management of sialoblastoma with surgery and brachytherapy. Pediatr Blood Cancer 2010;55(7):1427–30.
114. Stones DK, Jansen JC, Griessel D. Sialoblastoma and hepatoblastoma in a newborn infant. Pediatr Blood Cancer 2009;52(7):883–5.
115. Takahama A Jr, Leon JE, de Almeida OP, et al. Nonlymphoid mesenchymal tumors of the parotid gland. Oral Oncol 2008;44(10):970–4.
116. Walterhouse DO, Pappo AS, Baker KS, et al. Rhabdomyosarcoma of the parotid region occurring in childhood and adolescence. A report from the Intergroup Rhabdomyosarcoma Study Group. Cancer 2001;92(12):3135–46.
117. Valencerina Gopez E, Dauterman J, Layfield LJ. Fine-needle aspiration biopsy of alveolar rhabdomyosarcoma of the parotid: a case report and review of the literature. Diagn Cytopathol 2001;24(4):249–52.
118. BenJelloun H, Jouhadi H, Maazouzi A, et al. Rhabdomyosarcoma of the salivary glands. Report of 3 cases. Cancer Radiother 2005;9(5):316–21 [in French].
119. Luna MA, Tortoledo ME, Ordonez NG, et al. Primary sarcomas of the major salivary glands. Arch Otolaryngol Head Neck Surg 1991;117(3):302–6.

Pediatric Lingual and Other Intraoral Lesions

Brian D. Kulbersh, MD*, Brian J. Wiatrak, MD

KEYWORDS

- Pediatric lesions • Lingual lesions • Oral cavity • Oral cavity malformations
- Anatomic development

KEY POINTS

- Sore throats and dysphagia are one of the more common presenting symptoms in patients seen by pediatricians.
- Many systemic diseases have manifestations in the oral cavity, and may be diagnosed by recognition of these characteristics.
- Most embryonic development of the oral cavity occurs between the fourth and eighth week of gestation.

EMBRYOLOGY AND ANATOMY OF THE ORAL CAVITY

The oral cavity is bounded anteriorly by the lips, laterally by the cheeks, and superiorly by the hard and soft palate. The posterior border is defined by the circumvallate papillae and the junction of the hard and soft palate. The oral cavity is further divided into two parts. The vestibule is defined as the area between the teeth and lips and the oral cavity proper is defined as the area posterior to the teeth and alveolar ridge.[1]

The Lips

In the fourth week of development the lower lip is formed as the mandibular prominences merge. In weeks 6 to 8 of development the medial frontonasal and lateral maxillary prominences merge to form the upper lip.

The lips are innervated by branches of the facial nerve. The buccal branch provides motor innervation to the upper lip and the marginal mandibular branch provides motor innervations to the lower lip.[2] Sensory innervation to the upper and lower lips is provided by the infraorbital nerve and the mental nerve, respectively.

Pediatric ENT Associates, Children's of Alabama, Birmingham, AL, USA
* Corresponding author. 1600 7th Avenue South, Birmingham, AL 35233.
E-mail address: Brian.kulbersh@childrensal.org

Otolaryngol Clin N Am 48 (2015) 175–190
http://dx.doi.org/10.1016/j.otc.2014.09.012
0030-6665/15/$ – see front matter © 2015 Elsevier Inc. All rights reserved.

The Tongue

In the fourth week of gestation development of the tongue begins when two paired lateral lingual swellings and one central tuberculum impar appear on the floor of the oral cavity and pharynx. These two structures fuse and form the anterior two-thirds of the tongue. The posterior third of the tongue develops from a second median swelling known as the hypobranchial eminence or the copula.[3] The glossopharyngeal and vagus nerves provide sensation and motor innervations to the posterior third of the tongue, whereas the trigeminal and chorda tympani nerves supply the anterior two-thirds of the tongue.[4]

A V-shaped groove separates the anterior two-thirds and posterior one-third of the tongue. This groove is called the sulcus terminalis. The foramen cecum is a blind depression in the midline of the apex of the sulcus terminalis. The thyroid gland originates from the foramen cecum and migrates inferiorly.

The Palate

In the twelfth week of development the palate is formed from fusion of the primary and secondary palates. The primary palate is formed from the intermaxillary segment by the merger of two medial nasal swellings.

Beginning at the seventh week gestation the secondary palate is formed by the fusion of two palatal processes.[5] The hard palate initially occurs in the midline anteriorly and proceeds posteriorly with the fusion of the horizontal palatal shelves.

The anterior two-thirds of the palate functions to separate the nasal cavity from the oral cavity, whereas the soft palate provides a barrier between the nasopharynx and the oropharynx. Proper functioning of the soft palate plays a key role in deglutition and normal articulation in speech.

INFECTIONS AND INFLAMMATORY DISEASES OF THE ORAL CAVITY

Sore throats and dysphagia are one of the more common presenting symptoms in patients seen by pediatricians. There are many causative organisms from localized viral, bacterial, and fungal infections to more systemic diseases that manifest in the oral cavity.

Viral Infections

Many viruses can cause dysphagia and orpharyngitis. In the oral cavity, herpetic infection is the most common type of viral illness.

Herpes simplex virus

There are two forms of herpes simplex virus infections. Herpes simplex virus 1 is a primary severe infection affecting the oral mucosa. Herpes simplex virus 2 is a secondary infection that is more common and affects the genitalia.

Primary herpetic infection classically presents in children younger than 5 years old. After a brief prodrome of constitutional symptoms, stomatitis develops with a tingling sensation of the oral mucosa followed by erythema and edema. Vesicles then develop and rupture turning into ulcers that heal spontaneously within 10 to 14 days.[6] A gray pseudomembrane then covers the ulcers, which may coalesce or become secondarily infected with oral bacteria. There may be associated fever and flulike symptoms with rare progression to herpes or meningoencephalitis. Treatment involves antiviral drugs, such as acyclovir either topically or parentally.[7]

Once primary infection has occurred with herpes simplex virus, the virus may lie dormant in the regional neuroganglia until activated. Fever, excessive sun exposure, stress, or immunodeficiency can result in activation of the virus. A burning or tingling sensation signals the formation of mucosal erythema and vesicle formation shortly after. The vesicles usually rupture within the first day leaving a superficial ulceration that spontaneously heals within 10 to 14 days. These ulcers usually reoccur in the same sites on the vermillion border of the lips or intraorally on the mucosa of the gingival.

Herpes zoster
Herpes zoster, or shingles, presents as skin or mucosal vesicles along the distribution of the trigeminal nerve and can involve the mucosa of the lips and oral mucosa. This is classically seen in patients who are immunocompromised. This is thought to be caused by the reactivation of the varicella virus that is dormant in the sensory ganglia. Vesicles usually resolve within 10 days and patients are treated symptomatically.

Herpangia
This usually occurs in young children caused commonly by coxsackievirus A. It is characterized by the sudden onset of fever, malaise, with an intense sore throat.[8] Multiple small vesicles are usually located in the posterior oral cavity, which ruptures to form small ulcers. This condition spontaneously resolves in 7 to 10 days.[9]

Hand-foot-and-mouth disease
This viral illness mimics herpangia in every respect. It is also caused by the coxsackievirus A. Vesiculaopapular lesions on the palms of the hand and soles of the feet differentiate this illness from herpangia.[10] Spontaneous resolution usually occurs within a week.

Papilloma
Human papilloma virus types 6, 14, and 22 usually infect the mucosa of the upper aerodigestive system. Although papilloma of the larynx are more common and problematic, papilloma may also occur on the soft palate, tonsillar pillars, and uvula (**Fig. 1**).[11] Excision is recommended to avoid risk of distal seeding into the supraglottis and glottis.

Infectious mononucleosis
This infection is caused by the Epstein-Barr virus and usually effects adolescents and young adults. It is characterized by malaise, fatigue, and generalized lymphadenopathy. The tonsils become hypertrophic and erythematous with a gray membrane (**Fig. 2**). Airway compromise is a possible morbidity, especially in small children,

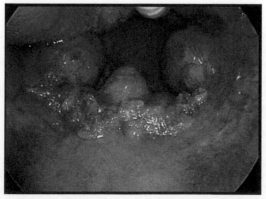

Fig. 1. Papillomas seen here on the soft palate, caused by the human papilloma virus, are amenable to local excision.

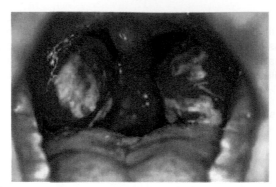

Fig. 2. Tonsils in the setting of mononucleosis. Note the hypertrophic appearance with gray pseudomembrane.

and the airway must be managed immediately via endotracheal intubation. Usually supportive treatment is all that is required, with some patients requiring intravenous steroids in cases of worsening respiratory obstruction.

Bacterial Infections

Bacterial infections of the oral cavity are rare and usually occur as the result of normal oral flora that becomes pathologic when the host defense is impaired because of immunodeficiency. Approximately 80% of the oral flora is anaerobic streptococci and diphtherias.

Gingivitis

Gingivitis is caused by oral bacteria manifesting as tender swelling and bleeding of the gingivae. It is usually seen in patients with poor oral hygiene, wearing dental appliances, or that are immunosuppressed.

Acute necrotizing ulcerative gingivitis is caused by an anaerobic spirochete. Also known as Vincent infection, the gingival papillae necrotize to produce a psuedomembrane with exposure of the dental roots and loosening of the teeth. The gingivae are very painful and hemorrhagic and symptoms include high fever, halitosis, and malaise. Treatment includes local debridement of necrotic tissues, mouthwash, and penicillin.[12]

Ludwig cellulitis

A bacterial infection precipitated by poor oral hygiene or dental extractions can result in a rapidly progressive cellulitis of the sublingual and submandibular space. This manifests rapidly with erythematous skin, pitting edema, trismus, and high fever. If inadequately treated, Ludwig cellulitis can result in airway compromise and the need for fiberoptic intubation or tracheostomy. Treatment includes surgical drainage in combination with broad-spectrum antibiotics.

Streptococcal infection

Pharyngotonsillitis is most commonly caused by respiratory viruses with symptoms including rhinosinusits, sneezing, and cough. Approximately 20% to 30% of patients with symptoms of sore throat, fever, and lymphadenopathy are attributed to bacterial infection (**Fig. 3**). The most common bacterial cause is group A β-hemolytic *Streptococcus pyogenes*.[13] Early detection and treatment is necessary given the systemic complications of streptococcal infections including scarlet fever, rheumatic fever,

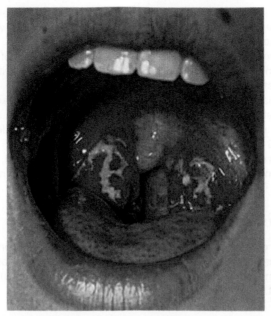

Fig. 3. Tonsils in the setting of group B streptococcal infection. Tonsils appear enlarged and erythematous with purulent discharge.

septic arthritis, and glomerulonephritis. The treatment of choice for streptococcal tonsillitis is penicillin-based antibiotics and rehydration.[14]

Diphtheria

Pharyngitis caused by the pathogen *Corynebacterium diptheriae* is very rare in the United States as a result of widespread immunization. However, cases have been reported in immunosuppressed children and recent immigrants. Diphtheria is characterized by high fever and sore throat with hypertrophic erythematous tonsils. A thick yellow gray pseudomembrane on the pharyngeal mucosa is pathognomonic for diphtheria. Delayed treatment may result in airway obstruction and neurologic and cardiac complications. Immediate treatment with intravenous penicillin and anitioxin is necessary.

Fungal Infections

Oral candidiasis is common in milk-fed infants, especially those infants who have taken broad-spectrum antibiotics. It presents with erythematous macules on the oral mucosa with a white membranous exudates that does not bleed with debridement. Treatment includes oral nystatin or ketoconazole.

Systemic Disease

Many systemic diseases have manifestations in the oral cavity, and may be diagnosed by recognition of these characteristics. Children with significant immunodeficiency, such as AIDS and leukemia, are at an increased risk for recurrent viral and bacterial infections of the oral cavity. Angular chelitis, hairy leukoplakia, and Kaposi sarcoma are three oral manifestations or systemic diseases that affect these children.

Common childhood viral infections, such as measles and varicella (chicken pox), also have oral manifestations. Koplik spots, nontender red lesions with a pale center, on the buccal mucosa are pathognomonic for measles.

Behçet syndrome is a systemic disease characterized by ulcers of the genitalia and urethra, uveitis, iridocyclitits, and recurrent ulcers of the oral cavity. Treatment includes systemic steroids and varied mouthwashes.[15]

Kawasaki disease is a disease of uncertain cause. It is characterized by 4 to 5 days of high fever; facial rash; and erythematous and painful lips, tongue, and oral mucosa. Other conditions resulting in tongue edema and erythema include iron deficiency anemia, vitamin B and C deficiency, and Sjögren syndrome.

Granulomatous diseases in the oral mucosa are exceedingly rare, but there can be oral manifestations in children with tuberculosis, Wegener granulomatosis, and leprosy.

CONGENITAL MALFORMATIONS OF THE ORAL CAVITY

Most embryonic development of the oral cavity occurs between the fourth and eighth week of gestation. Anomalies present at birth result from errors in embryogenesis during this time frame or as a result of intrauterine events that affect embryonic or fetal development.

The Lips

Clefting anomalies are far more common in the upper lip than the lower lip as a result of a more complex fusion in embryogenesis. Cleft upper lip and palate malformations are described in detail elsewhere in this issue.

Astomia results from complete fusion of the upper and lower lips. Microstomia refers to a small oral aperture. This condition is sometimes associated with other more serious conditions and syndromes, such as holoprosencephaly (**Fig. 4**). Macrostomia results from lateral clefting of the oral cavity stoma and requires surgical creation of new oral commissures to create a more normal stoma.

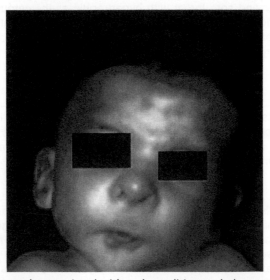

Fig. 4. Microstomia can be associated with such conditions as holoproscencephaly.

Lip pits may be present in association with a larger syndrome (Van der Woude) or as paired pits arising from secondary notching of the lip epithelium. These congenital pits are usually located in the paramedian location of the lower lip.[16] Lip pits may be associated with salivary glands at the base of the structure and often secrete a mucosalivary discharge (**Fig. 5**).

Labial frenula may develop abnormally and cause feeding and speech issues with the upper and lower lips. When the labial frenula extend over the alveolar ridge to the interdental papilla, it can result in abnormal eruption of teeth and periodontal disease. In these cases, surgical division is recommended to prevent spreading of the medial incisors or bone loss.

The Tongue

Maldevelopment of the lingual frenulum results in ankyloglossia or tongue tie. Physical findings that require surgical intervention include notching of the protruding tongue tip, inability of the tongue to contact the maxillary alveolar ridge, and restriction of tongue protrusion beyond the mandibular alveolus (**Figs. 6** and **7**).

Macroglossia can cause a wide range of symptoms from drooling and swallowing dysfunction to speech dysfunction and airway obstruction. Generalized macroglossia is more commonly associated with such syndromes as Down syndrome and Beckwith-Wiedemann syndrome.[17] Focal enlargement of the tongue is more characteristic of congenital tumors, such as hemangiomas or lymphangiomas. Rarely, tongue reduction surgery is indicated and is performed via a dorsal wedge resection and resection of the lateral margins of the tongue.

Other congenital anomalies of the tongue include bifid tongue, fissured tongue, geographic tongue, and median rhomboid glossitis. Geographic tongue is a chronic disorder of the filiform papillae. These appear as red lesions with white borders and tend to recur. Median rhomboid glossitis is an absence of papilla in the region of the embryonic tuberculum impar.[18]

Lingual thyroid tissue usually presents as a mass in the posterior midline of the tongue with symptoms of dysphagia, dysphonia, and occasional dyspnea. The thyroid develops from the floor of the pharynx at the foramen cecum and migrates inferiorly to reach its normal location in the inferior neck. Complications with this descent process can result in the development of a thyroglossal duct cyst or thyroid tissue at the base of the tongue.[19] Radionuclide scanning is important to determine if this is the only

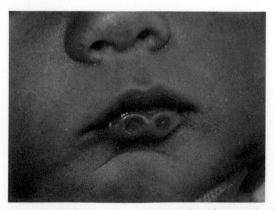

Fig. 5. Lip pits are most commonly found on the lower lip. They can be isolated entities or associated with larger syndromes.

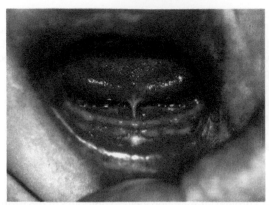

Fig. 6. Ankyloglossia, or "tongue tie," is routinely found in infants with difficulty latching on while feeding.

functioning thyroid tissue in the body. Excision should be avoided unless the mass is causing airway obstruction. If the lingual thyroid is resulting in symptoms for the patient, the mass can be reduced by administration of thyroid hormone.

The most common cysts of the oral cavity are the cysts and pseudocysts of the major and minor salivary glands. Mucoceles are pseudocysts because they lack an epithelial lining. These are formed by secretions dissecting into the soft tissues around the salivary gland and present as smooth, translucent masses that most commonly occur in the buccal mucosa. Surgical resection or unroofing of the mucocele is considered the gold standard for treatment (**Fig. 8**).

Ranulas are also pseudocysts that are frequently associated with the sublingual glands. Large ranulas can dissect through the sublingual space and mylohyoid muscle of the floor of the mouth into the neck. These "plunging ranulas" require complete excision, which includes removal of the sublingual gland to prevent recurrence (**Fig. 9**). A combined transoral-transcervial approach is frequently required.[20]

True cysts of the floor of mouth are rare but can be very troublesome in infancy. Foregut duplication cysts account for about one-third of duplications and arise from remnants of the stomach and first and second parts of the duodenum. They are classified as choristomas-containing tissues ectopic to their site of origin (**Fig. 10**). Oral

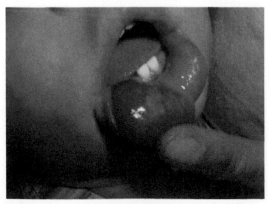

Fig. 7. Mucoceles are pseudocysts that develop from blocked salivary gland ducts. Surgical excision is usually required.

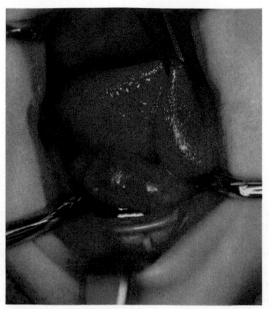

Fig. 8. Ranulas are also pseudocysts that are frequently associated with the sublingual glands.

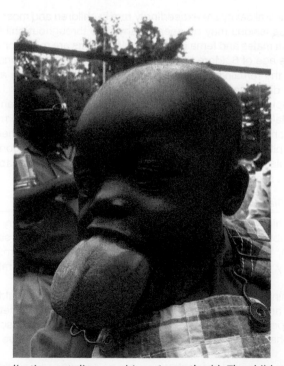

Fig. 9. Foregut duplication cyst discovered in a 4 month old. The child required tracheostomy and urgent decompression of the cyst to avoid airway compromise.

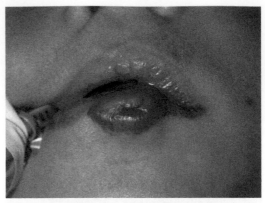

Fig. 10. Oral cavity hemangiomas can usually be treated with oral propranolol with good results. Surgical excision is required in cases of ulceration or bleeding.

cavity duplications may alternately reflect abnormal cellular migration because the primitive foregut and the pharyngeal arches are in close proximity.[21] When large enough these can be diagnosed in utero and perinatal planning can result in the need for an ex utero intrapartum treatment procedure to prevent airway compromise. Alternatively, the cyst can be marsupialized and definitive surgical excision can occur at a later time.

NEOPLASMS OF THE ORAL CAVITY

Neoplasms of the oral cavity are exceedingly rare in children and most of those tumors are benign. These lesions may be seen at any time throughout childhood and have equal incidence in males and females.[22] Vascular lesions are most common in children younger than the age of 6. More than two-thirds of oral cavity lesions arise from soft tissue, whereas the remaining third are derived from the mandible and maxilla. The latter of these is discussed elsewhere in this issue.

Malignant neoplasms arising in the oral cavity account for less than 5% of all childhood masses. Malignant tumors in this area are more often mesodermal in origin than ectodermal, which conflicts with the occurrence of tumors in all other sites.[22]

However, despite their infrequency, there is a wide variety of congenital and acquired oral neoplasms. As a result the otolaryngologist must be able to recognize these and have a systematic plan for evaluation and treatment.

Evaluation and Diagnosis

Evaluation of a child with an oral cavity mass begins with a full history. Important data that should be obtained include age of onset of mass; change in size; presence or absence of pain, bleeding, or inflammation; presence of other similar lesions; and any family history. Any problems with speech, swallowing, or respiration should also be documented.

Physical examination should focus on the head and neck and should account for the site, size, color, and texture of the mass. One should also note whether the mass is fixed or mobile, pedunculated or sessile, tender or painless, circumscribed or diffuse. A flexible nasopharyngoscopy can be used for evaluation of tongue base masses if necessary.

Some masses, such as hemangiomas, can be identified by history and physical alone. For other lesions, imaging provides additional data for diagnosis. Computed tomography and MRI scans may be indicated especially for preoperative surgical planning. Lesions that continue to enlarge, cause persistent symptoms, or are still difficult to diagnosis should undergo biopsy if they are easily accessible to ensure proper treatment.

BENIGN SOFT TISSUE ORAL CAVITY NEOPLASMS
Hemangiomas

Hemangiomas are the most common head and neck tumor in childhood. Hemangiomas and lymhpangiomas account for approximately 30% of oral cavity tumors in children with most occurring in the lip, cheek, and tongue in order of frequency (see **Fig. 10**).

Hemangiomas are classified as juvenile, capillary, cavernous, or mixed. They are usually not present at birth and have a rapid proliferation phase until 12 months of age.[23] At that time, they begin a slow involuting phase that can last up to age 6. Mucosal hemangiomas are raised and red, whereas submucosal hemangiomas appear blue or purple. Extensive replacement of the lip and the tongue by hemangiomas has been described. Macroglossia secondary to circumscribed hemangiomas within the tongue itself can be differentiated by a more systemic process but the circumscribed vascular nature of the mass.

Because hemangiomas have a natural involuting course, conservative management is usually recommended. Active management is warranted when complications arise from uncontrolled hemorrhage, pain, ulceration, infection, or airway obstruction.[24]

Treatment of oral cavity hemangiomas begins with medical therapy. Propranolol is the drug of choice for first-line treatment. Although the exact mechanism of action is not completely known, there are countless examples in the literature of significant reduction in size and color changes in children treated with propranolol during the proliferation phase for at least 6 months. In addition to propranolol, oral or systemic corticosteroids have been shown to be effective in 30% to 60% of hemangiomas.[24] In addition to medical therapy, surgical excision, carbon dioxide laser treatment, cryosurgery, and sclerosing agents have all been used in the management of large oral cavity hemangiomas.

Vascular Malformations

Unlike hemangiomas, vascular malformations are present at birth and grow proportionately with the child. Vascular malformations fluctuate in size in response to infection, trauma, and hormonal changes in the patient, and can cause skeletal abnormalities as a result of mass effect on surrounding bones.

Vascular malformations are described by the type of vessel involved. They are subdivided into capillary, venous, arterial, lymphatic, or in some instances a combination of two vessels. Capillary, venous, and lymphatic malformations are classified as low-flow lesions, whereas arterial and arteriovenous malformations are classified as high-flow lesions (**Fig. 11**). Appearance of physical examination and imaging with MRI can help to differentiate between the two classes.[25]

Treatment of vascular malformations depends on the particular class of lesion. Lymphatic malformations often involve the oral cavity, specifically the tongue and floor of mouth. Infections, such as upper respiratory infections, cause significant and rapid enlargement of the size of lymphatic malformations. When these are located in the tongue and floor of mouth, rapid treatment is necessary to prevent possible airway compromise (**Fig. 12**). Microcystic lymphatic malformations, those containing cysts smaller than 2 cm^3, are treated with surgical excision as the primary treatment.[26] If

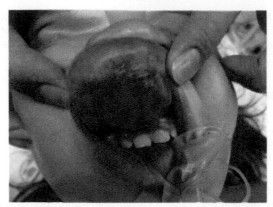

Fig. 11. Vascular malformations do not respond to propranolol. Embolization, sclerotherapy, and surgical excision are the most accepted treatment modalities.

the microcystic lymphatic malformation is in an area that is not amenable to surgical excision or has recurred following attempted surgical excision, rapamycin has recently become an option for these lesions. A 6-month course of treatment with rapamycin has been shown to slow the growth or shrink the size of these difficult masses.[27] Macrocystic lymphatic malformations that consists of isolated or multiple cysts greater than 2 cm^3 are treated via surgical excision or sclerotherapy with any number of sclerosing agents.[26]

Venous, arterial, and mixed malformations can be treated with different modalities. These lesions are much more vascular than their lymphatic counterparts, which makes surgical excision difficult because of potential blood loss. The goal of treatment is complete removal of the lesion; however, it is important to not sacrifice normal anatomy given the benign nature of these malformations.

Venous malformations have been successfully treated with sclerotherapy in the lips, tongue, and cheeks. Under fluoroscopic guidance, the contents of the mass are drawn off via syringe, and a sclerosing agent (ethanol, sodium tetradecyl sulfate, OK432) is then injected into the mass. The goal of this treatment is scarring of the walls of the malformation to prevent reaccumulation. Multiple treatments are usually necessary

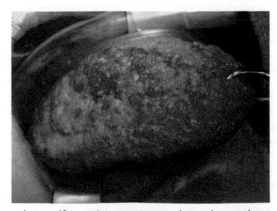

Fig. 12. Lymphovascular malformation treatment depends on the primary vessel type involved. This case required sclerotherapy and partial glossectomy.

for larger lesions, and can be complicated by necrosis of the surrounding tissues and interim or long-term neural injury from reaction to the sclerosing agents.[25]

Arterial and arteriovenous malformations are considered high-flow lesions, which makes surgical excision problematic. Embolization of these lesions with the help of an interventional radiologist is the first-line treatment. Surgical excision after embolization is often required, but incomplete excision of an arteriovenous malformations may lead to increased collateral flow and enlargement of the lesion.[28]

Cystic Lesions

Mucoceles present as soft, painless, smooth masses that are commonly found in the oral cavity. They usually appear on the tongue and floor of mouth, but can occasionally appear in the valeculla resulting in airway obstruction.

A ranula is a mucocele that develops on the floor of mouth. These cysts appear as mucosal covered, translucent bluish white mass. Ranulas form as a result of obstruction of the sublingual gland duct. Ranulas can present with an accompanying neck mass. A computed tomography scan helps define the relationship between the two masses. If the ranula tracks down through the mylohyoid muscle and into the neck it is referred to as a "plunging ranula." Complete surgical excision, with removal of the sublingual gland, is the recommended treatment.

Fibrous Tumors

These benign, but locally aggressive tumors derive from the musculoaponeuroses. The most common of these tumors are referred to as desmoids or fibromatosis tumors. Fifteen percent to 30% of pediatric desmoids tumors occur in the head and neck. Although they are histologically benign, they are locally aggressive and can erode or even invade surrounding soft tissue and bony structures.[29] Aggressive surgical treatment with wide local excision is recommended, but patients must have close follow-up given the high recurrence rate seen in desmoid tumors.

Epithelial Tumors

A variety of benign epithelial masses are found in the oral cavity. Oral squamous papillomas of the tongue, palate, and lips are the most common mucosal lesions. Unlike squamous papillomas found in other parts of the body, oral cavity papillomas do not show a potential for premalignant transformation. They respond well to local surgical excision.

A white sponge nevus is a rare familial form of epithelial hyperplasia of the oral mucosa. The lesion occurs either at birth or later in childhood as a diffuse, whitish, thickened lesion usually presenting on the buccal mucosa, lips, or tongue.[30] The lesion can progress but is essentially benign and requires no specific treatment.

Approximately 20% of head and neck dermoids appear in the oral cavity. Dermoids present in the anterior floor of mouth at birth or may not manifest themselves until the second or third decade of life. Complete surgical excision is the treatment of choice.

Miscellaneous Tumors

Granular cell tumors occur throughout the body, but in the oral cavity they are found in the tongue. They are a result of a benign proliferation of neurogenic elements of the Schwann cell. Granular cell tumors present as a firm subcutaneous nodule within the tongue. A congenital granular cell tumor located on the alveolar ridge is called epulis of newborn.[31] Recurrence of these lesions is rare following complete surgical excision.

Neural Tumors

Multiple endocrine neoplasia syndrome type II (Sipple syndrome) is characterized by hyperparathyroidism; medullary thyroid carcinoma; pheochromocytoma; and multiple neuromas of the lip, also known as "bumpy lip syndrome." Neurofibromas can be seen in the oral cavity as a symptom of neurofibromatosis type 1 or as solitary lesions. The plexiform type may be difficult to control locally.

MALIGNANT TUMORS OF THE ORAL CAVITY

Malignant tumors of the oral cavity are exceedingly rare in the pediatric population. They account for less than 10% of all tumors in children. As a result, there are very little reliable data with regard to incidence, treatment recommendations, or prognosis. The three most common groups of malignant masses are (1) rhabdomyosarcoma, (2) sarcomas, and (3) epidermoid carcinomas.

Rhabdomyosarcoma

Rhabdomyosarcoma is an embryonic malignant neoplasm of skeletal muscle. It is the most common soft tissue malignancy of childhood and the most common sarcoma of the head and neck in children. Rhabdomyosarcoma has two age peaks, the first between 2 and 6 years of age, and the second in adolescence. Within the oral cavity, the most common sites of involvement are the tongue, palate, and cheeks.

Rhabdomyosarcoma usually presents as a mass that initially has a benign polypoid appearance but soon undergoes rapid growth, ulceration, and bleeding. Given the rapid growth of these tumors, metastatic disease, most commonly to the lungs and bones, is common at the time of diagnosis. There are three subtypes of rhabdomyosarcoma: (1) embryonal, (2) alveolar, and (3) botyroid. Most head and neck rhabdomyosarcomas are embryonal.[32]

Treatment of rhabdomyosarcoma is largely determined by primary site of involvement. Complete surgical excision is reserved for only smaller lesions to avoid functional or cosmetic morbidity. Surgery is usually reserved for diagnostic biopsy. Before the use of adjuvant chemotherapy and radiation, survival rates were less than 10% at 5-year survival. However, now local therapy with local excision, chemotherapy, and radiation has yielded remission rates as high as 87% for certain subtypes.[33] Within the oral cavity, aggressive surgical excision is rarely used given the possible functional consequences, and chemoradiation is the treatment of choice. Recent data suggest patients who are disease-free at 2 years will remain in remission. However, those that recur in less than 2 years have a poor chance of long-term survival.[34]

Oral Sarcomas

Specific oral sarcomas reported in the pediatric population include fibrosarcoma, leiomyosarcoma, angiosarcoma, Kaposi sarcoma, and reticulum cell sarcoma. Sarcomas usually present as a bulky, infiltrating submucosal mass. Kaposi sarcoma of the oral cavity is very rare, but the presence should alert the physician to the possibility of AIDS for that patient. Treatment consists of some combination of surgery, chemotherapy, and radiation, but prognosis is poor.

Epidermoid Carcinoma

This is an extremely rare tumor in children. Squamous cell carcinomas in the oral cavity in adults are usually the result of prolonged tobacco or alcohol abuse. In children, the incidence of this is most likely related to genetic factors or immunodeficiency. Oral squamous cell carcinomas in children have been linked to organ transplant recipients who are immunosuppressed. Pediatric tumors are treated in similar fashion as their adult counterparts but have been shown to be more virulent with poorer prognosis.

REFERENCES

1. Crelin ES. Development of the upper respiratory system. Clin Symp 1976;28(3): 1–30.
2. Winning TA, Townsend GC. Oral mucosal embryology and histology. Clin Dermatol 2000;18(5):499–511.
3. Emmanouil-Nikoloussi EN, Kerameos-Foroglou C. Developmental malformations of human tongue and associated syndromes (review). Bull Group Int Rech Sci Stomatol Odontol 1992;35(1–2):5–12.
4. Vidic B, Melloni BJ. Applied anatomy of the oral cavity and related structures. Otolaryngol Clin North Am 1979;12(1):3–14.
5. Whetzel TP, Saunders CJ. Arterial anatomy of the oral cavity: an analysis of vascular territories. Plast Reconstr Surg 1997;100(3):582–7 [discussion: 588–90].
6. Levin LS, Johns ME. Lesions of the oral mucous membranes. Otolaryngol Clin North Am 1986;19(1):87–102.
7. Brunell PA. Indications for oral acyclovir in children. Pediatr Infect Dis J 1993; 12(11):970.
8. Porter SR, Scully C. Aphthous stomatitis: an overview of aetiopathogenesis and management. Clin Exp Dermatol 1991;16(4):235–43.
9. Cherry JD, Jahn CL. Herpangina: the etiologic spectrum. Pediatrics 1965;36(4): 632–4.
10. Richardson HB Jr, Leibovitz A. "Hand, foot, and mouth disease" in children; an epidemic associated with coxsackievirus a-16. J Pediatr 1965;67:6–12.
11. Derkay CS, Wiatrak B. Recurrent respiratory papillomatosis: a review. Laryngoscope 2008;118(7):1236–47.
12. Dowling BT. Acute ulcerative gingivitis (Vincent's infection). Old ideas and current concepts. Bull N Z Soc Periodontol 1968;25:2–9 contd.
13. Tuner K, Nord CE. Emergence of beta-lactamase producing anaerobic bacteria in the tonsils during penicillin treatment. Eur J Clin Microbiol 1986;5(4):399–404.
14. Van Asselt GJ, Mouton RP. Detection of penicillin tolerance in Streptococcus pyogenes. J Med Microbiol 1993;38(3):197–202.
15. Lehner T. Pathology of recurrent oral ulceration and oral ulceration in Behcet's syndrome: light, electron and fluorescence microscopy. J Pathol 1969;97(3): 481–94.
16. Krauel L, Francisco Jose Parri, Angeles M. Sancho, et al. Van der Woude syndrome and lower lip pits treatment. J Oral Maxillofac Surg 2008;66(3):589–92.
17. Rimell FL, Shapiro AM, Shoemaker DL, et al. Head and neck manifestations of Beckwith-Wiedemann syndrome. Otolaryngol Head Neck Surg 1995;113(3): 262–5.
18. Drezner DA, Schaffer SR. Geographic tongue. Otolaryngol Head Neck Surg 1997;117(3 Pt 1):291.
19. Williams JD, Sclafani AP, Slupchinskij O, et al. Evaluation and management of the lingual thyroid gland. Ann Otol Rhinol Laryngol 1996;105(4):312–6.
20. Matt BH, Crockett DM. Plunging ranula in an infant. Otolaryngol Head Neck Surg 1988;99(3):330–3.
21. Batsakis JG, el-Naggar AK, Hicks MJ. Epithelial choristomas and teratomas of the tongue. Ann Otol Rhinol Laryngol 1993;102(7):567–9.

22. Bhaskar SN. Oral tumors of infancy and childhood. A survey of 293 cases. J Pediatr 1963;63:195–210.
23. Burrows PE. Hemangiomas and vascular malformations. Can Assoc Radiol J 1995;46(2):143.
24. Musumeci ML, Schlecht K, Perrotta R, et al. Management of cutaneous hemangiomas in pediatric patients. Cutis 2008;81(4):315–22.
25. Glade RS, Richter GT, James CA, et al. Diagnosis and management of pediatric cervicofacial venous malformations: retrospective review from a vascular anomalies center. Laryngoscope 2010;120(2):229–35.
26. Boardman SJ, Cochrane LA, Roebuck D, et al. Multimodality treatment of pediatric lymphatic malformations of the head and neck using surgery and sclerotherapy. Arch Otolaryngol Head Neck Surg 2010;136(3):270–6.
27. Luo Y, Lei Liu, Donna Rogers, et al. Rapamycin inhibits lymphatic endothelial cell tube formation by downregulating vascular endothelial growth factor receptor 3 protein expression. Neoplasia 2012;14(3):228–37.
28. Palafox D, Sierra-Juarez MA, Cordova-Quintal PM. High flow arteriovenous malformation in the neck. Acta Otorhinolaryngol Esp 2014;65(5):324–5.
29. Masson JK, Soule EH. Desmoid tumors of the head and neck. Am J Surg 1966; 112(4):615–22.
30. Cummings CW. Cummings otolaryngology head & neck surgery. 4th edition. Philadelphia: Elsevier Mosby; 2005.
31. Bluestone CD, Simons JP, Healy GB. Bluestone and Stool's pediatric otolaryngology. 5th edition. Philadelphia (PA): WB Sanders Company; 1996.
32. Raney RB Jr, Crist WM, Maurer HM, et al. Prognosis of children with soft tissue sarcoma who relapse after achieving a complete response. A report from the Intergroup Rhabdomyosarcoma Study I. Cancer 1983;52(1):44–50.
33. van Grotel M, Nowak P, Meeuwis CA, et al. Long-term remission after non-radical surgery combined with brachytherapy in an infant with a chemo-resistant rhabdomyosarcoma of the tongue. Med Pediatr Oncol 2003;41(6):558–61.
34. Kraft SM, Singh V, Sykes KJ, et al. Differentiating between congenital rhabdomyosarcoma versus fibromatosis of the pediatric tongue. Int J Pediatr Otorhinolaryngol 2010;74(7):781–5.

Prenatal Diagnosis of Obstructive Head and Neck Masses and Perinatal Airway Management

The Ex Utero Intrapartum Treatment Procedure

Patrick C. Walz, MD[a,b], James W. Schroeder Jr, MD[c],*

KEYWORDS

- EXIT procedure • *Ex utero* intrapartum treatment
- Congenital high airway obstruction • Teratoma • Lymphatic malformation
- Congenital airway obstruction

KEY POINTS

- The ex utero intrapartum treatment (EXIT) procedure allows partial delivery of a fetus with prenatally diagnosed airway obstruction in a controlled fashion, allowing continued placental function while the fetal airway is secured.
- The EXIT procedure requires input from a coordinated multidisciplinary team including representatives from anesthesiology, maternal-fetal medicine, neonatology, nursing, respiratory therapy, and pediatric otolaryngology.
- Despite advancements in the procedure, patients requiring EXIT are uniformly critically ill.
- Extensive counseling regarding the risks of the procedure, the appropriateness of the procedure, and alternative management strategies should be reviewed with the family before deciding whether to proceed.

INTRODUCTION

Neonatal airway obstruction that is diagnosed at delivery creates an emergent situation with high morbidity. This obstruction may be either intrinsic (due to abnormalities in laryngotracheal development) or extrinsic (from a congenital head and neck mass or anatomic deformation). Every situation requires an individualized approach to secure

[a] Department of Pediatric Otolaryngology, Ann and Robert H. Lurie Children's Hospital of Chicago, 225 E. Chicago Ave, Box 23, Chicago, IL 60611-2991, USA; [b] Department of Otolaryngology Head and Neck Surgery, The Ohio State University, 9000 Olentangy River Rd, Suite 4000, Columbus, OH 43212, USA; [c] Department of Otolaryngology-Head and Neck Surgery and Medical Education, Northwestern University Feinberg School of Medicine, Chicago, IL, USA
* Corresponding author.
E-mail address: JSchroeder@luriechildrens.org

Otolaryngol Clin N Am 48 (2015) 191–207
http://dx.doi.org/10.1016/j.otc.2014.09.013
0030-6665/15/$ – see front matter © 2015 Elsevier Inc. All rights reserved.

the airway that often uses specialized equipment and personnel. In the last 20 years, advances and innovations have been made in prenatal imaging, maternal and fetal anesthesia, and fetal surgery that have significantly altered the management of patients with congenital airway obstruction. Owing to widespread use of prenatal ultrasonography,[1,2] patients with airway obstruction can now be prenatally diagnosed. Often the degree of obstruction can also be estimated. With advances in fetal surgery, congenital malformations that were previously considered to be untreatable or lethal can be ameliorated, leading to improved neonatal viability.[3] Advances in maternal-fetal anesthesia have enabled a transition from the light anesthesia and increased uterine tone typical of traditional cesarean section to the deep anesthesia and uterine relaxation that facilitates maintenance of uteroplacental circulation and fetal anesthesia.[4–6] The confluence of these advances has allowed development of the ex utero intrapartum treatment (EXIT) procedure, whereby prenatally diagnosed patients with airway obstruction undergo partial delivery and, while maintained on placental support, undergo airway instrumentation to secure the airway before completion of delivery and umbilical cord clamping.

Development of the Ex Utero Intrapartum Tracheoplasty Procedure

Although the EXIT procedure was initially developed for the management of congenital diaphragmatic hernia (CDH), allowing a controlled intrapartum setting in which a previously placed tracheal clip, plug, or balloon could be removed and the airway assessed,[3] the procedure quickly was adopted for the management of congenital airway obstruction. There are multiple published reports and case series describing intrapartum airway management,[7–10] but these reports used either vaginal delivery or standard cesarean delivery techniques without consideration for the maintenance of amniotic fluid volume to prolong uteroplacental circulation. Contemporaneous with the initial descriptions of EXIT for the management of congenital diaphragmatic hernia was the initial description of the operation on placental support (OOPS), which discussed the need for uterine relaxation and used subtotal delivery of the fetus, although no specific mention of maintenance of uterine volume is made.[11] Although this report by Skarsgard and colleagues[11] represents the first description of controlled intrapartum airway management of congenital airway compression, the first description of the EXIT procedure as it is known today is credited to Mychaliska and colleagues[12] in 1997, in which they present CDH data that include 2 reports of EXIT for lymphatic malformations of the neck and oropharynx. Whether because of the dubious nature of Skarsgard's chosen acronym (OOPS) or true differences in surgical technique, the preferred terminology has remained EXIT in subsequent literature.

Expansion of Indications for Procedure

Following the initial description of EXIT, its indications have expanded to include 4 broad categories: EXIT to airway, EXIT to resection, EXIT to extracorporeal membranous oxygenation (ECMO), and EXIT to separation.[1] Specific indications within these categories are outlined in **Table 1**. As the focus herein is on the role of the otolaryngologist–head and neck surgeon in EXIT, the remaining discussion is limited to EXIT procedures performed for congenital head and neck anomalies producing either intrinsic or extrinsic airway obstruction. This review presents the preoperative and perioperative assessment and management of patients with prenatally diagnosed airway obstruction, indications and contraindications for the EXIT procedure, technical details of the procedure, and outcomes.

| Table 1 | | | |
| Indications for ex utero intrapartum treatment (EXIT) procedure | | | |
	Obstruction Source	Examples	
EXIT to airway	Extrinsic	Teratoma (cervical, pharyngeal, epignathus)[13,22,23,25,28]	
		Lymphatic/vascular malformation[11–13,33]	
		Congenital giant ranula[21]	
		Severe micrognathia[1]	
	Intrinsic	Congenital high airway obstruction syndrome (CHAOS)[23,40–42,48]	
	Iatrogenic	Tracheal clipping or Balloon occlusion in congenital diaphragmatic hernia[3]	
EXIT to resection		Thoracic/mediastinal masses[1]	
		Congenital cystic adenomatoid malformations (CCAM)[1]	
		Bronchopulmonary sequestration[1,56]	
		Fetal lobar interstitial tumor[56]	
		Mediastinal teratoma[1]	
EXIT to ECMO		Severe congenital heart disease[1,57,58]	
		Severe congenital diaphragmatic hernia[1]	
EXIT to separation		Conjoined twins[53]	

Abbreviation: ECMO, extracorporeal membranous oxygenation.

TREATMENT GOALS AND PLANNED OUTCOMES
Goals

Stated simply, the goal of the EXIT procedure is to convert what was formerly an emergent procedure, establishing a neonatal airway, into a controlled procedure. This overarching goal is achieved by using a multidisciplinary team approach whereby each team member accomplishes individual objectives.

Radiology and maternal-fetal medicine

The goals of the radiologist and maternal-fetal medicine specialist are to accurately diagnose fetal pathophysiology and aid in the selection of appropriate candidates for EXIT. This prenatal diagnostic information was initially obtained using 2-dimensional ultrasonography. Advances in ultrasound technology now allow for 3-dimensional and 4-dimensional imaging, which provide additional detail and 3-dimensional renderings of fetal anatomy. Detailed imaging has sometimes identified patients who do not require EXIT and who can be managed by means of traditional delivery.[2] If airway obstruction is suspected based on findings identified on ultrasonography, a fetal magnetic resonance (MR) image is obtained to further delineate the anatomy.[1] MR imaging has been shown to have greater than 90% sensitivity for predicting the etiology of obstructive lesions in these situations.[13] Ultrasonography can have an intraoperative role in confirmation of fetal position, ultrasound-guided cyst decompression, and mapping of placental edges before hysterotomy so as to avoid maternal hemorrhage.

Anesthesia

The goals of the anesthesia team are to achieve a deep plane of anesthesia while maintaining uterine relaxation and maternal blood pressure and blood flow to the uterus. In addition, the anesthesia team must consider the impact of the maternal anesthetic on the fetus. In contrast to cesarean delivery, the transmission of anesthetic to the fetus is desired in the EXIT procedure, as the fetus may require multiple stimulating interventions to secure the airway. To achieve these goals, multiple anesthetic techniques have been published. All, at their root, include achieving a deep general anesthetic; either by use an inhaled anesthetic titrated to 2 to 3 minimum alveolar concentration (MAC), or by using a combination of intravenous anesthetics (such as propofol and a narcotic), with a lower MAC of inhaled anesthetic gas. In addition, ephedrine is used as needed to support maternal blood pressure, and nitroglycerin is added as needed to augment uterine relaxation.[4–6]

Obstetrics

The goals of the maternal-fetal medicine team are to maintain uteroplacental circulation, ensure safe delivery of the fetus, limit maternal blood loss, and ensure maternal safety. Achieving these goals requires the careful planning of the hysterotomy incision using a hemostatic stapler.[14,15] Also, preincision mapping of placental edges so it can be avoided helps prevent maternal hemorrhage and continue placental circulation.[16,17] In addition, securing the amniotic membranes to the uterine wall and using amnioinfusion will aid in the maintenance of uterine amniotic fluid volume, which contributes to the long-term maintenance of placental circulation.[15] Following successful fetal airway instrumentation, the obstetric team works in concert with the anesthesia team to complete delivery of the fetus, repair the uterus, and reverse uterine relaxation.[3,12,15]

Otolaryngology

The goal of the otolaryngology team is to secure the fetal airway. Following partial delivery of the fetus, a preplanned algorithm (see later description) is followed in an ascendingly invasive manner as needed.

Neonatology

The goal of the neonatology team is to stabilize the neonate following delivery. This task is made difficult in part by the potential pulmonary problems that may accompany EXIT deliveries. There are published case reports describing pulmonary hypoplasia thought to be due to extreme fetal neck flexion, caused by a congenital neck mass compressing the lungs against the thoracic outlet.[18–20] The presence of an experienced neonatology team is essential to the care of the critically ill neonate. In addition, the neonatal team must ensure adequate sedation and analgesia of the neonate. Recent literature suggests that the pain response is intact in the late-term fetus, and early exposure to painful stimuli may alter the development of central pathways.[5]

Indications and Contraindications

Indications

The EXIT procedure may be considered in cases where there is a prenatally diagnosed upper airway obstruction that would be lethal or potentially lethal if traditional delivery were undertaken. Primarily, these obstructions are caused by head and neck teratoma, lymphatic/vascular malformations, severe micrognathia, and congenital high airway obstruction syndrome (CHAOS). Other unique indications, such as congenital giant ranula[21] and fetal epignathus,[22] have also been described. Not every prenatally diagnosed head and neck mass requires EXIT. Specific indications have been suggested as criteria for use of the EXIT procedure. These criteria include the diagnosis of a teratoma, mass size greater than 5 cm, polyhydramnios or absence of fetal gastric fluid suggesting obstruction of the alimentary canal, or signs of intrinsic airway obstruction such as hyperexpanded lungs or flattened diaphragm.[23,24] Ultimately, any airway anticipated to be difficult based on review of prenatal imaging also warrants consideration by the EXIT team.

Teratoma Teratoma is a germ cell tumor that can occur in the fetal head and neck.[25] Teratomas can present from mandible to clavicle, and can extend into the tongue and floor of the mouth.[26] These tumors are characterized by components from all germ cell layers and rarely have malignant potential.[26,27] Typically they originate near midline and tend to compress the aerodigestive tract against the spine, rather than distorting the location of the airway.[28] When compared with all patients with obstructive head and neck masses, patients with teratoma are more likely to require surgical intervention during EXIT,[13,19] likely because of the solid incompressible nature of teratoma that makes exposure of the larynx with direct laryngoscopy difficult. Teratomas also have a propensity for intratumoral hemorrhage. For these reasons, even if there is no airway obstruction at birth, intubation to secure the airway and excision of the lesion as soon as possible has been recommended.[25] Though typically isolated anomalies, teratoma can be associated with chondrodystrophia fetalis, imperforate anus, hypoplastic left heart, mandibular hypoplasia, and Patau syndrome.[26,29]

Lymphatic/vascular malformation Lymphatic malformation (LM) is the most common head and neck indication for EXIT,[17] and occurs most frequently in the head and neck. These lesions tend to be more infiltrative than teratoma in tissues, and tend toward displacement of the aerodigestive tract rather than compression of the lumen against the spine.[28] LMs demonstrate a bimodal distribution with respect to timing of appearance in fetal development, with important implications for incidence of associated chromosomal anomalies, location of the malformation, and outcome.[17,26] LMs identified early in the second trimester arise most commonly in the posterior triangle of the neck, are associated with chromosomal anomalies in 60% of cases, have multiple associated structural anomalies, and are associated with hydrops and a high mortality.[26] However, LMs identified in the third trimester or diagnosed at birth arise in a more anterior position, are rarely associated with chromosomal anomalies, and have a much lower mortality.[26] Use of the de Serres staging[30] and Cologne Disease Score for LMs have been used to predict complications and clinical outcomes.[31–33] After establishment of a secure airway and safe delivery, LMs can be managed with surgical excision or sclerotherapy.[33–35]

Severe micrognathia The micrognathic (underdeveloped) and retrognathic (retrodisplaced) mandible caused by mandibular hypoplasia can displace the tongue base, obstructing the aerodigestive tract. In the most severe cases, the obstruction is to a degree that endotracheal intubation and respiration are likely impossible. As a result of fetal inability to swallow amniotic fluid, polyhydramnios develops during gestation.[36,37] Only the most severe cases of mandibular hypoplasia require EXIT. Management by endotracheal intubation over a flexible fiberoptic bronchoscope by itself or via an intubating laryngeal mask airway such as the Air-Q (Mercury Medical, Clearwater, FL, USA) can be used in most cases of micrognathia to secure the airway.[38] The jaw index has been developed to diagnose micrognathia, measuring the ratio of the difference of the anterior and posterior mandibular diameter to the biparietal diameter.[39] Micrognathia is diagnosed with 100% specificity and 98.1% sensitivity when the jaw index is less than 23.[39] Several investigators have applied the jaw index and have identified several factors that increase the likelihood for requiring perinatal intervention such as EXIT. These factors include objective findings of a jaw index less than the fifth percentile and findings suggestive of esophageal obstruction (ultrasonography suggesting polyhydramnios or the absence of a gastric bubble), or MR imaging evidence of glossoptosis.[17,37]

Congenital high airway obstruction syndrome CHAOS encompasses a spectrum of disease from laryngeal web to complete laryngeal and/or tracheal stenosis. It is defined radiographically by a triad of ultrasonographic findings: large echogenic lungs, flattened or everted diaphragm, and dilated airways distal to the site of obstruction.[40,41] With complete obstruction, ascites and, ultimately, hydrops develop from lymphatic and cardiac compression, with the potential for fetal demise.[15] As a result, fetuses with CHAOS require frequent monitoring so that intervention may be undertaken at the time ascites is found to develop.[15] In some cases, a small tracheoesophageal fistula or pinpoint tracheal/laryngeal lumen allows for decompression of the hyperinflated lungs, with cessation of the progression to hydrops.[40] However, if no such "release valve" exists and the patient progresses toward ascites and polyhydramnios, fetoscopic intervention can be undertaken and wire tracheoplasty performed to create a route for decompression.[40,42] Whereas CHAOS is most frequently a sporadic finding, laryngotracheal atresia can be associated with chromosomal anomalies or Fraser syndrome (laryngeal anomalies, cryptophthalmos, syndactyly, genitourinary tract malformations, craniofacial anomalies, orofacial clefting, mental retardation, and musculoskeletal anomalies).[15,40] There is also a suggestion of a possible autosomal dominant inheritance pattern.[43,44] In the presence of other anomalies, prenatal and perinatal mortality increase,[40] a situation that must be thoroughly reviewed during preoperative counseling. Whereas CHAOS was previously fatal, EXIT has allowed the controlled delivery of affected fetuses, confirmation of the diagnosis with bronchoscopy, and establishment of the airway with tracheostomy. EXIT has transitioned CHAOS from a uniformly lethal condition to a surgically manageable disease. CHAOS remains a condition with the potential for significant long-term morbidity, including ventilator dependence and the need for airway reconstruction.[26]

Contraindications

The EXIT procedure is a high-risk procedure for two patients. As such, a thorough consideration of the risks, both maternal and fetal, must be weighed against the likelihood of achieving the potential benefits. Instances in which the balance of risks to benefits is shifted more toward incurring additional maternal and fetal risk with low likelihood of benefit represent contraindications to proceeding with EXIT.

Maternal No absolute contraindications to EXIT exist from a maternal standpoint. From a technical standpoint, uterine anomalies and placental position may significantly increase the technical difficulty of the procedure, but these considerations do not represent absolute contraindications. Moreover, the concern for increased risk of maternal complications has been discussed as a relative contraindication to EXIT. Reports have demonstrated a significant increase in maternal blood loss and superficial wound infection in comparison with cesarean section, but no difference was appreciated in hematocrit change or incidence of endometritis or in overall infectious complications.[45] These findings suggest that the statistically significant differences may not have clinical significance. More recent reports have demonstrated that EXIT represents a safe option with risks similar to those of cesarean section.[19,23] In the obstetric literature, a recent publication suggests that the benefits of EXIT far outweigh maternal risks.[14]

Fetal Fetal considerations represent the more likely source of contraindications to EXIT. Critical evaluation of prenatal imaging may suggest that the neonatal airway would be attainable after delivery with the use of direct laryngoscopy or laryngeal mask airway, without need for placental support. In a recent report from Lazar and colleagues,[19] one-third of patients referred for EXIT did not require the procedure because of minimal tracheal involvement. On the opposite end of the spectrum, cases of CHAOS with complete tracheal agenesis may not allow successful tracheostomy to be performed,[42] making EXIT delivery a futile exercise. Moreover, consideration of the viability of the neonate, accounting not only for the gravity of the airway anomaly but also considering any other concomitant anomalies, should be carefully weighed before electing to proceed with EXIT. Certain causes of obstruction (eg, cervical teratoma and LM) are associated with other chromosomal abnormalities. When present, the mortality of EXIT increases to more than 36%.[17] This risk must be assessed and considered in discussions with the family. However, the mortality of non-EXIT delivery in patients with obstructive head and neck lesions is approximately 80%,[46] a factor that must be considered when deciding to offer EXIT.

Special consideration must also be taken in the case of a multiple fetal pregnancy. If the EXIT procedure is performed for the benefit of one fetus with an obstructed airway, but will expose the other nonobstructed fetus to a significant level of risk, the procedure should be subject to an additional level of scrutiny. In this case and in any case where the ratio of risks to benefits is not clear, an independent ethical consultation should be considered.

PREOPERATIVE PLANNING AND PREPARATION

The importance of preoperative team planning for an EXIT cannot be overstated. The early prenatal diagnosis of a potentially obstructive head and neck lesion enables all involved medical professionals to be assembled, and an EXIT to be initiated that optimizes the chance of a successful outcome. This preparation begins with the imaging. The initial screening ultrasonographic examination is typically followed by higher-resolution ultrasonography and fetal MR imaging using HASTE (half-Fourier acquisition single-shot turbo spin-echo) sequences developed to optimally image fetal anatomy and minimize motion artifact.[1,14,17,47] These images can be reviewed and the nature, location, and extent of airway obstruction delineated. Identification of EXIT candidates typically occurs in the weeks following the standard obstetric 20-week sonogram.[26]

After identifying a patient as a candidate for EXIT, a frank and thorough discussion with the family must be undertaken wherein the risks and benefits of the procedure are discussed. Family counseling must include risks of the procedure to both fetus and mother, alternatives to EXIT (comfort care, standard delivery with urgent airway intervention), and review of risks of alternative management strategies.

After the maternal-fetal medicine, neonatology, otolaryngology, and anesthesia teams and the family agree to proceed with EXIT, a planned date between 34 and 37 weeks' gestation is selected.[26] The idea is to initiate EXIT before the beginning of natural labor. In the weeks leading up to the EXIT, the team regularly meets to coordinate the timing, equipment, and personnel required. In 2012, Stefini and colleagues[33] published a flow chart identifying the teams, procedures, and planned durations during the critical periods of the EXIT procedure that could be useful in preoperative planning. The entire EXIT team should consider gathering for a rehearsal in the operating room before EXIT to address any logistical issues. This aspect is particularly important because the delivery room/operating suite will be more crowded than usual, with specialized equipment and staff from multiple medical specialties. Coordinating the sequence and timing of movements of people and equipment around the surgical field is critical to avoid complications.

PATIENT POSITIONING

When preparing for EXIT, careful consideration must be given to the layout of the operating room and the positioning of the patient. Several previous reports have described configurations allowing appropriate access to the mother and fetus.[1,33,47,48]

The number of personnel ranges from 6 to 15 in the schemes describing a singleton delivery to 21 team members for an EXIT twin delivery.[48] The suggested personnel are listed in **Table 2**. Given the volume of equipment and personnel, an organized layout with dedicated maternal personnel and neonatal personnel is suggested. Furthermore, the room design should allow for a separate surgical setup in the primary operating suite or in an adjacent room should immediate surgical intervention on the neonate be required.[1,15]

In addition to accounting for the number of personnel involved, the fact that obstetrics, otolaryngology, neonatology, and, possibly, pediatric anesthesia may, at various points in the procedure, require simultaneous access to the maternal abdomen should be noted. The standard lithotomy position with a slight leftward tilt to improve maternal venous return is recommended, and each team should understand its relative positioning around the patient.

PROCEDURAL APPROACH

With appropriate preparation, planning, and setup, the EXIT procedure can be performed in a controlled fashion. There are many technical considerations regarding maternal and fetal anesthesia that maximize safe access to the fetus while minimizing maternal blood loss. These aspects are well described in the literature,[5,14,18,47] and although the details are beyond the scope of this review, the points pertinent to the otolaryngologist's role are highlighted.

Access

After obtaining a deep plane of endotracheal anesthesia, the maternal-fetal medicine team proceeds with their approach to the uterus, typically via Pfannentiel skin incision. After entering the peritoneum and obtaining visual access to the uterus, a sterile ultrasonogram is used to confirm placental location to ensure that the hysterotomy incision avoids the placenta. The position of the fetus is also confirmed to allow appropriate access to the head and neck. In cases of polyhydramnios, amnioreduction is performed before hysterotomy to avoid drastic volume changes that could lead to placental abruption and loss of placental support. Ultrasonography is also useful in cases of macrocystic LMs or cervical teratomas with a large cystic component, as these can be drained before hysterotomy to facilitate delivery.[1] Sufficient time must

Table 2 Personnel for EXIT		
Specialty	**Maternal**	**Fetal**
Anesthesia	1	1–2
Obstetrics/Gynecology	2–3	
Otolaryngologist		2–3
Pediatric surgeon		1
Neonatologist		2
Scrub nurse	1	1
Circulating nurse	1	1
Respiratory therapist[a]		1
Ultrasonographer[a]	1	

[a] Not recommended by all investigators, but add valuable insight and technical skills to the EXIT team.

be allowed for uteroplacental transfer of inhaled anesthetic, a process that typically requires 1 hour to achieve 70% of maternal levels.[26] When all preparatory goals have been accomplished, uterine incision is made sharply and extended with a hemostatic stapling device (U.S. Surgical Corp, Norwalk, CT, USA). Following hysterotomy, the fetus' head and shoulders are delivered, maintaining uterine volume by keeping the bulk of the fetus within the uterus. At this point intramuscular fentanyl, atropine, and paralytic are applied to the fetus.[15,18] These measures ensure that the neonate will not make a respiratory effort, which could hasten the loss of placental support. To further maintain uterine distension, amnioinfusion with warm saline solution is initiated.

Intrapartum Treatment

At this point, the fetus is attached to pulse oximetry and heart rate monitors by the fetal anesthesia and neonatology teams. Concurrent with initiation of monitoring, the otolaryngologist begins the airway assessment according to a predetermined algorithm (**Fig. 1**) of increasingly invasive options used to secure the airway. Typically the progression of maneuvers includes:

1. Direct laryngoscopy with intubation
2. Rigid bronchoscopy with intubation
3. Retrograde intubation
4. Tracheostomy

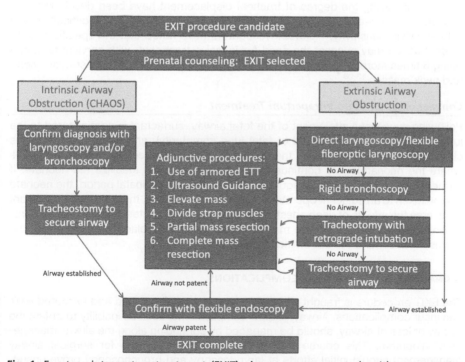

Fig. 1. Ex utero intrapartum treatment (EXIT) airway management algorithm, a stepwise approach to perinatal airway management. Note the differences between management of intrinsic and extrinsic congenital airway obstruction. Adjunctive procedures can and should be used at any point in the treatment of airway obstruction if deemed clinically appropriate. ETT, endotracheal tube.

Additional procedures that may improve the likelihood of obtaining a secure airway can also be included in the algorithm. These actions include use of flexible fiberoptic or rigid laryngoscopy with Seldinger intubation,[1] ultrasound guidance,[1,17] elevation of the obstructing mass off the airway during laryngoscopy or bronchoscopy to alleviate obstruction,[26] neck incision with release of strap muscles,[26] partial mass resection to allow for visualization of the airway,[17] or complete excision of obstructing mass during EXIT followed by securing the airway.[25] If complete excision of the mass is required, uteroplacental circulation has been shown to be maintainable for up to 2.5 hours.[49] Although tracheostomy is traditionally considered the most stable airway, this is not necessarily so during the EXIT procedure. Efforts are made to obtain an orotracheal airway if possible during the EXIT procedure, even when dissection in the neck and retrograde intubation are required.[50] Laje and colleagues[50] cite the more tenuous nature of tracheostomy in neonates with giant neck masses, with the distance between skin and trachea increased and, following resection of the mass, destabilized skin folds, which also make maintaining a patent tracheostoma difficult as the reason for preferential avoidance of tracheostomy.

Several factors must be considered in the development of the algorithm, as individual instances may alter the utility of some interventions. For instance, in the case of CHAOS resulting from laryngeal atresia, attempts at obtaining the airway in a transoral fashion would not be successful. As such, the first airway intervention after confirmation of the diagnosis with bronchoscopy would be tracheostomy. In an effort to help predict likelihood of requiring invasive procedures to secure the airway, predictive indices quantifying the degree of tracheal displacement have been developed.[28] In this model, tracheal displacement greater than 12 mm predicted a difficult airway with excellent sensitivity.[28] Other investigators have noted that the specific causes of obstruction may suggest the need for invasive treatment, with cervical teratoma being 5 times more likely to require surgical intervention than other obstructive head and neck masses.[13,28]

Completion of Ex Utero Intrapartum Treatment

Following successful attainment of the fetal airway, surfactant is administered to the lungs (given the high likelihood of fetal lung immaturity), and the umbilical cord is clamped and cut. At this point, the neonate is taken to a secondary operating table where the neonatologists continue their assessments and stabilize the neonate. If further surgical intervention is required in the immediate perinatal period, the neonate can be taken to an adjacent operating room. During this time, the maternal teams work to reverse the effects of deep anesthesia rapidly, reversing uterine relaxation and promoting contraction to minimize maternal blood loss. The placenta is delivered, the uterus repaired, and the abdominal incision closed.

MANAGEMENT OF POTENTIAL COMPLICATIONS

The EXIT procedure is fraught with risk, and even a well-planned and executed EXIT can incur complications. Airway-related complications, such as inability to obtain the airway or loss of airway, should be managed by continuing along the airway management algorithm. This course will provide contingency plans for surgical airway management should initial efforts at laryngoscopy and bronchoscopy prove unsuccessful. In addition to technical difficulties in visualizing and securing the airway owing to the expected airway obstruction, disruption of the obstructing mass, especially in the case of teratoma,[25] can lead to hemorrhage into the mass and further obstruction of the airway. In this scenario, prevention is the most effective management, with gentle delivery and minimal manipulation of the mass. Should hemorrhage occur, resection of the mass while on placental support may be necessary.

Another potential complication of the EXIT procedure is premature loss of placental support.[47] Constant monitoring of fetal vital signs and uterine relaxation aid in maintenance of placental support, but the EXIT team must maintain communication to transition to more emergent airway procedures should impending loss of placental support be suspected. The need for uterine relaxation increases the risk of uterine hemorrhage. While avoiding the placenta during hysterotomy and using hemostatic staples for hysterotomy to minimize blood loss, attention must be given to ensuring that maternal hemodynamics and uterine blood flow remain sufficient to support both maternal and fetal circulation.

POSTPROCEDURAL CARE

Successful airway protection and delivery do not ensure an uneventful postnatal period. The severe extension of the neck forced by large cervical neck masses can compress the developing lungs against the thoracic inlet, leading to pulmonary hypoplasia.[18–20] In this situation the neonatology team is essential for further care, stabilization, and mechanical ventilation.

Once the fetal airway is secured, the child will likely require mechanical ventilation, possibly because of underlying respiratory failure, pulmonary prematurity, or congenital abnormality. Even in the absence of these comorbidities, the effect of intrapartum fetal muscle relaxant will likely persist after delivery. As such, the neonatology team should be prepared with the equipment to provide oxygenation and ventilation to the neonate after delivery.

Another consideration following delivery is whether further surgical intervention is necessary. In the setting of congenital high airway obstruction, perinatal interventions are complete after tracheostomy and administration of surfactant. In cases of cervical teratoma and LMs, however, it must be determined whether the obstructive lesion should be resected immediately or in delayed fashion.[18,25]

REHABILITATION, RECOVERY, AND OUTCOMES

The rehabilitative potential of the individual patient is highly variable, and is contingent less on the specific maneuvers performed during EXIT and more on the underlying abnormality and associated anomalies in the neonate. Outcomes reported in longterm analyses of EXIT deliveries are extremely variable, ranging from no long-term sequelae to long-term hospitalization, neurovascular compromise, tracheostomy, and ventilator dependence. Attempting to identify factors that affect outcome will assist with appropriate preoperative counseling. Recent literature has attempted to delineate fetal outcomes following EXIT procedures based on the specific pathologic conditions managed.

Congenital High Airway Obstruction Syndrome

In an analysis of the largest CHAOS series to date, the group from Philadelphia[42] identified development of prenatal hydrops as a risk factor for fetal demise and noted that, for patients who survived to the time of EXIT, 66% (4 of 6) survived beyond 13 months. The group from University of California at San Fransisco[40] also recently reported survival beyond 1 year of all (4/4) CHAOS deliveries that progressed to the point of EXIT. In each cohort, a significant proportion of the initial population for whom EXIT was offered did not survive to term because of either fetal demise or elective termination.[40,42] Of EXIT deliveries, one airway could not be obtained at EXIT owing to agenesis of the trachea extending to within 1.5 cm of the carina.[42] The other early mortality was related to a tracheostomy complication. Of the surviving CHAOS cohort (n = 9), 2 patients underwent laryngotracheal reconstruction procedures and are tracheostomy free, 5 tolerate an oral diet, and 2 are verbal.[40,42]

Teratoma

Following EXIT for teratoma, the postnatal clinical course is dictated primarily by the degree of pulmonary hypoplasia, as most deaths following EXIT result from respiratory failure.[50] In Laje and colleagues'[50] recent disease-specific review of 17 EXIT procedures for teratoma, they describe a neonatal mortality rate of 23% with all mortalities attributable to severe pulmonary hypoplasia, with no mortality occurring while on placental support. Additional smaller series experienced modest improvements in survival,[16,19] although small sample size limits the generalizability of these results. In Lazar's series,[19] all patients were tracheostomy free and developmentally normal after a median follow-up of 5.4 years.

With respect to resection of the teratoma, early intervention is recommended for several reasons. First, intratumoral hemorrhage may lead to cardiovascular compromise or increased airway compression, and increase the difficulty of mass resection.[50] Moreover, between 1% and 5% of teratomas demonstrate malignant components.[51,52] Of course, intervention at an earlier age can increase morbidities associated with prematurity. These risks must be weighed to identify the appropriate time for intervention.

Avoidance of tracheostomy at EXIT does not preclude the potential need for later tracheostomy in the management of cervical teratoma. Five of 17 patients in the series of Laje and colleagues[50] required tracheostomy during EXIT, and an additional 5 required subsequent tracheostomy either at the time of resection or after failure to wean from mechanical ventilation. Eventual decannulation is possible, but significant tracheomalacia may persist following resection, perhaps a result of compression of the airway during gestation, leading to long-term tracheostomy dependence.[50]

Compression of the pharynx can reduce the ability to swallow, leading to microgastria and resultant feeding issues, which can necessitate the need for surgical intervention. This situation occurred in the minority of cases in 2 series, with 3 of 21 cases requiring gastrostomy tube and/or fundoplication.[19,50] Invasive teratomas or issues related to resection of these lesions can compromise nearby structures, leading to difficulties such as hypothyroidism or cranial nerve deficits.[19,50]

Lymphatic and Venous Malformation

More limited disease-specific outcome information is available following EXIT for LM. The available data suggest that if the airway can be obtained during EXIT, long-term survival is likely.[16,19] Owing to the developmental characteristics of LMs, surrounding rather than displacing neurovascular structures, resection or sclerotherapy can result in neurovascular injury more often than with other congenital masses. Although resection and/or sclerotherapy are the mainstays of treatment,[33–35] recurrences with the need for multiple procedures are often encountered.[18]

Maternal Outcomes

Maternal outcomes following EXIT are more predictable. No maternal deaths following EXIT have been reported. Whereas initial reports suggested increased maternal blood loss in comparison with traditional cesarean section,[45] more recent reports have found no statistical increase in blood loss and no change in hematocrit.[26,45,53] The theoretic risk of uterine rupture or dehiscence with a subsequent pregnancy following EXIT does not seem to be different relative to following cesarean section, although the numbers are still small and may not reflect true risk.[54] In addition, fertility does not seem to be affected following EXIT.[54] Some literature reviewing maternal outcomes includes patients who underwent open maternal-fetal surgery (OMFS) in whom the pregnancy continued after the operation. These findings must be interpreted with care with regard to EXIT, as OMFS is known to result in higher uterine rupture and uterine dehiscence during the ongoing pregnancy, and carries the potential for similar risks and decreased fertility in subsequent pregnancies.[54]

ADDITIONAL CONSIDERATIONS

An experienced pediatric otolaryngologist is no stranger to managing an urgent or emergent difficult airway in a neonate. The EXIT procedure is no exception. However, there are some important unique aspects to the EXIT procedure that should be considered. Although most of the technical aspects of securing the airway during the EXIT, either through laryngoscopy, bronchoscopy, or surgical means, are similar to securing the airway in other difficult or challenging cases, the environment in which the surgeon is performing these procedures is drastically different and bears mentioning. First of all, the pressure is amplified by the fact that the surgeon is performing in a crowded room being watched by 15 to 30 people. The surgeon may be standing between the mother's legs with the mother in the lithotomy position, and must be prepared to experience (smell, touch, and sight) the rush of amniotic fluid and maternal blood, often to a level with which the surgeon is not accustomed. Knee-high obstetric boots are recommended. The fetus will be a grayish color, slippery, and covered in white vernix, so careful handling of the fetus with sterile towels is imperative. The fetus will also not be breathing, moving, or making any attempt to ventilate. Seeing a patient in this state can be very anxiety provoking. However, the surgeon should take the time to make careful and planned movements despite the lack of respiratory effort and the poor color in this case as the patient is oxygenated via placental circulation. Fetal oxygenation while on placental support is normally around 75%.[5] Rushing though the initial assessment may lead to oral or hypopharyngeal bleeding that may limit future success. Positioning the fetus also can be challenging. The fetus may be partially removed from the uterus with legs and, possibly, one arm still inside, and laying on the mother's lower abdomen or side. It is often not possible to use carefully placed surgical towels to improve visualization. However, the surgeon must work with the obstetrician and other members of the otolaryngology team to achieve the best positioning possible.

Specific jobs must be assigned beforehand, and a checklist is helpful for this task. Every task must be assigned, even the relatively simple ones such as drying the neonate or placing monitors. Those responsible for transferring the neonate to the neonatology team should also be assigned surgical towels and prepared to achieve this task safely.

Although these comments seem very basic, any misstep can have significant consequences in the maelstrom of an EXIT delivery with many medical teams taking charge at different times. Consider these unique aspects of the EXIT environment when planning your role in the EXIT team. Make a detailed plan and treatment algorithm based on the specific details of the case, and practice your approach with the otolaryngology team and then with the entire EXIT team in the room several times before the actual event to maximize the chances of a favorable outcome.

Future Directions in Fetal Surgery

Future directions for improvement of neonatal care include advancements in fetal surgery to correct fetal problems with a high likelihood for fetal demise. For instance, the downstream effects of tracheal agenesis can potentially be alleviated via fetal tracheostomy or wire puncture to allow the hyperinflated lungs to decompress, thereby preventing or mitigating the severity of hydrops. In fact, this procedure has been attempted in several patients with CHAOS, with modest success.[40,55] In addition, advancements in fetal surgery may allow for in utero resection of obstructive masses, obviating EXIT in some circumstances. Moreover, improvements in maintenance of uteroplacental circulation with alterations in anesthetic regimens may afford a more consistent time frame for more definitive intrapartum interventions.

SUMMARY

The EXIT procedure holds the potential to convert some formerly dire situations into manageable problems. The procedure does so by allowing a controlled, stepwise approach to intrapartum airway management, with improved survival and the potential for improved postnatal development. Although a significant risk of morbidity and mortality still exists, this technique has helped advance the frontier of care for complex congenital airway obstruction into the perinatal period.

REFERENCES

1. Dighe MK, Peterson SE, Dubinsky TJ, et al. EXIT procedure: technique and indications with prenatal imaging parameters for assessment of airway patency. Radiographics 2011;31:511–26.
2. Ruano R, Benachi A, Aubry MC, et al. The impact of 3-dimensional ultrasonography on perinatal management of a large epignathus teratoma without ex utero intrapartum treatment. J Pediatr Surg 2005;40:e31–4.
3. Harrison MR, Adzick NS, Flake AW, et al. Correction of congenital diaphragmatic hernia in utero VIII: response of the hypoplastic lung to tracheal occlusion. J Pediatr Surg 1996;31:1339–48.
4. Chang LC, Kuczkowski KM. The ex utero intrapartum treatment procedure: anesthetic considerations. Arch Gynecol Obstet 2008;277:83–5.
5. Ngamprasertwong P, Vinks AA, Boat A. Update in fetal anesthesia for the ex utero intrapartum treatment (EXIT) procedure. Int Anesthesiol Clin 2012;50:26–40.
6. Kuczkowski KM. Ex utero intrapartum treatment (EXIT) procedure versus standard cesarean section. Ann Fr Anesth Reanim 2007;26(11):1003–4 France.
7. Kelly MF, Berenholz L, Rizzo KA, et al. Approach for oxygenation of the newborn with airway obstruction due to a cervical mass. Ann Otol Rhinol Laryngol 1990;99: 179–82.
8. Langer JC, Tabb T, Thompson P, et al. Management of prenatally diagnosed tracheal obstruction: access to the airway in utero prior to delivery. Fetal Diagn Ther 1992;7:12–6.
9. Catalano PJ, Urken ML, Alvarez M, et al. New approach to the management of airway obstruction in "high risk" neonates. Arch Otolaryngol Head Neck Surg 1992;118:306–9.
10. Thompson DM, Kasperbauer JL. Congenital cystic hygroma involving the larynx presenting as an airway emergency. J Natl Med Assoc 1994;86:629–32.
11. Skarsgard ED, Chitkara U, Krane EJ, et al. The OOPS procedure (operation on placental support): in utero airway management of the fetus with prenatally diagnosed tracheal obstruction. J Pediatr Surg 1996;31:826–8.
12. Mychaliska GB, Bealer JF, Graf JL, et al. Operating on placental support: the ex utero intrapartum treatment procedure. J Pediatr Surg 1997;32:227–30 [discussion: 230–1].

13. Steigman SA, Nemes L, Barnewolt CE, et al. Differential risk for neonatal surgical airway intervention in prenatally diagnosed neck masses. J Pediatr Surg 2009;44: 76–9.
14. Abraham RJ, Sau A, Maxwell D. A review of the EXIT (Ex utero Intrapartum Treatment) procedure. J Obstet Gynaecol 2010;30:1–5.
15. Moldenhauer JS. Ex utero intrapartum therapy. Semin Pediatr Surg 2013;22:44–9.
16. Liechty KW, Crombleholme TM, Weiner S, et al. The ex utero intrapartum treatment procedure for a large fetal neck mass in a twin gestation. Obstet Gynecol 1999;93:824–5.
17. MacArthur CJ. Prenatal diagnosis of fetal cervicofacial anomalies. Curr Opin Otolaryngol Head Neck Surg 2012;20:482–90.
18. Olutoye OO, Olutoye OA. EXIT procedure for fetal neck masses. Curr Opin Pediatr 2012;24:386–93.
19. Lazar DA, Olutoye OO, Moise KJ Jr, et al. Ex-utero intrapartum treatment procedure for giant neck masses—fetal and maternal outcomes. J Pediatr Surg 2011;46:817–22.
20. Liechty KW, Hedrick HL, Hubbard AM, et al. Severe pulmonary hypoplasia associated with giant cervical teratomas. J Pediatr Surg 2006;41:230–3.
21. Chan DF, Lee CH, Fung TY, et al. Ex utero intrapartum treatment (EXIT) for congenital giant ranula. Acta Paediatr 2006;95:1303–5.
22. Chung JH, Farinelli CK, Porto M, et al. Fetal epignathus: the case of an early EXIT (ex utero intrapartum treatment). Obstet Gynecol 2012;119:466–70.
23. Hirose S, Farmer DL, Lee H, et al. The ex utero intrapartum treatment procedure: looking back at the EXIT. J Pediatr Surg 2004;39:375–80 [discussion: 375–80].
24. Billmire DF, Grosfeld JL. Teratomas in childhood: analysis of 142 cases. J Pediatr Surg 1986;21:548–51.
25. Taghavi K, Berkowitz RG, Fink AM, et al. Perinatal airway management of neonatal cervical teratomas. Int J Pediatr Otorhinolaryngol 2012;76:1057–60.
26. Marwan A, Crombleholme TM. The EXIT procedure: principles, pitfalls, and progress. Semin Pediatr Surg 2006;15:107–15.
27. Muscatello L, Giudice M, Feltri M. Malignant cervical teratoma: report of a case in a newborn. Eur Arch Otorhinolaryngol 2005;262:899–904.
28. Lazar DA, Cassady CI, Olutoye OO, et al. Tracheoesophageal displacement index and predictors of airway obstruction for fetuses with neck masses. J Pediatr Surg 2012;47:46–50.
29. Gundry SR, Wesley JR, Klein MD, et al. Cervical teratomas in the newborn. J Pediatr Surg 1983;18:382–6.
30. de Serres LM, Sie KC, Richardson MA. Lymphatic malformations of the head and neck. A proposal for staging. Arch Otolaryngol Head Neck Surg 1995;121: 577–82.
31. Wiegand S, Eivazi B, Zimmermann AP, et al. Evaluation of children with lymphatic malformations of the head and neck using the cologne disease score. Int J Pediatr Otorhinolaryngol 2009;73:955–8.
32. Wittekindt C, Michel O, Streppel M, et al. Lymphatic malformations of the head and neck: introduction of a disease score for children, Cologne Disease Score (CDS). Int J Pediatr Otorhinolaryngol 2006;70:1205–12.
33. Stefini S, Bazzana T, Smussi C, et al. EXIT (Ex utero Intrapartum Treatment) in lymphatic malformations of the head and neck: discussion of three cases and proposal of an EXIT-TTP (Team Time Procedure) list. Int J Pediatr Otorhinolaryngol 2012;76:20–7.

34. Ogita K, Suita S, Taguchi T, et al. Outcome of fetal cystic hygroma and experience of intrauterine treatment. Fetal Diagn Ther 2001;16:105–10.
35. Kuwabara Y, Sawa R, Otsubo Y, et al. Intrauterine therapy for the acutely enlarging fetal cystic hygroma. Fetal Diagn Ther 2004;19:191–4.
36. Baker PA, Aftimos S, Anderson BJ. Airway management during an EXIT procedure for a fetus with dysgnathia complex. Paediatr Anaesth 2004;14:781–6.
37. Morris LM, Lim FY, Elluru RG, et al. Severe micrognathia: indications for EXIT-to-airway. Fetal Diagn Ther 2009;26:162–6.
38. Barch B, Rastatter J, Jagannathan N. Difficult pediatric airway management using the intubating laryngeal airway. Int J Pediatr Otorhinolaryngol 2012; 76(11):1579–82 Ireland: 2012 Elsevier Ireland Ltd.
39. Paladini D, Morra T, Teodoro A, et al. Objective diagnosis of micrognathia in the fetus: the jaw index. Obstet Gynecol 1999;93:382–6.
40. Saadai P, Jelin EB, Nijagal A, et al. Long-term outcomes after fetal therapy for congenital high airway obstructive syndrome. J Pediatr Surg 2012;47: 1095–100.
41. Shimabukuro F, Sakumoto K, Masamoto H, et al. A case of congenital high airway obstruction syndrome managed by ex utero intrapartum treatment: case report and review of the literature. Am J Perinatol 2007;24:197–201.
42. Roybal JL, Liechty KW, Hedrick HL, et al. Predicting the severity of congenital high airway obstruction syndrome. J Pediatr Surg 2010;45:1633–9.
43. Vanhaesebrouck P, De Coen K, Defoort P, et al. Evidence for autosomal dominant inheritance in prenatally diagnosed CHAOS. Eur J Pediatr 2006;165:706–8.
44. Baker DC Jr, Savetsky L. Congenital partial atresia of the larynx. Laryngoscope 1966;76:616–20.
45. Noah MM, Norton ME, Sandberg P, et al. Short-term maternal outcomes that are associated with the EXIT procedure, as compared with cesarean delivery. Am J Obstet Gynecol 2002;186:773–7.
46. Neidich MJ, Prager JD, Clark SL, et al. Comprehensive airway management of neonatal head and neck teratomas. Otolaryngol Head Neck Surg 2011;144: 257–61.
47. Zadra N, Giusti F, Midrio P. Ex utero intrapartum surgery (EXIT): indications and anaesthetic management. Best Pract Res Clin Anaesthesiol 2004;18:259–71.
48. Elliott R, Vallera C, Heitmiller ES, et al. Ex utero intrapartum treatment procedure for management of congenital high airway obstruction syndrome in a vertex/breech twin gestation. Int J Pediatr Otorhinolaryngol 2013;77:439–42.
49. Hirose S, Sydorak RM, Tsao K, et al. Spectrum of intrapartum management strategies for giant fetal cervical teratoma. J Pediatr Surg 2003;38:446–50 [discussion: 446–50].
50. Laje P, Johnson MP, Howell LJ, et al. Ex utero intrapartum treatment in the management of giant cervical teratomas. J Pediatr Surg 2012;47:1208–16.
51. Kerner B, Flaum E, Mathews H, et al. Cervical teratoma: prenatal diagnosis and long-term follow-up. Prenat Diagn 1998;18:51–9.
52. Jordan RB, Gauderer MW. Cervical teratomas: an analysis. Literature review and proposed classification. J Pediatr Surg 1988;23:583–91.
53. Bouchard S, Johnson MP, Flake AW, et al. The EXIT procedure: experience and outcome in 31 cases. J Pediatr Surg 2002;37:418–26.
54. Zamora IJ, Ethun CG, Evans LM, et al. Maternal morbidity and reproductive outcomes related to fetal surgery. J Pediatr Surg 2013;48:951–5.
55. Kohl T, Hering R, Bauriedel G, et al. Fetoscopic and ultrasound-guided decompression of the fetal trachea in a human fetus with Fraser syndrome and

congenital high airway obstruction syndrome (CHAOS) from laryngeal atresia. Ultrasound Obstet Gynecol 2006;27:84–8 [discussion: 88].

56. Cass DL, Olutoye OO, Cassady CI, et al. EXIT-to-resection for fetuses with large lung masses and persistent mediastinal compression near birth. J Pediatr Surg 2013;48:138–44.

57. Auguste TC, Boswick JA, Loyd MK, et al. The simulation of an ex utero intrapartum procedure to extracorporeal membrane oxygenation. J Pediatr Surg 2011;46: 395–8.

58. Stoffan AP, Wilson JM, Jennings RW, et al. Does the ex utero intrapartum treatment to extracorporeal membrane oxygenation procedure change outcomes for high-risk patients with congenital diaphragmatic hernia? J Pediatr Surg 2012;47:1053–7.

Congenital Lesions of Epithelial Origin

Susannah E. Hills, MD, John Maddalozzo, MD*

KEYWORDS

- Midline cervical cleft • Dermoid cyst • Pilomatrixoma • Foregut duplication
- Preauricular pit dermoid

KEY POINTS

- Congenital lesions of the epithelium have varied presentations, including clefts, cysts, sinuses and pits, and masses.
- Management ranges from simple observation for asymptomatic lesions to surgical excision with complex repair.
- Nasal dermoids may take a multidisciplinary approach with neurosurgical involvement for intracranial extension.
- Syndromes associated with these lesions must also be considered in the evaluation of the pediatric patient with these defects.

INTRODUCTION

Most masses of the head and neck in children are benign in nature. Most commonly, these lesions are congenital, inflammatory, or infectious in cause. Defects of epithelial origin are the result of failure of fusion during embryologic development, failure of involution of primordial remnants during embryologic development, and defects of ectodermal development during childhood.

CONGENITAL MIDLINE CERVICAL CLEFT
Epidemiology

Congenital midline cervical cleft (CMCC) is a rare developmental defect of the anterior neck with fewer than 100 cases reported in the literature.[1] These defects account for less than 2% of congenital cervical malformations.[2] There is some predilection for caucasian female children, and it can occur as a concomitant lesion with thyroglossal duct cysts and branchial cleft anomalies with an incidence of 1.7% in this population.[3]

Division of Otolaryngology, Ann & Robert H. Lurie Children's Hospital of Chicago, 225 East Chicago Avenue, Box 25, Chicago, IL 60611-2605, USA
* Corresponding author. Division of Otolaryngology - Head and Neck Surgery, Ann & Robert H. Lurie Children's Hospital of Chicago, Northwestern University Feinberg School of Medicine, 225 East Chicago Avenue, Box 25, Chicago, IL 60611-2605.
E-mail address: jpmaddal@luriechildrens.org

Otolaryngol Clin N Am 48 (2015) 209–223
http://dx.doi.org/10.1016/j.otc.2014.09.014
0030-6665/15/$ – see front matter © 2015 Elsevier Inc. All rights reserved.

No familial inheritance pattern has been identified, and they are thought to be a sporadic defect.[2]

Cause/Embryology

Although the exact cause of CMCC is unknown, it is generally thought to be the result of failure of midline fusion of the branchial arches.[4] In normal embryologic development, during the third and fourth week of gestation, mesenchymal tissue migrates between the branchial arches, pushing the ectoderm outward and resulting in fusion of the arches. A disruption in this process results in a midline defect. Failure of fusion of the second (hyoid) arches results in CMCC, whereas defects of the first (mandibular) arches result in clefts of the lower lip, tongue, and mandible, as well as CMCC.

Presentation

CMCCs are present at birth, although they become more apparent over time. They may be overlooked or misdiagnosed early on.[5] These lesions may present at any point in the anterior midline neck from the mandible to the sternum.[1] There are 3 primary anatomic components in these lesions: a superior skin tag, a midline cleft of moist atrophic epidermis lacking adnexal structures, and a caudal sinus or duct at the inferior aspect of the cleft, which may drain mucous.[1] The senior author has operated on many of these lesions, and in his experience, the skin tag associated with this lesion may present at the superior or inferior aspect of the defect. It is also noted that CMCCs are associated with a subcutaneous amorphous fibrous cord that traverses the sternum to the midline of the mandible. This cord as well as a paucity of dermis contributes to a contracture that results in a wry neck. In the senior author's experience, there is nearly always a subcutaneous cord along the tract of the cleft, which may extend as high as the mandible and as low as the sternum. This cord is the result of maldevelopment of the median raphe of the strap muscles.[5] CMCC may be a solitary deformity or may be accompanied by other lesions, such as thyroglossal duct cyst, branchial cleft cyst, ectopic bronchogenic cyst, cleft lip, mandible, or tongue, absence of hyoid bone or thyroid cartilage, cleft sternum, or congenital heart disease.[1]

With time, the cleft heals with a scar, resulting in a web.[1] The web may ultimately result in neck contracture, limited mobility, and functional impairment, or torticollis. In more severe cases, this webbing can result in micrognathia, or a bony spur of the mandible or sternum (**Fig. 1**).

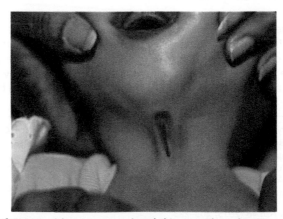

Fig. 1. Example of CMCC without an associated skin tag. The subcutaneous cord and associated contracture are evident.

Diagnosis

The diagnosis is typically made by clinical presentation. Early in life CMCC will present with a midline cleft associated with a cord, and possibly a skin tag and a caudal sinus or duct. Over time, webbing or contracture may also be evident. Imaging is generally not necessary in the management of these lesions; however, the authors advocate ultrasound to rule out synchronous thyroglossal duct cyst or branchial cleft anomaly.[5]

These lesions may be associated with other midline defects. Therefore, it is also important to inquire about signs of congenital heart disease. It is important to examine the sternum, mandible, and tongue for signs of cleft as well.

Management

Surgical excision is the treatment for CMCC. The entire tract, as well as the superior skin tag and the inferior sinus, must be excised to avoid drainage and recurrence of contracture. It is also necessary to dissect and excise the subcutaneous fibrous cord. The most frequently used technique for repair is multiple Z-plasties designed for lengthening of scar and release of contracture.[6] A single Z-plasty can be used as well (**Figs. 2–4**). The senior author has noted that small lesions less than 2 cm in size with lax adjacent skin can be excised and repaired primarily, without Z-plasty. These small lesions still require resection of the fibrous cord, and they represent a minority of cases.

The age of repair should be early, during infancy, to avoid contracture and cosmetic deformity.[1]

PILOMATROXIMA
Epidemiology

Pilomatrixoma is a benign neoplasm of the dermis, occurring most frequently in children and young adults. It is reported that 40% occur before the age of 10 years and 60% occur before the age of 20 years.[7] However, there is a second smaller peak of onset in the elderly. There is a female preponderance of these lesions as well.

Although extremely rare, malignant degeneration (pilomatrix carcinoma) of these lesions may also occur. There are fewer than 80 reported cases. Pilomatrix carcinoma is most common in the head and neck, with a male predominance and predominance among the elderly.[8]

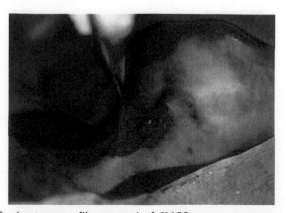

Fig. 2. Excision of subcutaneous fibrous cord of CMCC.

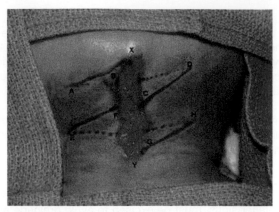

Fig. 3. Design of double Z-plasty closure for midline cleft.

Cause

Pilomatrixoma is a benign tumor of ectodermal origin. They arise from matrix cells of the outer root sheath of the hair follicle.[9] These lesions represent a disturbance of the hair follicle cycle in which development into mature hair fails to take place.[10] The vast majority of cases are solitary, sporadic neoplasms. However, the lesion may also be associated with Gardner syndrome, myotonic muscular dystrophy (Steinert disease), sarcoidosis, skull dysostosis, Rubinstein-Taybi syndrome, and Turner syndrome.[11]

Presentation

These lesions generally present in the first 2 decades of life as a gradually enlarging, painless, mobile subcutaneous mass. They often have a hard nodular surface, and overlying skin may demonstrate a bluish discoloration.[9] These lesions may also demonstrate a "tent sign," whereby stretching the skin over the surface of the lesion allows the nodular surface to become more apparent.[8] Calcifications may be seen as yellow or white flecks seen through the skin surface. These lesions generally slide freely over the underlying tissues.

Pilomatrixoma most frequently presents in the head and neck. The most common sites of presentation are reported to be the neck, cheek, and periorbital skin, followed by the scalp (**Figs. 5** and **6**).[8,9] Two percent to 10% of cases will have multiple lesions.

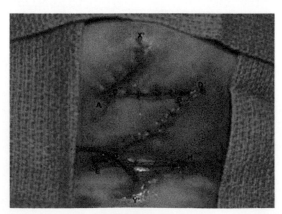

Fig. 4. Completed double Z-plasty closure of midline cleft.

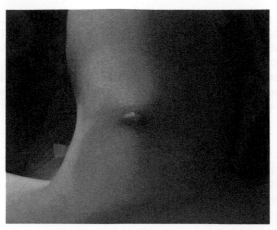

Fig. 5. Pilomatrixoma of anterior neck. The "tent sign," or stretching of the overlying skin, make the nodularity of the lesion apparent.

Histology

Histopathologic examination of pilomatroxima demonstrates a well-circumscribed intradermal nodule with a capsule of compressed fibrous tissue.[10]

There are distinct peripheral and central components of the tumor. The peripheral zone consists of small, uniform, darkly staining basaloid cells originating from the hair matrix cells, whereas the central portion is composed of remnants of cells that have lost their nuclei called "ghost cells" or "shadow cells."[8] These "ghost cells" are thought to be the product of apoptosis.

Calcification or ossification is also common and can be seen in 69% to 89% of cases.[10]

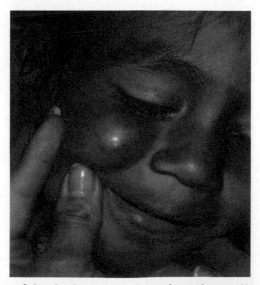

Fig. 6. Pliomatrixoma of the cheek overlying the malar eminence. Note the blue discoloration of the skin overlying the lesion.

Management

Imaging is generally not necessary in the workup of these superficial, benign lesions. However, pilomatrixoma in the parotid or preauricular region may warrant imaging, particularly if parotid dissection is anticipated.

Complete surgical excision is curative for these lesions (**Figs. 7–9**). No additional therapy is needed if the lesion is removed in its entirety. Recurrence can occur, requiring additional surgery if excision is incomplete.[10]

DERMOID
Epidemiology

Dermoid cysts are relatively rare. In a study by Orozco-Covarrubias and colleagues,[12] 75 cases of pediatric dermoids presenting to dermatology were identified over an 18-year period, representing 3 per 10,000 general pediatric patients.

Cause

Dermoid cysts are benign neoplasms derived from ectoderm and mesoderm. These lesions form from epithelial rests found along embryonic fusion lines. Histology will typically identify a keratinizing squamous epithelium along with dermal derivatives, such as hair follicles, smooth muscle, sweat and sebaceous glands, and fibroadipose tissue.[13]

Presentation

Congenital dermoid cysts are present at birth (**Figs. 10–12**), although only 40% are noted in the newborn period.[12] Roughly 70% are diagnosed by age 5 years.[14,15] Approximately 7% of dermoids occur in the head and neck,[16] with the most common site being along the outer third of the eyebrow.[12] **Table 1** lists head and neck locations of dermoid cysts. Dermoid cysts generally follow a pattern of slow growth during the first few years of life, thereafter remaining largely unchanged.[12]

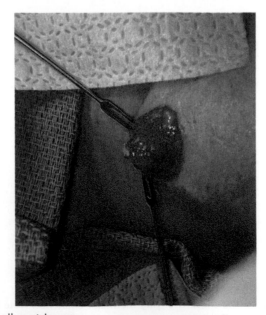

Fig. 7. Excision of pilomatrixoma.

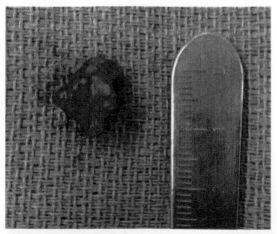

Fig. 8. Excised pilomatrixoma. Note granular, calcified appearance of the lesion.

Particular note should be made of midline dermoid cysts, which may be associated with dysraphism (cranial or spinal) or have intracranial extension.[17] On the neck, they are most frequently found in 1 of 2 locations; one is the parahyoid region, where they mimic thyroglossal duct cysts. The second location is suprasternal, where they insinuate themselves between the strap muscles and onto the trachea. Nasal dermoids are the most common of the midline dermoid cysts as well as the midline congenital malformations.[12] These cysts develop during ossification of the frontonasal plate and are the result of failure of closure of the neuropore.[12]

The most widely accepted theory of formation was presented by Grunwald in 1910, later termed the "cranial theory," which postulated that dermal attachments follow the neurectodermal tract as it recedes and can form a sinus or a cyst through connection with the skin overlying the dorsum of the nose.[18] The intracranial tract passes through the foramen cecum or cribriform plate to the base of the frontal fossa, adhering to the leaves of the falx cerebri.[19]

Nasal dermoid present as a swelling over the nasal dorsum, often associated with a sinus opening or punctum, which may extrude sebaceous material.[20] Recurrent

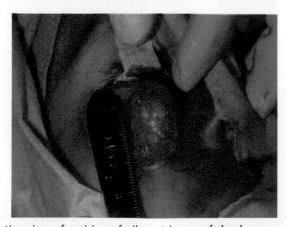

Fig. 9. Intraoperative view of excision of pilomatrixoma of cheek.

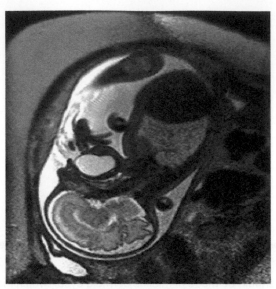

Fig. 10. Prenatal MRI showing dermoid cyst of the floor of mouth. (*Courtesy of* Dr Glenn Green, Ann Arbor, MI.)

infection is not uncommon. Hair protruding through the punctum is a pathognomonic feature of nasal dermoids.

Management

The approach to a dermoid is largely dependent on the location of the cyst. Most dermoids require only simple excision without disruption of the cyst wall. Another option is simple observation, although these lesions will continue to grow and are likely to ultimately require excision.

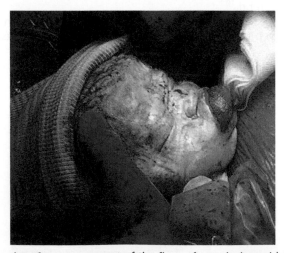

Fig. 11. EXIT procedure for management of the floor of mouth dermoid cyst in the MRI of **Fig. 10.** The airway was initially managed with oral intubation, with transoral resection of the lesion the following day. (*Courtesy of* Dr Glenn Green, Ann Arbor, MI.)

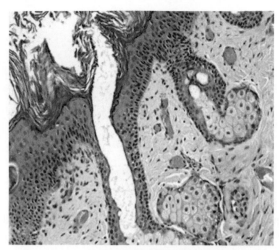

Fig. 12. Histology of floor of mouth dermoid cyst demonstrated in figures above. Adnexal structures such as sweat and sebaceous glands and fibroadipose tissue are evident.

Special consideration should be given to midline nasal dermoids (**Figs. 13** and **14**). Midline lesions have a higher risk of intracranial extension and require imaging to determine if such extension is present. The nasal dermoid requires dissection down to the upper lateral nasal cartilages and/or nasal bones and may require a combined approach to resection with neurosurgery.

FOREGUT DUPLICATION CYST
Epidemiology

Foregut duplication cysts of the oral cavity were first reported in 1927 by Toyama and Schultz.[21] Before 2004, there were only 21 reported cases of oral cavity enteric

Table 1				
Head and neck locations of dermoid cysts				
	Pryor et al,[13] 2005		Orozco-Covarrubias et al,[12] 2013	
Location	No.	%	No.	%
Orbit	30	61	52	71
Medial canthus	8	16		
Lateral canthus/brow	22	45	50	68
Neck	9	18	1	1
Scalp	4	8	17	23
Nose	3	6	3	4
Dorsum	1	2		
Intranasal	1	2		
Intranasal/intracranial	1	2		
Ear			2	3
Intracranial			1	1
Middle ear/NP			1	1
Total	49		73	

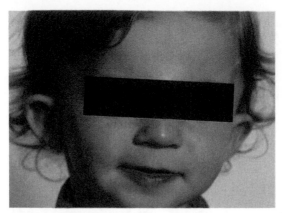

Fig. 13. Frontal view of nasal dermoid. Note the pit of the anterior midline nasal dorsum and the associated glabellar fullness.

in the literature,[22] and oral cavity duplications constitute 0.3% of all duplication cysts.[23]

Cause

The embryologic foregut gives rise to the pharynx, lower respiratory tract, esophagus, stomach, duodenum, and hepatobiliary tract. Enteric duplication cysts occur anywhere along the alimentary tract from the oral cavity to the rectum (**Fig. 15**). Foregut duplication cysts arise from remnants of the stomach and the first and second parts of the duodenum. Midgut duplications are most common, and foregut duplications account for about one-third of all duplications.[22,24]

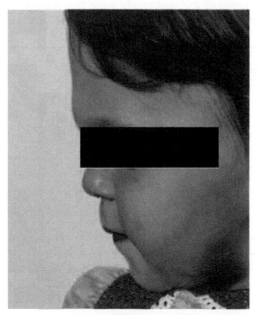

Fig. 14. Lateral view of nasal dermoid. Glabellar fullness is particularly pronounced on this view.

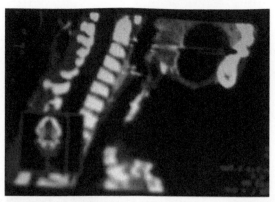

Fig. 15. Foregut duplication cyst of the floor of mouth demonstrated with CT scan.

Enteric duplications are embryologic in origin, although the exact mechanism of formation is unknown. In 1952, Veeneklaas[25] postulated a theory that foregut duplication cysts arise from abnormal notochord attachment. In the 1970s, a second theory arose that foregut duplications may arise from small inclusions of epithelium retained along the lines of primordial fusion within the upper aerodigestive tract.[26]

Presentation

Foregut duplications are typically diagnosed in asymptomatic neonates and small children, although they may be undetected until adulthood.[27] These lesions may result in swallowing difficulties. The most concerning potential symptom of these lesions is airway obstruction.[27]

Management

The first step in the management of a foregut duplication of the mouth or upper aerodigestive tract is ensuring there is a secure airway. In the event of airway compromise, intubation or, in rare cases, tracheostomy may be indicated. There have been reported cases of obstructive foregut duplication cysts identified in utero, which have required an EXIT procedure to secure the airway.[22]

The mainstay of treatment is surgical excision. **Figs. 16** and **17** demonstrate excision of floor of the mouth duplication cysts. **Fig. 18** presents histology of cyst.

PREAURICULAR SINUS/PIT
Epidemiology

The preauricular sinus was first described by Heusinger in 1864.[28] There is an incidence that varies among races and is reported between 0.02% and 5%. These preauricular sinuses are transmitted by an incomplete, dominant, autosomal gene of variable penetrance.[29–32]

Cause

Development of the external ear begins during the fourth week of gestation (**Fig. 19**):

- The first hillock forms the tragus.
- The second hillock gives rise to the crus of the helix.
- The third hillock forms the remainder of the helix.
- The fourth hillock develops into the antihelix.

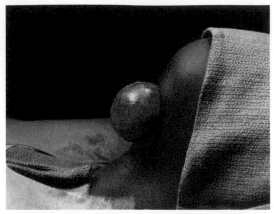

Fig. 16. Submental approach to excision of foregut duplication cyst of the floor of mouth.

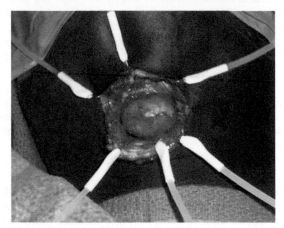

Fig. 17. Interaoperative exposure with submental approach to foregut duplication cyst of the floor of mouth.

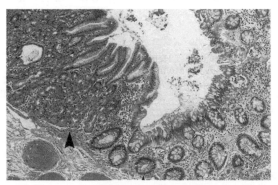

Fig. 18. Histology of the floor of mouth lesion excised in figures above. The deep crypts and abundant goblet cells are reflective of colonic mucosa, defining this lesion as foregut duplication cyst.

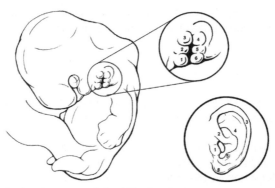

Fig. 19. Embryologic development of the hillocks of His.

- The fifth hillock produces the antihelix.
- The sixth hillock creates the lower helix and lobule.

By the twelfth week, the 6 hillocks of His from the first and second branchial arches fuse, forming the auricle. Preauricular pits and sinuses are thought to derive from failure of fusion of the hillocks.

Presentation

These deformities can be unilateral (80%) or bilateral. They typically present as a small opening at the anterior crus of the helix near its attachment by the tragus. These lesions may mimic type I or type II first branchial cleft anomalies, which are duplications of the external auditory canal. A complete otologic examination is indicated to look for a potential sinus opening in the external auditory canal.

These lesions can be associated with congenital malformations, particularly deafness and renal anomalies in a disease process known as branchio-oto-renal syndrome. Therefore, a complete history including possible hearing and renal function problem should be obtained.

Management

Most of these lesions are asymptomatic, in which case observation is an appropriate option. However, if there is a history of recurrent infection, complete surgical excision is indicated to prevent recurrent skin infection and skin breakdown. If the tract is incompletely excised, recurrence is very likely. Excision of the cartilaginous attachment to the helix at the base of the tract is also advocated as well to decrease the chance of recurrence.

In the instance of recurrence, the natural fistula opening becomes occluded, and the cyst secondarily fistulizes through the skin. Resulting ulceration and necrosis will often require excision of the overlying affected skin with local flap reconstruction.

SUMMARY

Congenital lesions of the epithelium of the head and neck have varied clinical presentations, including clefts, cysts, sinuses and pits, and masses. Management ranges from simple observation for asymptomatic preauricular pits and small dermoids to surgical excision with complex repair of cervical clefts, larger dermoids, duplication cysts, and pilomatrixoma. Nasal dermoids require special consideration with possible neurosurgical involvement for intracranial extension. It is also important to recognize possible syndromic associations of these lesions and to evaluate for other related medical conditions, such as hearing loss and renal anomalies in the setting of a preauricular pit.

REFERENCES

1. Sinopidis X, Kourea HP, Panagidis A, et al. Congenital midline cervical cleft: diagnosis, pathologic findings, and early stage treatment. Case Rep Pediatr 2012; 2012:951040.
2. McInnes CW, Benson AD, Verchere CG, et al. Management of congenital midline cervical cleft. J Craniofac Surg 2012;23(1):e36–8.
3. Gargan TJ, McKinnon M, Mulliken JB. Midline cervical cleft. Plast Reconstr Surg 1985;76:225–9.
4. Kakodkar K, Patel S, Maddalozzo J. Congenital midline cervical cleft. Otolaryngology 2013;3(2).
5. Maddalozzo J, Frankel A, Holinger LD. Midline cervical cleft. Pediatrics 1993; 92(2):286–7.
6. Habal MB, Scheuerle J. Lateral facial clefts: closure with W-plasty and implications of speech and language development. Ann Plast Surg 1983;11(3):182–7.
7. Julian CG, Bowers PW. A clinical review of 209 pilomatricomas. J Am Acad Dermatol 1998;39(2 Pt 1):191–5.
8. O'Connor N, Patel M, Umar T, et al. Head and neck pilomatricoma: an analysis of 201 cases. Br J Oral Maxillofac Surg 2011;49(5):354–8.
9. Danielson-Cohen A, Lin SJ, Hughes CA, et al. Head and neck pilomatrixoma in children. Arch Otolaryngol Head Neck Surg 2001;127(12):1481–3.
10. Lan MY, Lan MC, Ho CY, et al. Pilomatricoma of the head and neck: a retrospective review of 179 cases. Arch Otolaryngol Head Neck Surg 2003;129(12): 1327–30.
11. Yencha MW. Head and neck pilomatricoma in the pediatric age group: a retrospective study and literature review. Int J Pediatr Otorhinolaryngol 2001;57(2):123–8.
12. Orozco-Covarrubias L, Lara-Carpio R, Saez-De-Ocariz M, et al. Dermoid cysts: a report of 75 pediatric patients. Pediatr Dermatol 2013;30(6):706–11.
13. Pryor SG, Lewis JE, Weaver AL, et al. Pediatric dermoid cysts of the head and neck. Otolaryngol Head Neck Surg 2005;132(6):938–42.
14. Crawford JK, Webster JR. Congenital dermoid cysts of the nose. Plast Reconstr Surg 1952;9:235–60.
15. Brownstein MH, Helwig EB. Subcutaneous dermoid cysts. Arch Dermatol 1973; 107:237–9.
16. New GB, Erich JB. Dermoid cysts of the head and neck. Surg Gynecol Obstet 1937;65:48–55.
17. Hanikeri M, Waterhouse N, Kirkpatrick N, et al. The management of midline transcranial nasal dermoid sinus cysts. Br J Plast Surg 2005;58:1043–50.
18. Pratt LW. Midline cysts of the nasal dorsum: embryologic origin and treatment. Laryngoscope 1965;75:968–80.
19. Wardinsky TD, Pagon RA, Kropp RJ, et al. Nasal dermoid sinus cysts: association with intracranial extension and multiple malformations. Cleft Palate Craniofac J 1991;28:87–95.
20. Bartlett SP, Lin KY, Grossman R, et al. The surgical management of orbitofacial dermoids in the pediatric patient. Plast Reconstr Surg 1993;91(7):1208–15.
21. Toyama T. Occurrence of stomach mucosa in the base of tongue. J Kyoto Med Univ 1927;1:13–7.

22. Kong K, Walker P, Cassey J, et al. Foregut duplication cyst arising in the floor of mouth. Int J Pediatr Otorhinolaryngol 2004;68(6):827–30.
23. Lipsett J, Sparnon AL, Byard RW. Embryogenesis of enterocystomas-enteric duplication cysts of the tongue. Oral Surg Oral Med Oral Pathol 1993;75(5): 626–30.
24. Carachi R, Azmy A. Foregut duplications. Pediatr Surg Int 2002;18(5–6):371–4.
25. Veeneklaas GM. Pathogenesis of intrathoracic gastrogenic cysts. AMA Am J Dis Child 1952;83(4):500–7.
26. Gorlin RJ, Jirasek JE. Oral cysts containing gastric or intestinal mucosa. An unusual embryological accident or heterotopia. Arch Otolaryngol 1970;91(6): 594–7.
27. Davis PL 3rd, Gibson KG, Evans AK. Foregut duplication cysts in siblings: a case report. Int J Pediatr Otorhinolaryngol 2010;74(11):1331–4.
28. Heusinger H. Fisteln von noch nicht beobachteter form. Arch Pathol Anat 1864; 29:358.
29. Gur E, Yeung A, Al-Azzawi M, et al. The excised preauricular sinus in 14 years of experience: is there a problem? Plast Reconstr Surg 1998;102(5):1405–8.
30. His W. Anatomie menschlichen embryonen, vol. 3. Leipzig (Germany): F.C.W. Vogel; 1885. p. 211.
31. Bloom D, Carvalho D, Edmonds J, et al. Neonatal dermoid cyst of the floor of the mouth extending to the midline neck. Arch Otolaryngol Head Neck Surg 2002; 128(1):68–70.
32. Fraser L, Howatson AG, MacGregor FB. Foregut duplication cyst of the pharynx. J Laryngol Otol 2008;122(7):754–6.

Imaging of Pediatric Head and Neck Masses

Jessica S. Stern, MD[a,b,*], Daniel T. Ginat, MD, MS[c],
Jennifer L. Nicholas, MD, M.H.A[a,b], Maura E. Ryan, MD[a,b]

KEYWORDS

• Imaging • Pediatrics • Head and neck masses

KEY POINTS

- Ultrasound is often the initial imaging examination for evaluation of pediatric neck masses. Doppler interrogation is useful for evaluating vascularity.
- MRI and CT are complementary modalities, particularly in evaluating the deep cervical structures.
- CT is helpful in evaluating infectious and inflammatory processes, as well as in providing information regarding calcification.
- MRI is useful in characterization of soft tissue lesions, and evaluation of enhancement characteristics.
- Minimizing the risks of radiation and sedation must be considered in the imaging work up of a pediatric neck mass.

INTRODUCTION

Imaging is often an essential component in evaluating pediatric neck masses and can be helpful in characterizing congenital, inflammatory, vascular, and neoplastic lesions.[1] In some cases, characteristic imaging appearances can be diagnostic. In other instances, imaging may not yield a definitive diagnosis, but can be helpful in narrowing the differential diagnosis, defining lesion extent, assessment for metastatic disease, and in follow-up evaluation for treatment response or recurrence.

Imaging workup must consider the risks and benefits associated with various modalities, particularly the risks of sedation and radiation. Ultrasound is typically the initial imaging performed for evaluation of a palpable pediatric neck mass as it utilizes no radiation, requires no sedation or intravenous contrast, is easily accessible, and is

a Department of Medical Imaging, Ann & Robert H. Lurie Children's Hospital of Chicago, Northwestern University, 225 East Chicago Avenue, Box 9, Chicago, IL 60611, USA; b Department of Radiology, Feinberg School of Medicine, Northwestern University, Chicago, IL, USA; c Department of Radiology, Pritzker School of Medicine, University of Chicago Medical Center, 5841 S. Maryland Avenue, Chicago, IL 60637, USA
* Department of Medical Imaging, Ann & Robert H. Lurie Children's Hospital of Chicago, Northwestern University, 225 East Chicago Avenue, Box 9, Chicago, IL 60611.
E-mail address: JStern@luriechildrens.org

Otolaryngol Clin N Am 48 (2015) 225–246
http://dx.doi.org/10.1016/j.otc.2014.09.015
0030-6665/15/$ – see front matter © 2015 Elsevier Inc. All rights reserved.

relatively low in cost. Ultrasound can provide information about lesion size, location, cystic or solid nature; additionally, it can assess for vascular flow with Doppler interrogation. Cross-sectional imaging with multidetector computed tomography (MDCT) and MRI may be required for further assessment, particularly when the deeper cervical soft tissues are involved. MRI and CT have complimentary roles in lesion characterization and assessment of extent of disease.[2] However, both these modalities often require intravenous (IV) contrast, sedation in younger children, and with CT, exposure to radiation.

IMAGING TECHNIQUES
Ultrasound

Ultrasound of the pediatric neck is usually performed with the patient in the supine position, with his or her neck extended. A high-frequency linear transducer provides good resolution of superficial structures and is therefore useful for evaluation of most palpable masses in the pediatric neck. Ample ultrasound gel and/or a stand-off pad may improve visualization of lesions very close to the surface. Doppler imaging provides visualization of arterial and venous flow, and can be used to evaluate the presence and distribution of flow within a mass. The examination should also include assessment of the submandibular, parotid, and thyroid glands, when indicated. Identifying a normal thyroid gland is important in the preoperative workup of some congenital neck masses such as thyroglossal duct cyst or ectopic thyroid.[3]

One of the primary advantages of ultrasound is its ability to distinguish between solid and cystic masses. Simple cystic masses are anechoic (ie, nearly black) and demonstrate posterior acoustic enhancement. This phenomenon is sometimes referred to as increased through transmission, making the tissues behind the cyst appear brighter than the adjacent soft tissues due to the increased velocity of sound waves through fluid in the cyst relative to soft tissues. However, complex cystic masses with internal debris or hemorrhage may have more intermediate echogenicity, and may approximate the echogenicity of soft tissue. Doppler interrogation can also help distinguish cysts, which should not demonstrate internal flow, from solid lesions or vessels. Doppler imaging can also elucidate how flow is distributed within a mass (centrally, peripherally, or evenly throughout), and whether the flow is normal, increased, or decreased, all which may have diagnostic significance.

Ultrasound is also practical for evaluating palpable lymph nodes. Normal lymph nodes are typically ovoid to reniform in shape, are slightly hypoechoic when compared to the surrounding soft tissues with a hyperechoic region that represents the fatty hilum of the lymph node. On color Doppler interrogation, there is flow in normal lymph nodes, which is relatively increased near the hilum. Reactive lymph nodes are typically less than 1 cm in greatest diameter (short:long ratio <0.5).[4] In the pediatric population, however, lymph node morphology and clinical course are also important considerations (**Fig. 1**).

On ultrasound, malignant lymph nodes may be increased in size (>1–1.5 cm in greatest diameter) and may have lost their characteristic reniform shape, appearing more round in morphology. Malignant lymph nodes may show decreased internal echogenicity with loss of the echogenic fatty hilum.[5] Size alone cannot be used as a reliable criterion for distinguishing benign from reactive lymph nodes in children, but there is an increased risk of malignancy in lymph nodes measuring more than 3 cm in longest diameter.[6,7] Evaluation with a high-frequency linear transducer may reveal internal reticulation.[8] Findings suspicious for malignant infiltration of lymph nodes on color and power Doppler imaging include the presence of peripheral, subcapsular vessels with distortion or displacement of the intranodal vessels and focal areas of

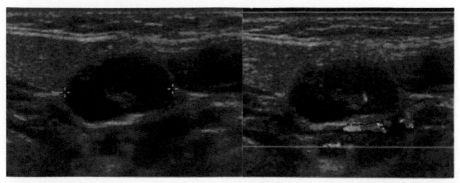

Fig. 1. Normal lymph node on ultrasound. The image on the left demonstrates a normal reniform lymph node, with a central area of hyperechogenicity representing the fatty hilum. Color Doppler interrogation is shown in the image on the right, demonstrating vascular flow in the region of the hilum.

absent perfusion.[1,2,9] Any or all of these characteristics warrant consideration of fine needle aspiration (FNA) or biopsy (**Fig. 2**).

Necrosing lymph nodes tend to become increasingly hypoechoic and may initially show increased flow, but central flow may become decreased as the lymph node becomes more necrotic. As the lymph node degenerates to an abscess, the node becomes more anechoic centrally and can develop a hyperechoic rind that typically demonstrates increased flow. As the necrotic lymph node becomes more liquid in composition, there may be posterior acoustic enhancement/increased through transmission, as is seen in cysts.

Although an excellent screening tool, there are several limitations of ultrasound imaging. Deep structures of the neck, particularly the retropharyngeal soft tissues, are not well-visualized with ultrasound. The short length of the neck in infants and toddlers can present technical challenges for the sonographer, and patient motion can also make the acquisition of diagnostic-quality images challenging. As image

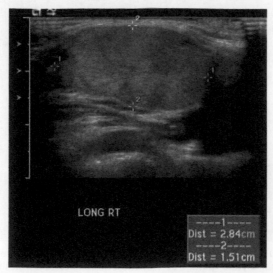

Fig. 2. Lymph node metastasis from papillary thyroid carcinoma on ultrasound.

quality is highly dependent on sonographic technique, ultrasound is best performed by sonographers with experience scanning children, and may require the interpreting physician to be present during at least part of the examination.

Ultrasound is also limited in its ability to accurately diagnosis the specific histology of masses in children by imaging characteristics alone. There is overlap in the imaging features of many congenital and acquired lesions. For example, complex, previously infected thyroglossal duct cysts may demonstrate heterogenous or intermediate echogenicity mimicking other midline lesions such as dermoid cysts (most commonly), epidermal inclusion cysts, vellus hair cysts, lymph nodes, or scar tissue (**Fig. 3**).[10]

Although calcifications may be readily identified on ultrasound by characteristic posterior acoustic shadowing, ultrasound does not visualize bony structures well. Also, as a result of posterior acoustic shadowing, which occurs because sound waves cannot penetrate calcifications, evaluation of structures deep to large calcifications is limited.

Computed Tomography

MDCT should be performed helically with acquisition of images in the axial plane in soft tissue and bone algorithms, and reconstructions in coronal and sagittal planes. The technique should be optimized to provide the lowest radiation dose possible while acquiring diagnostic quality images, according to the ALARA (as low as reasonably achievable) principle, utilizing age-stratified pediatric protocols. Intravenous contrast

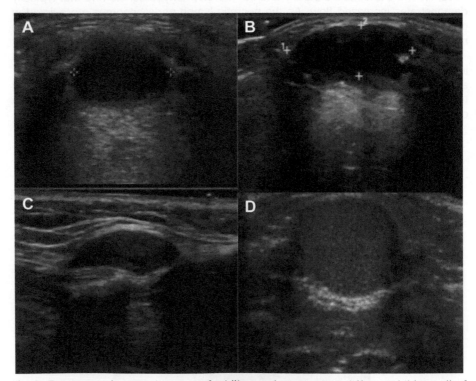

Fig. 3. Transverse ultrasound images of midline neck masses in 4 different children, all of whom had a normal thyroid gland. All 4 of these lesions were surgically removed. (A–C) Pathology-proven thyroglossal duct cysts. (D) Dermoid cyst.

is usually recommended for the workup of a neck mass, assuming no contraindications such as allergy or renal impairment. Intravenous contrast is useful for evaluation for abscess, delineating lesion margins, assessment of lesion vascularity, distinguishing between vessels and lymph nodes, and detection of abnormally enhancing lymph nodes. In particular, cases in which sialoliths or other calcifications are suspected, precontrast imaging through the region of interest is recommended, as contrast may obscure calcifications. In the workup of some thyroid lesions, iodinated contrast should be avoided because of the avid uptake of iodine by the thyroid gland.

The advantages of CT in the evaluation of neck lesions are high-resolution delineation of anatomy, osseous structures, and airspaces, as well as detection of calcification and fat. It is widely available and provides rapid image acquisition, particularly with newer multichannel scanners, reducing the need for anesthesia compared with MRI. However, sedation may still be required in young patients to minimize motion artifact. Additionally, in contrast to ultrasound, CT imaging is far less operator dependent.

The primary drawback of CT is that it requires exposure to ionizing radiation, which is particularly relevant in children, who are more radiosensitive than adults. This is an especially important consideration in patients requiring multiple examinations for long-term follow-up. Additionally, there are risks associated with iodinated CT contrast including allergic reaction and nephrotoxicity, which are uncommon but potentially serious.

MRI

A typical pediatric neck MRI protocol includes multiplanar T1, fat-suppressed T2 or short tau inversion recovery (STIR) sequences, diffusion-weighted images (DWI), and postcontrast, fat-suppressed T1 weighted sequences.[11] Compared with CT, MRI protocols are more complex, and may require tailoring to specific pathologies. T1 weighted images are helpful for delineation of anatomy. Fat appears bright on T1 and T2 weighted images, and fat suppression is helpful for elucidating underlying lesions on T2 weighted and postcontrast sequences. Various fat-suppression sequences are available, which vary by technique and manufacturer, including STIR, iterative decomposition of water and fat with echo asymmetry and least-squares estimation (IDEAL), and Dixon.[12,13] Time of flight or time-resolved magnetic resonance angiography (MRA) is recommended for suspected vascular lesions.[14] Diffusion-weighted imaging can increase the conspicuity of lymph node metastases and may play a role in differentiating tumor recurrence from post-treatment changes.[15] High field strength MRI systems such as 3T can provide higher signal-to-noise ratio and/or shorter scan times, which may be particularly advantageous in evaluating small lesions in children.

The superior soft tissue contrast capability and lack of ionizing radiation exposure make MRI an ideal modality for evaluating many masses in pediatric patients, particularly when intracranial extension is a consideration.[11] However, these advantages must be weighed against the disadvantages of relatively long scan times often necessitating sedation, as well as the increased cost and resource utilization compared with CT and ultrasound.

CROSS-SECTIONAL IMAGING FEATURES OF PEDIATRIC NECK MASSES
Congenital Lesions

Branchial cleft cysts
Congenital cystic lesions such as branchial cleft cysts are often well depicted on CT examinations. In some cases, however, branchial cleft cysts and associated sinus

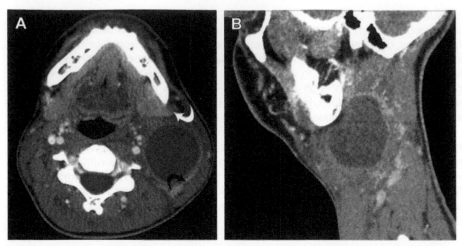

Fig. 4. Second branchial cleft cyst. Axial (*A*) and recontructed sagittal (*B*) contrast-enhanced CT images show a unilocular low density collection at the angle of the mandible, postero-lateral to the submandibular gland (*curved white arrow*), and anteriomedial to the SCM (*curved black arrow*).

tracts may be collapsed, rendering them difficult to identify on any imaging modality. Uncomplicated branchial cleft cysts appear as hypoattenuating lesions with a thin wall (**Fig. 4**). In cases of infected branchial cleft cysts, CT demonstrates a hypoattenuating cystic lesion, which may have a thickened wall, and inflammatory changes in the surrounding soft tissues (**Fig. 5**).

MRI may be helpful in evaluating atypical features of branchial cleft cysts, which can result from intracapsular hemorrhage or solidification of cystic fluid, appearing as abnormal signal intensities of the contents (**Fig. 6**). In particular, intracystic hemorrhage can demonstrate hyperintensity on T1 and T2 weighted images, while solidification of cystic fluid displays homogeneous hypointensity on T2 weighted images without enhancement.[16] Atypical branchial cleft cysts can be difficult to differentiate from cystic malignancies even on MRI, and tissue sampling may ultimately be necessary.[17]

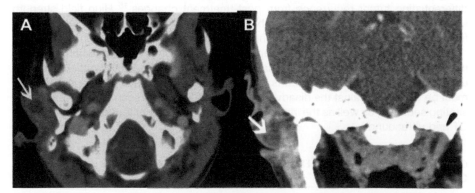

Fig. 5. First branchial cleft cyst. Axial (*A*) and recontructed coronal (*B*) contrast enhanced CT images demonstrate a low-density periauricular cyst (*white arrows*) adjacent to the external auditory canal (EAC) with inflammatory changes of the surrounding soft tissues.

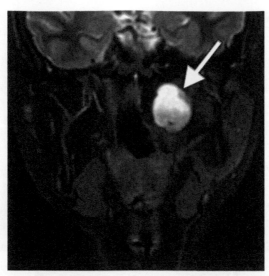

Fig. 6. Branchial cleft cyst. Recurrent branchial cleft cyst 2 years after resection demonstrating mural thickening (*arrow*), an atypical feature likely related to prior infection.

Dermoid and epidermoid/cholesteatoma

Subcutaneous and calvarial epidermoids typically appear as well-defined nonenhancing cystic lesions with high T2 signal and variable degrees of restricted diffusion (**Fig. 7**).[18,19] Although dermoids can also have a cystic appearance similar to epidermoids, dermoids tend to occur in the midline and may contain fat components and/or calcification. When multiple globules of fat are present, a sac of marbles appearance can result, with corresponding high T1 signal, and hypoattenuation on CT. Multiplanar high-resolution MRI enables detection of intracranial extension of a sinus tract associated with nasal dermoids (**Fig. 8**), which is useful for surgical planning.[20,21]

Teratoma

Teratomas of the head and neck can cause respiratory compromise due to mass effect, necessitating urgent surgical intervention. Imaging plays an important role in the assessment of these lesions, especially in preparation for surgery.[22] The presence of hypodense fat on CT (**Fig. 9**) with corresponding T1 hyperintensity on MRI can be a helpful feature, but is not always present.[22] Teratomas may also contain calcification, which is well visualized by CT. Teratomas demonstrate variable degrees of cystic and solid enhancing components (**Fig. 10**) and thus can be difficult to distinguish from other complex partially enhancing lesions, such as venolymphatic malformations.

Thyroglossal duct cyst

Thyroglossal duct cysts appear as thin-walled hypodense cystic lesions that may occur anywhere along the course of the thyroglossal duct, with thin enhancement of the cyst wall. Superimposed infection in a thyroglossal duct cyst may result in a thickened enhancing wall and inflammatory change in the adjacent tissues (**Figs. 11** and **12**).

Vascular Lesions

Venolymphatic malformations

Venolymphatic malformations typically appear as multicystic transpatial masses, most commonly occurring in the posterior cervical triangle. They often contain

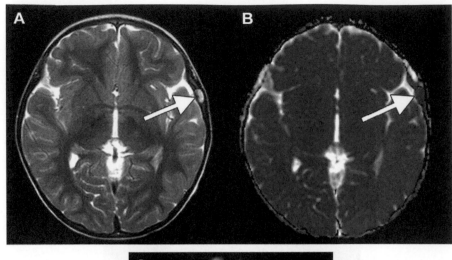

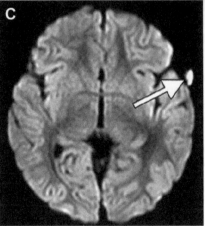

Fig. 7. Epidermoid. Axial T2 MRI (*A*) shows a hyperintense focus in the left temporal calvarium (*arrow*). Diffusion weighted imaging (DWI) and apparent diffusion coefficient (ADC) images show corresponding restricted diffusion within the lesion (*arrows*).

hemorrhage fluid levels related to prior hemorrhage or infection (**Figs. 13** and **14**), as well as phleboliths, which manifest as low signal foci on MRI[23] and hyperdense calcific foci on CT. Venolymphatic malformations may be heterogeneous in appearance, and may be difficult to distinguish from some neoplastic lesions. These lesions are characterized by a low-flow pattern of vascularity on time-resolved magnetic resonance angiography.[24]

Infantile hemangioma

Proliferating infantile hemangiomas typically appear as well-circumscribed masses with high signal on T2 weighted images, and demonstrate prominent enhancement and vascularity with conspicuous flow voids (**Fig. 15**). However, involuting hemangiomas can display focal areas of high signal on T1 weighted images due to fatty replacement.[23] Large (>5 cm) facial hemangiomas, particularly in the V3 distribution, may be associated with other abnormalities of the posterior fossa, as well as abnormalities of

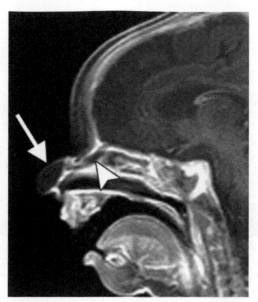

Fig. 8. Dermoid cyst. Sagittal postcontrast T1 MRI shows a cystic mass in the midline of the nasal dorsum (*arrow*) associated with a sinus tract (*arrowhead*) that extends to the anterior cranial fossa.

head and neck vasculature in patients with PHACE (posterior fossa, hemangioma, arterial, cardiac/aortic, and eye anomalies) syndrome.[25] Thus, MRI and magnetic resonance angiograhy of the brain and neck are useful for evaluating associated intracranial anomalies in such cases.

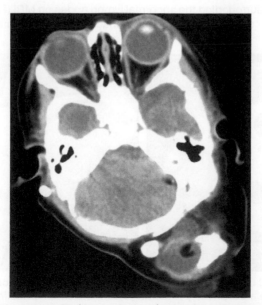

Fig. 9. Teratoma. Noncontrast CT demonstrates a heterogeneous mass containing fat and calcification in the left posterior cervical/suboccipital soft tissues.

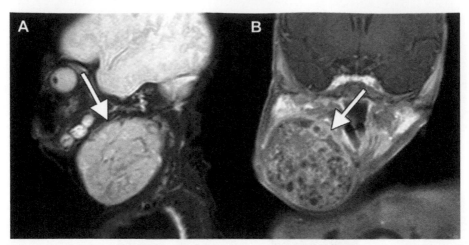

Fig. 10. Immature teratoma. Sagittal fat-suppressed T2 (A) and coronal fat-suppressed coronal postcontrast T1 (B) magnetic resonance images show a bulky T2 hyperintense, heterogeneously enhancing mass in the right neck (*arrows*). No discernible fat is evident in this immature, less differentiated lesion.

Infectious and Inflammatory Lesions

Cervical lymphadenitis

Contrast-enhanced CT is useful in the evaluation of infectious and inflammatory processes in the neck, which typically demonstrate infiltration of the fat planes in the involved areas, usually with associated enhancing lymphoid tissue (**Fig. 16**). Infectious cervical lymphadenitis can be focal, particularly if bacterial, versus diffuse, particularly if viral in etiology. The presence of periadenitis associated with bacterial lymphadenitis is a helpful feature, which appears as ill-defined T2 hyperintensity and enhancement surrounding the abnormal lymph nodes on MRI (**Fig. 17**). Mycobacterial (tuberculous or nontuberculous) lymphadenopathy demonstrates clustered

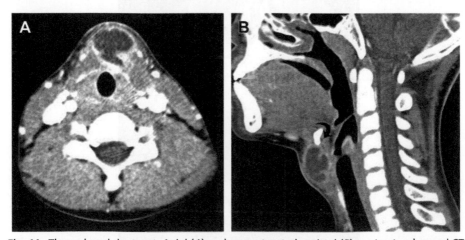

Fig. 11. Thyroglossal duct cyst. Axial (A) and reconstructed sagittal (B) contrast-enhanced CT images demonstrate a peripherally enhancing cyst in the anterior midline neck, embedded in the strap musculature. The collection abuts the hyoid bone, extending slightly into the posterior hyoid space (*black curved arrow*).

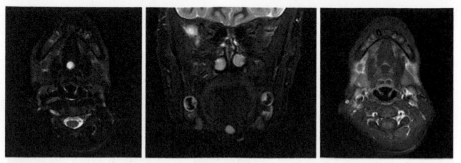

Fig. 12. Thyroglossal duct cyst. Axial T2 weighted (L), coronal T2 weighted (*middle*), and axial postcontrast T1 weighted magnetic resonance images demonstrate a circumscribed rounded cystic lesion at the tongue base demonstrating thin peripheral enhancement on postcontrast images, consistent with a thyroglossal duct cyst.

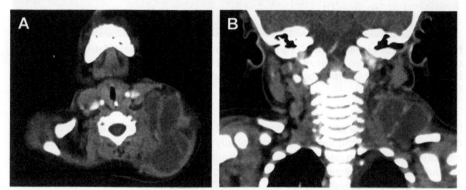

Fig. 13. Venolymphatic malformation. Axial (*A*) and reconstructed coronal (*B*) contrast-enhanced CT images demonstrate a large, multilocular low density lesion in the posterior cervical space.

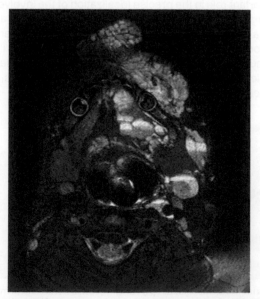

Fig. 14. Venolymphatic malformation. Axial fat-suppressed T2-weighted magnetic resonance images show a multicystic, transpatial mass in the left neck and submandibular region that contains multiple hemorrhage fluid levels.

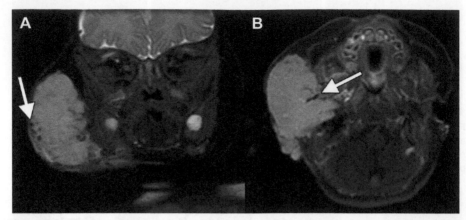

Fig. 15. Infantile hemangioma. Coronal fat-suppressed T2 (*A*) and axial fat-suppressed post-contrast T1 (*B*) magnetic resonance images show a bulky mass in the right face subcutaneous tissues that invades the masticator and parotid spaces and contains prominent flow voids (*arrows*).

lymph nodes with peripheral rim enhancement and central hypodense necrosis, adjacent inflammatory change, and occasionally calcifications. Furthermore, diffusion weighted imaging can be useful for differentiating malignant from benign lymph nodes in adults and some older children[26]; however, this correlation has not yet been well established in young children.

Abscess

Although head and neck infections are generally not difficult to diagnose clinically, imaging plays an important role in the precise localization of the involved space for timely incision and drainage if necessary.[27,28] CT is helpful in identifying abscess formation, which presents as a hypodense collection with a complete peripheral rim of enhancement (**Fig. 18**). A focal collection without enhancement or with an incomplete rim of enhancement is indicative of phlegmon. In particular, multiplanar MRI sequences are useful for depicting the extent of head and neck abscesses, which appear as peripherally enhancing fluid collections (**Fig. 19**).

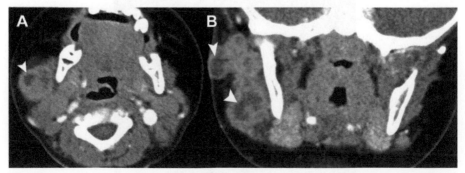

Fig. 16. Mycobacterial adenitis. Axial (*A*) and reconstructed reformatted (*B*) contrast-enhanced CT images demonstrate multiple enlarged lymph nodes in the left neck with heterogeneous enhancement. Areas of central low density (*white arrowheads*) represent nodal necrosis.

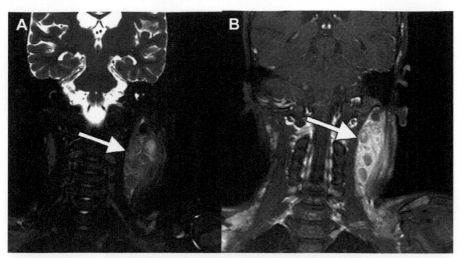

Fig. 17. Infectious cervical lymphadenitis. Coronal fat-suppressed T2 (*A*) and fat-suppressed postcontrast T1 (*B*) magnetic resonance images show a cluster of enlarged left cervical lymph nodes with abnormal signal and enhancement (*arrows*) with associated surrounding inflammatory changes. The patient improved following administration of antibiotics.

Ranula

CT imaging demonstrates ranulas as low-density cystic lesions involving the sublingual space. Simple ranulas present as circumscribed, thin-walled cystic lesions confined to the sublingual space. Plunging ranulas (eg, diving or cervical ranula) extend beyond the sublingual space, either through the mylohyoid muscle, or around the posterior mylohyoid muscle margin (**Fig. 20**). In cases of prior infection, the cyst contents may demonstrate increased attenuation. In active infection, CT demonstrates a thickened, enhancing wall and surrounding inflammation.

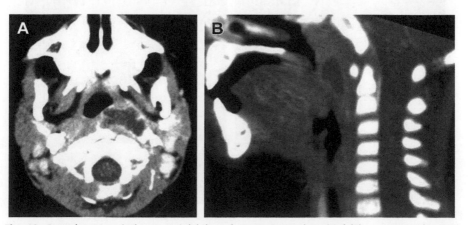

Fig. 18. Parapharyngeal abcess. Axial (*A*) and reconstructed sagittal (*B*) contrast-enhanced CT images demonstrate an irregular low-density collection in the left retropharyngeal soft tissues with thick rim enhancement and mild mass effect on the airway. Surrounding enlarged, enhancing nodes reflect reactive adenopathy.

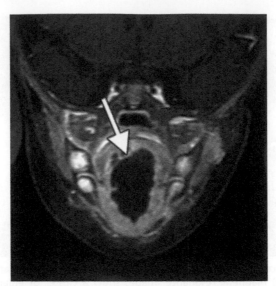

Fig. 19. Abscess. The patient is a 6-month-old female with fevers, high bandemia on white blood cell count, and floor of mouth swelling, leading to emergent intubation. Coronal fat-suppressed postcontrast T1 MRI shows a peripherally enhancing fluid collection centered in the root of the tongue (*arrow*).

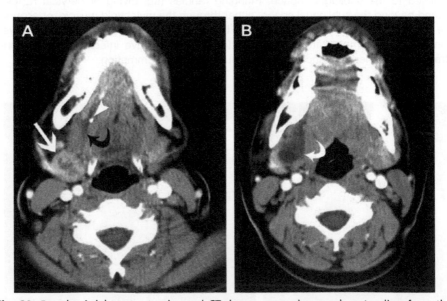

Fig. 20. Ranula. Axial contrast-enhanced CT shows a complex ranula extending from the sublingual compartment (*A, curved black arrow*) posteriorly into the submandibular space (*B, curved white arrow*). A punctate high density along Whartons duct is consistent with a sialolith (*A, white arrowhead*), and there are inflammatory changes of the left submandibular gland with heterogenous enhancement (*A, straight white arrow*).

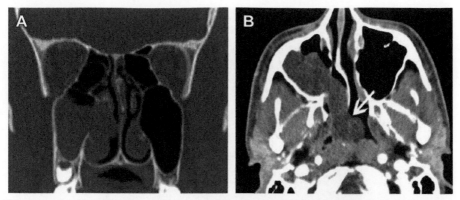

Fig. 21. Antrochoanal polyp. Contrast-enhanced CT with coronal bone windows (*A*) and reconstructed axial soft tissue images (*B*) shows a low density lesion partly filling the left maxillary sinus and posterior nasal cavity. There is extension through the choana into the nasopharynx (*white arrow*).

Sinonasal lesions

Sinonasal lesions are well delineated on CT. One example is an antrochoanal polyp, which appears as a lobulated hypodense lesion involving the maxillary antrum and nasal cavity, with extension through the choana (**Fig. 21**).

Langerhans cell histiocystosis

Involvement of the skull, maxillofacial bones, and hypothalamic–pituitary axis is fairly common in Langerhans cell histiocytosis.[29] CT typically demonstrates circumscribed rounded or oval lytic lesions involving the inner and outer tables of the calvarium, with a characteristic beveled edge configuration, and often a bony sequestrum. An associated enhancing soft tissue mass is present in some cases (**Fig. 22**).

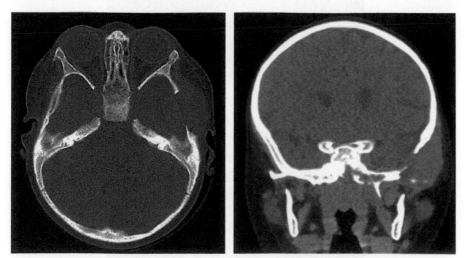

Fig. 22. Langerhans cell histiocytosis. Axial CT in bone algorithm (*left*) demonstrates a lytic lesion in the left temporal bone with a beveled edge configuration. Coronal CT in soft tissue algorithm (*right*) demonstrates an associated soft tissue mass traversing the inner and outer tables, with extracranial extension.

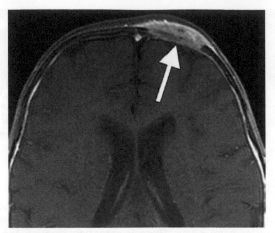

Fig. 23. Langerhans cell histiocytosis. Axial fat-suppressed postcontrast T1 weighted MRI shows an expansile enhancing lesion in the left frontal calvarium, with an associated soft tissue mass extending into the left frontal extracranial soft tissues (*arrow*).

On MRI, the skull lesions often have intermediate signal on T1 weighted images, intermediate-to-high signal on T2 weighted images; they demonstrate enhancement on postcontrast T1 weighted images. Furthermore, Langerhans cell histiocystosis can display diffusion restriction, a feature that can be seen with malignant lesions (**Fig. 23**).[20] The boundaries of the skull and extracranial head and neck lesions are well delineated on MRI, specifically with fat-suppressed postcontrast T1 weighted sequences, which are helpful in elucidating commonly associated soft tissue masses. Similarly, MRI is an excellent modality for evaluating intracranial involvement.[29,30]

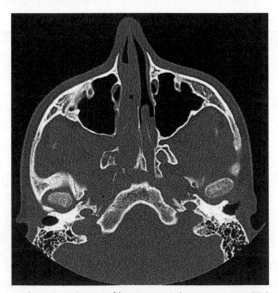

Fig. 24. Juvenile nasopharyngeal angiofibroma. Axial noncontrast CT image in bone algorithm demonstrates widening of the right pterygopalatine fossa with associated bony erosive changes.

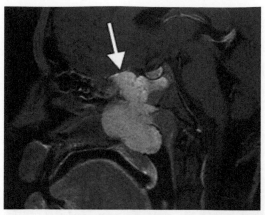

Fig. 25. JNA. Sagittal fat-suppressed T1 weighted MRI shows an enhancing mass in the left nasopharynx with extension into the anterior cranial fossa (*arrow*).

Benign Neoplasms

Juvenile nasopharyngeal angiofibroma

CT is a useful modality for delineating osseous detail, including bony anatomy, expansion, and erosion (**Fig. 24**). CT and MRI are complementary modalities in the evaluation of juvenile nasopharyngeal angiofibromas (JNA), as MRI is superior to CT for detecting intracranial extension of the tumor into soft tissues of the skull base.[31,32] On MRI, these lesions characteristically demonstrate low signal intensity on T1 weighted images, heterogeneous intermediate signal intensity on T2 weighted images, and avid enhancement with flow voids on contrast-enhanced MRI. These MRI features, along with the patient demographics, can help in differentiating a JNA from other nasopharyngeal tumors.[31,32] MRI is useful for preoperative planning by depicting extension of the tumor into the surrounding spaces (**Fig. 25**). MRI also plays an important role postoperatively for the detection of residual or recurrent tumor and monitoring the effects of radiotherapy.

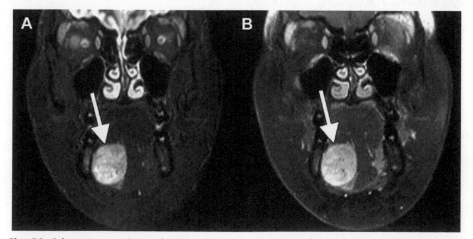

Fig. 26. Schwannoma. Coronal STIR (*A*) and fat–suppressed postcontrast T1 (*B*) magnetic resonance images show a well-defined T2 hyperintense, homogeneously enhancing mass in the right tongue (*arrows*).

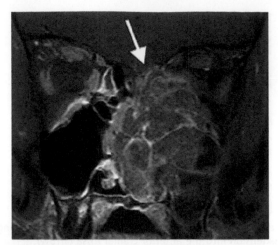

Fig. 27. Rhabdomyosarcoma. Coronal post-contrast fat-suppressed T1 MRI shows a sinosnasal mass with intracranial invasion (*arrow*) that demonstrates multiple lobular components with more intense peripheral enhancement suggestive of the "botryoid sign".

Schwannoma

MRI is sensitive and specific for the diagnosis of extracranial head and neck schwannomas and should be considered the imaging modality of choice for evaluating the associated nerve of origin.[33,34] Schwannomas typically appear as ovoid or fusiform masses with high T2 signal and avid enhancement on MRI (**Fig. 26**).

Malignant Neoplasms

Rhabdomyosarcoma

MRI findings of rhabdomyo sarcoma are most helpful in staging and assessing therapeutic response.[35] In particular, multiplanar postcontrast T1 weighted sequences are useful for identifying intracranial extension (**Fig. 27**). The presence of multiple ring enhancing components within the tumors that resemble bunches of grapes (botryoid sign) is helpful in suggesting rhabdomysarcoma.[36]

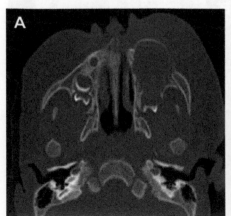
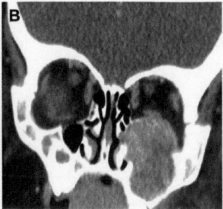

Fig. 28. Maxillary alveolar sarcoma. Contrast enhanced CT with axial bone windows (*A*) and reconstructed coronal soft tissue images (*B*) demonstrate an expansile, solid mandibular lesion with extension into the orbit.

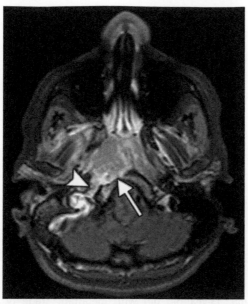

Fig. 29. Nasopharyngeal carcinoma. Axial fat-suppressed post-contrast T1 weighted MRI shows a right nasopharyngeal mass with associated erosion of the clivus (*arrow*) and extension into the right hypoglossal canals (*arrowhead*).

CT is beneficial for evaluation of osseous erosion and expansion associated with sarcomas and other malignant lesions (**Fig. 28**).

Nasopharyngeal carcinoma

Children often have enlargement of the nasopharyngeal soft tissues due to benign hypertrophy of adenoids.[37] Consequently, pediatric nasopharyngeal carcinoma may not be suspected clinically until late into the disease process. MRI is useful for screening patients with suspected nasopharyngeal carcinoma and has been found to be more sensitive than endoscopy.[38] Nasopharyngeal carcinoma typically appears as an enhancing mass centered in the posterolateral aspect of the nasopharynx

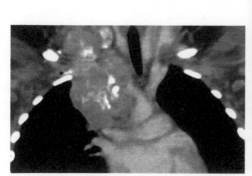
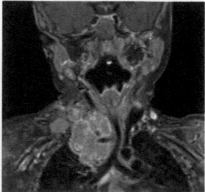

Fig. 30. Neuroblastoma. Coronal contrast-enhanced CT (L) and contrast-enhanced T1-weighted fat-suppressed MRI demonstrate a heterogeneously enhancing solid lower cervical/upper mediastinal soft tissue mass, consistent with neuroblastoma.

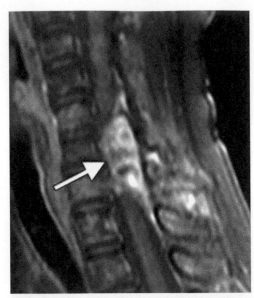

Fig. 31. Neuroblastoma. 13-year-old girl with metastatic stage IV neuroblastoma and new-onset bilateral leg paresthesias and weakness. Sagittal fat-suppressed post-contrast T1 MRI shows epidural extension of an enhancing lesion (*arrow*).

(**Fig. 29**). Invasion of the central skull base and extension into the adjacent parapharyngeal space, the pterygopalatine fossa, and the masticator space are not uncommon features of pediatric nasopharyngeal carcinoma and are readily depicted on MRI.

Neuroblastoma

On MRI, neuroblastoma is typically isointense to hypointense to muscle on T1 weighted images and hyperintense on T2 weighted images, and it demonstrates enhancement (see **Fig. 30**).[39] Heterogneous signal characteristics can be attributable to necrosis and hemorrhage. MRI is superior to CT for staging, particularly with respect to identifying bone marrow infiltration and intraspinal extension of tumor (**Fig. 31**).[40] Additionally, MRI is better than CT for post-treatment follow-up of midline or paraspinal neuroblastomas.[40] Ultimately, the evaluation of patients with neuroblastoma may require a multimodality approach, including metaiodobenzylguanidine (MIBG) nuclear scans.

REFERENCES

1. Friedman ER, John SD. Imaging of pediatric neck masses. Radiol Clin North Am 2011;49(4):617–32, v.
2. American College of Radiology. ACR appropriateness criteria: neck mass/ adenopathy. Available at: www.acr.org/~/media/ACR/Documents/AppCriteria/ Diagnostic/NeckMassAdenopathy.pdf. Accessed January 10, 2014.
3. Gupta P, Maddalozzo J. Preoperative sonography in presumed thyroglossal duct cysts. Arch Otolaryngol Head Neck Surg 2001;127(2):200–2.
4. Ahuja AT, Ying M. Sonographic evaluation of cervical lymph nodes. AJR Am J Roentgenol 2005;184(5):1691–9.
5. Lloyd C, McHugh K. The role of radiology in head and neck tumours in children. Cancer Imaging 2010;10:49–61.

6. Oguz A, Karadeniz C, Temel EA, et al. Evaluation of peripheral lymphadenopathy in children. Pediatr Hematol Oncol 2006;23(7):549–61.
7. Yaris N, Cakir M, Sözen E, et al. Analysis of children with peripheral lymphadenopathy. Clin Pediatr (Phila) 2006;45(6):544–9.
8. Ahuja A, Ying M. Sonography of neck lymph nodes. Part II: abnormal lymph nodes. Clin Radiol 2003;58(5):359–66.
9. Tschammler A, Ott G, Schang T, et al. Lymphadenopathy: differentiation of benign from malignant disease–color Doppler US assessment of intranodal angioarchitecture. Radiology 1998;208(1):117–23.
10. Sidell DR, Shapiro NL. Diagnostic accuracy of ultrasonography for midline neck masses in children. Otolaryngol Head Neck Surg 2011;144(3):431–4.
11. Robson CD. Imaging of head and neck neoplasms in children. Pediatr Radiol 2010;40(4):499–509.
12. Ma J, Jackson EF, Kumar AJ, et al. Improving fat-suppressed T2-weighted imaging of the head and neck with 2 fast spin-echo dixon techniques: initial experiences. AJNR Am J Neuroradiol 2009;30(1):42–5.
13. Barger AV, DeLone DR, Bernstein MA, et al. Fat signal suppression in head and neck imaging using fast spin-echo-IDEAL technique. AJNR Am J Neuroradiol 2006;27(6):1292–4.
14. Kadom N, Lee EY. Neck masses in children: current imaging guidelines and imaging findings. Semin Roentgenol 2012;47(1):7–20. http://dx.doi.org/10.1053/j.ro.2011.07.002.
15. Thoeny HC, De Keyzer F, King AD. Diffusion-weighted MR imaging in the head and neck. Radiology 2012;263(1):19–32.
16. Hu S, Hu CH, Yang L, et al. Atypical imaging observations of branchial cleft cysts. Oncol Lett 2014;7(1):219–22.
17. Goyal N, Zacharia TT, Goldenberg D. Differentiation of branchial cleft cysts and malignant cystic adenopathy of pharyngeal origin. AJR Am J Roentgenol 2012;199(2):W216–21.
18. Suzuki C, Maeda M, Matsumine A, et al. Apparent diffusion coefficient of subcutaneous epidermal cysts in the head and neck comparison with intracranial epidermoid cysts. Acad Radiol 2007;14(9):1020–8.
19. Ginat DT, Mangla R, Yeaney G, et al. Diffusion-weighted imaging for differentiating benign from malignant skull lesions and correlation with cell density. AJR Am J Roentgenol 2012;198(6):W597–601.
20. Zapata S, Kearns DB. Nasal dermoids. Curr Opin Otolaryngol Head Neck Surg 2006;14(6):406–11.
21. Bloom DC, Carvalho DS, Dory C, et al. Imaging and surgical approach of nasal dermoids. Int J Pediatr Otorhinolaryngol 2002;62(2):111–22.
22. Green JS, Dickinson FL, Rickett A, et al. MRI in the assessment of a newborn with cervical teratoma. Pediatr Radiol 1998;28(9):709–10.
23. Baker LL, Dillon WP, Hieshima GB, et al. Hemangiomas and vascular malformations of the head and neck: MR characterization. AJNR Am J Neuroradiol 1993;14(2):307–14.
24. Kramer U, Ernemann U, Fenchel M, et al. Pretreatment evaluation of peripheral vascular malformations using low-dose contrast-enhanced time-resolved 3D MR angiography: initial results in 22 patients. AJR Am J Roentgenol 2011;196(3):702–11.
25. Haggstrom AN, Garzon MC, Baselga E, et al. Risk for PHACE syndrome in infants with large facial hemangiomas. Pediatric 2010;126(2):e418–26.
26. Abdel Razek AA, Soliman NY, Elkhamary S, et al. Role of diffusion-weighted MR imaging in cervical lymphadenopathy. Eur Radiol 2006;16(7):1468–77.

27. Wang B, Gao BL, Xu GP, et al. Images of deep neck space infection and the clinical significance. Acta Radiol 2013;55(8):945–51.
28. Hoang JK, Branstetter BF 4th, Eastwood JD, et al. Multiplanar CT and MRI of collections in the retropharyngeal space: is it an abscess? AJR Am J Roentgenol 2011;196(4):W426–32.
29. D'Ambrosio N, Soohoo S, Warshall C, et al. Craniofacial and intracranial manifestations of langerhans cell histiocytosis: report of findings in 100 patients. AJR Am J Roentgenol 2008;191(2):589–97.
30. Koch BL. Langerhans histiocytosis of temporal bone: role of magnetic resonance imaging. Top Magn Reson Imaging 2000;11(1):66–74.
31. Lloyd G, Howard D, Phelps P, et al. Juvenile angiofibroma: Modern imaging and its influence on the surgical treatment of juvenile angiofibroma. J Laryngol Otol 1999;113:43–4.
32. Ludwig BJ, Foster BR, Saito N, et al. Diagnostic imaging in nontraumatic pediatric head and neck emergencies. Radiographics 2010;30:781–99.
33. Liu HL, Yu SY, Li GK, et al. Extracranial head and neck schwannomas: a study of the nerve of origin. Eur Arch Otorhinolaryngol 2011;268(9):1343–7.
34. Yasumatsu R, Nakashima T, Miyazaki R, et al. Diagnosis and management of extracranial head and neck schwannomas: a review of 27 cases. Int J Otolaryngol 2013;2013:973045.
35. Kim EE, Valenzuela RF, Kumar AJ, et al. Imaging and clinical spectrum of rhabdomyosarcoma in children. Clin Imaging 2000;24(5):257–62.
36. Hagiwara A, Inoue Y, Nakayama T, et al. The "botryoid sign": a characteristic feature of rhabdomyosarcomas in the head and neck. Neuroradiology 2001;43(4):331–5.
37. Stambuk HE, Patel SG, Mosier KM, et al. Nasopharyngeal carcinoma: recognizing the radiographic features in children. AJNR Am J Neuroradiol 2005;26(6):1575–9.
38. King AD, Vlantis AC, Bhatia KS, et al. Primary nasopharyngeal carcinoma: diagnostic accuracy of MR imaging versus that of endoscopy and endoscopic biopsy. Radiology 2011;258(2):531–7.
39. Papaioannou G, McHugh K. Neuroblastoma in childhood: review and radiological findings. Cancer Imaging 2005;5:116–27.
40. Kushner BH. Neuroblastoma: a disease requiring a multitude of imaging studies. J Nucl Med 2004;45(7):1172–88.

Index

Note: Page numbers of article titles are in **boldface** type.

A

Acinic cell carcinoma, 160, 163–164
Actinomyocosis, 139–140
Adenoid cystic carcinoma, 164–165
Airway management, perinatal, in prenatal diagnosis of obstructive masses of head and neck, **191–207**
Airway obstruction, neonatal, 191
Ameloblastoma, 109–110
    malignant, 110–111
Ankyloglossia, 182
Antrochoanal polp, 239
Arteriovenous malformations, diagnosis of, 39–40
    management of, 40–41
    staging of, 40

B

Behçet syndrome, 180
Branchial cleft, anatomy and pathophysiology of, 2
    anomalies of, and thymic cysts, **1–14**
        barium esophagram in, 7
        clinical presentation and examination in, 2–6
        computed tomography in, 6–7
        diagnostic procedures in, 6–7
        involving thyroid gland, 52–53
        literature on, 12, 13
        magnetic resonance imaging in, 7
        surgical technique in, 7–13
        ultrasound in, 7
    development of, 2, 3
    first, anomalies of, surgery in, 8–9
    fourth, anomalies of, 6
    second, anomalies of, 5
        surgery in, 9
    third, anomalies of, 5–6
        surgery in, 9
Branchial cleft cysts, cross-sectional imaging features of, 229–230, 231
Branchiogenic carcinoma, in brachial cleft cyst, controversy concerning, 10–13
Burkitt lymphoma, 66, 113
    clinical features of, 66
    staging for, 66

Otolaryngol Clin N Am 48 (2015) 247–255
http://dx.doi.org/10.1016/S0030-6665(14)00159-5
0030-6665/15/$ – see front matter © 2015 Elsevier Inc. All rights reserved.

oto.theclinics.com

Moving?

Make sure your subscription moves with you!

To notify us of your new address, find your **Clinics Account Number** (located on your mailing label above your name), and contact customer service at:

Email: journalscustomerservice-usa@elsevier.com

800-654-2452 (subscribers in the U.S. & Canada)
314-447-8871 (subscribers outside of the U.S. & Canada)

Fax number: 314-447-8029

Elsevier Health Sciences Division
Subscription Customer Service
3251 Riverport Lane
Maryland Heights, MO 63043

*To ensure uninterrupted delivery of your subscription, please notify us at least 4 weeks in advance of move.